Charity and Welfare

THE MIDDLE AGES SERIES

Ruth Mazo Karras, General Editor
Edward Peters, Founding Editor

A complete list of books in the series
is available from the publisher.

Charity and Welfare

Hospitals and the Poor in Medieval Catalonia

James William Brodman

PENN

University of Pennsylvania Press

Philadelphia

Publication of this volume was assisted by a subvention from the
Program for Cultural Cooperation between Spain's Ministry of Education and
Culture and United States Universities.

10 9 8 7 6 5 4 3 2 1

Published by
University of Pennsylvania Press
Philadelphia, Pennsylvania 19104-4011

Library of Congress Cataloging-in-Publication Data
Brodman, James
   Charity and welfare : hospitals and the poor in medieval Catalonia
/ James William Brodman.
      p.   cm. — (Middle Ages series)
   Includes bibliographical references and index.
   ISBN 0-8122-3436-7 (cloth : alk. paper)
      1. Charities — Spain — Catalonia — History.   2. Hospitals, Medieval —
Spain — Catalonia — History.   3. Social history — Medieval, 500–1500.
I. Title.   II. Series.
HV344.C37B76   1998
362.1'0946'70902 — dc21   97-45102
                                                               CIP

TO MARIAN

Contents

Preface

Hospitals, in the Middle Ages, were broadly conceived as institutions that received pilgrims and travelers, cared for the sick, and tended to individuals designated by society as being poor. In recent years, such institutions have begun to attract the attention of historians. Some scholars have come upon hospitals incidentally; these include those who study marginality and marginal groups, since the latter were frequently clients of hospitals and caritative institutions. Others have become interested in various examples of laic or nonclerical associations, such as confraternities, parish institutions, and municipal councils, and have subsequently discovered and addressed the assistance such organizations rendered to the poor. More directly tied to hospitals are the efforts of those who examine the origins and character of medical practice because this includes consideration of the settings within which the healing arts were actually practiced. In addition, among the historians of religion and the medieval Church, an interest in the Gregorian reform movement has been broadened to include a study of the various new orders, among which are caritative groups that operated and staffed hospitals. These scholars have been joined by local historians, whose analysis of urban archives has brought to light various types of civic institutions, which include hospitals and other institutions of municipal charity. Finally, contemporary society's debate over issues like welfare reform, care of children and the elderly, and the universality of health care has sparked an interest in the medieval response to these same subjects.

The first modern studies of European hospitals and charitable provision date from the late nineteenth century and, as in most history of this age, the attention was focused on the formation and development of institutions.[1] By the mid-twentieth century, some scholars began to consider the social context of medieval benevolence by exploring the legal framework within which charity was distributed.[2] Since 1970, there has been an explosion of interest in the subject along two principal lines of investigation. One thread of inquiry has centered on the study of particular urban societies and groups. This has produced illuminating studies of hospitals and charity for Italian communes like Venice, Genoa, and Florence, for the

English communities of York and Cambridge, and for Brussels and other urban centers of the Low Countries.[3] Social historians, on the other hand, have concentrated their attention on both ends of the social spectrum. Michel Mollat and his associates, such as Bronislaw Geremek, have introduced the subject of poverty and painted a picture of how the underclass fared in the world of medieval France.[4] Philippe Ariès, Shulamith Shahar, and others have addressed the nurturing of children, and John Boswell the phenomenon of their abandonment.[5] Prostitutes, lepers, slaves, and the aged have each found their historians.[6] Other scholars have tackled the issues of gender, social minorities, and power elites.[7] While much of this is peripheral to the study of hospitals per se, each of these topics deals in important ways with the methods, motives, and means of medieval caritative assistance.

Within Iberia, the modern study of hospitals, charity, and poor relief also began in the later nineteenth century, when Fermín Hernández Iglesias published a history of hospitals and Manuel de Bofarull a study of confraternities. In the decade before the outbreak of the Spanish Civil War, their interest was continued principally by the Catalan historians Joseph Maria Roca, Luis Batlle Prats, and César Martinell, whose focus remained chiefly institutional.[8] In 1944, as Spain was recovering from its recent conflict, and within the context of the Franco dictatorship, the Franciscan Pere Sanahuja and Antonio Rumeu de Armas both published histories of charity. The former focused on a single locality, Lleida, while the latter emphasized the national, or pan- Hispanic character of medieval assistance.[9] Both reflected the ethos of the era by emphasizing the religious and institutional aspects of medieval giving. Historians like José Tolivar Faes and Robert I. Burns, S.J., wrote in the 1960s about hospitals in Asturias and Valencia,[10] but general interest in the subject was not manifested until the convocation of a large conference at Lisbon in 1972.

The Lisbon Conference gathered historians from throughout Iberia who for the first time addressed a broad array of questions relating to poverty and relief in the Middle Ages. Michel Mollat, whose own studies of the subject at the University of Paris dated from 1962, was invited to deliver the keynote address. Twenty-seven *ponencías* followed. Given the locale of the conference, almost half of the presentations concerned Portugal; six dealt with Catalan subjects; another five were situated within the Crown of Castile; and three dealt with pan-Iberian topics. The poor in law and literature, institutions of charity, and the role of monarchs were among the topics addressed.[11] The impact of this assembly is evident from the flood of scholarship that followed in its wake. Within Castile in the 1980s, Luis Martínez García published several studies of hospitals at Burgos, and other scholars wrote of Valladolid, Alicante, and Córdoba. In 1986, Carmen López Alonso published an Iberian version of Mollat's general study of poverty and assistance.[12] But the primary focus of the new scholarship has been in eastern Spain, a region associated with the medieval Crown of Aragon, and especially Catalonia.

Several Catalan scholars, participants in the Lisbon conference and colleagues in the Department of Medieval History at the University of Barcelona, launched in 1975 an investigation of charitable institutions and their assistance to the poor of medieval Catalonia. This resulted in the publication of a collection of studies, *La pobreza y la asistencia a los pobres en la Cataluña medieval*.[13] Barcelona was the primary focus of this effort, which produced profiles of several of the city's medieval hospitals, studies of cathedral and parish charities, and a preliminary analysis of charitable bequests. The decade that followed led to major studies of hospitals and poor relief in Urgell, Girona, and Lleida within Catalonia, as well as to those of Valencia and Majorca. Although the initial focus of most of these publications was institutional, by the late 1980s scholars became more topical by turning to such subjects as food, gender, children, and class.

Much of the work to date has been of a provisional nature; typically, hospitals have been addressed only as part of a larger analysis of Catalan urban life in the later Middle Ages or else have been treated as isolated phenomena.[14] Archival collections that survive, particularly for hospitals and other charities from the fourteenth and fifteenth centuries, have not yet been systematically explored and only now are beginning to attract the attention of researchers. Towns like Tortosa, Tarragona, and Vic have yet to find their historians. The neighboring Kingdom of Aragon has attracted even less attention, and in the realms of Valencia and Majorca only the eponymous capital cities have received any significant study. Yet, despite these lacunae, this is an opportune time for a broad synthesis. Enough has been accomplished to reveal the broad outlines of Catalan charity, but the published research is diffuse, often difficult to access, and little known outside of Catalonia itself. This is unfortunate because eastern Spain belonged to the same Mediterranean world as the Italian city-states, which have by contrast received considerable attention from the outside world. The result has been a degree of distortion that attributes to Italian institutions a primacy and uniqueness that may not always be warranted. Consequently, the addition of Catalonia and eastern Spain to the map of medieval charitable provision will broaden the context and thus give us a truer picture of its genesis, character, and evolution.

This study, then, is motivated by several purposes. First of all, it seeks to be synoptic by placing the disparate studies produced over the past quarter-century and earlier into a broad and comparative structure that will enable us to understand the general contours of the development of organized charity and public policy toward the poor within Catalonia and in other regions of the Crown of Aragon. This will create an analytic framework for those who choose to pursue new research on Catalan themes and will permit Catalan material to be incorporated into an understanding of the European context of hospital development.

This work is, second, contextual, because it seeks to relate local developments to the mental and physical worlds shared by other European communities. Consequently, the institutions and practices of Catalonia will be compared with those of neighboring regions, like Castile and Languedoc, and also with the more distant societies of northern Europe and Italy. This broader perspective will assist in our understanding of the dynamic of hospital expansion and help us to understand the interplay of geography, ideology, and local institutions in the formation of a policy of assistance toward the poor.

Finally, questions of care inevitably raise issues of public policy because they involve the transfer of resources from one segment of the community to another. Just as contemporary society struggles with questions of welfare reform, managed health care, and assistance to the elderly, people of the Middle Ages had to make decisions about whom they wished to help, and for what reason(s). Their solutions were no easier than those of modern legislators. Natural catastrophes, demographics, societal resources, ideologies, and social prejudice each had a role to play. In formulating their responses, however, medieval authorities came to place great importance on the distinction between charity, that is, aid given gratuitously and indiscriminately to others, and welfare, which is assistance targeted toward certain groups for particular, desired ends. The emergence of a philosophy of welfare, moreover, implied the creation of criteria meant to distinguish the worthy and unworthy from among the great mass of the poor. Such concepts are only slowly returning to the contemporary debate over the reform of welfare. An understanding of the medieval context within which such ideas of charity, welfare, and the right to assistance were originally developed might bring a measure of perspective and sensitivity to the modern discussion.

This study will begin with a general consideration of poverty, because it was the essential condition that established a need for care and which provided a moral and practical justification for the assistance to be rendered to any individual. Chapter 1 will thus examine the notions of voluntary and involuntary poverty and the emergence of a separate and identifiable class of paupers who were deserving of society's assistance. Essential to our understanding of these ideas are the distinctions that developed after 1100 between the deserving and undeserving poor and between public motives based on ideas of charity and those proceeding from an intention to preserve a particular social order (welfare).

Chapters 2 and 3 define the basic modes of assistance toward the poor as the provision of food and shelter and establish the basic caritative infrastructure that was developed in Catalonia and elsewhere within the Crown of Aragon from the eleventh to the fifteenth century. Care is taken to sort out the sometimes vexing problems of chronology in the foundation of the various almshouses and shelters. A second question is one of initiative and how the patterns of institutional foundation and patronage change between the twelfth and fourteenth centuries.

Chapter 4 looks inside the hospital — at its governance, personnel, and patients, and the physical configuration of its space — in order to estimate the kind of care it was able to offer the needy. Also discussed is the transition from smaller institutions of the twelfth and thirteenth centuries to the larger general hospitals of the fifteenth century, a development in which Catalonia played a particularly important role.

Chapters 5 and 6 consider particular dimensions of care. Chapter 5 examines the emergence of shelters that specialized in the care of certain groups (for example, lepers and the insane), and then, with the emergence of medical practice, how many hospitals began to include medical assistance as part of the routine of care. Chapter 6 discusses how society regarded women and children who lived at its margins, the ways in which they were provided with assistance, and how this was meant to aid their reintegration into society.

Chapter 7 uses the question of public motivation to draw together the various themes of poor relief. After establishing the model for the development of Catalan hospitals in a comparative perspective, it turns to the issues of public policy and practice toward the poor. The discussion takes issue with Carmen López Alonso, Agustín Rubio Vela, and others who have argued that a fundamental shift took place in the fourteenth century from assistance predicated on religious values to one based on secular ideals. The reality, in fact, is more complex and nuanced and demonstrates that medieval assistance to the poor grew out of and depended on an interplay of motives and objectives. It combined elements of charity and welfare, the religious and the secular, and church and state.

The polyglot nature of the Crown of Aragon complicates decisions about how the names of persons and places should be rendered in the text. The town, for example, can be correctly identified in Castilian as Lérida or in Catalan as Lleida. The count-king who ruled between 1213 and 1276 can be Jaime I, Jaume I, or James I. There are no fixed conventions for deciding these matters, but the following rules govern decisions of orthography in this work. The names of persons and places, for the most part, are rendered in the native language. Because the setting for this study is Catalonia, Valencia, and Majorca, Catalan usage predominates. Consequently, monarchs are identified by their Catalan-Valencian names and numbers, not by their Aragonese designation. Thus, the Catalan count Pere II is also Pedro III of Aragon, Pere III is Pedro IV, Alfons II is Alfonso III, Alfons III is Alfonso IV, and so on. English equivalents are avoided as being even more ambiguous. Variants of some names are employed in bibliographical citations if the language of the work quoted is not Catalan. In some instances, however, when the English equivalent of a name is the better known and there is no ambiguity, it is employed. Thus, Catalonia is preferred to Catalunya, Florence to Firenze, and Ferdinand II to either Ferran or Fernando.

The same general system of money that was common in much of medieval Europe, based upon the Carolingian ratio of one pound (*libra*) to twenty sous (*solidi*), to two hundred forty pennies or diners (*denarii*), was used in the Crown of Aragon. The measure of value for each of these units varied from place to place; Barcelona, Valencia, Jaca, and Majorca each had its own independent coinage. The current study, however, is not intended to be statistical, and thus minor variations in the exchange among these currencies have been ignored. In addition to pounds, sous, and diners, other coins occasionally appear. The morabetin was worth between seven and nine sous; the *maravedí* about nine diners; the florin between eleven and seventeen sous; and the mazmodin around three and a half sous.

* * *

This study of hospitals has taken me over a decade to complete. During this time, I received assistance from several sources. I would like to acknowledge my debt here and express to each individual my gratitude and appreciation. The University of Central Arkansas was generous in its allotment of time and resources for this study, and the interlibrary loan staff of Torreyson Library was indispensable in finding articles from obscure journals. The Centre d'Estudis Medievals de Catalunya in Barcelona and its director, Maria Teresa Ferrer i Mallol, must be thanked for bibliographic assistance and for the use of an excellent collection of Catalan periodicals and monographs. The American Academy of Research Historians of Medieval Spain, the Society for Spanish and Portuguese Historical Studies, the North American Catalan Association, the Mid-American Medieval Association, and the Texas Medieval Association each provided opportunities for me to present and test sections of this study. I am particularly grateful to those whose reading of the manuscript provided both keen insights and practical advice. These include Charles Julian Bishko, who, a quarter-century after the completion of my doctoral work at the University of Virginia, remains a valued and trusted mentor, Gregory J. W. Urwin, my colleague at the University of Central Arkansas, and Teofilo F. Ruiz of Brooklyn College and Princeton. I also must acknowledge a debt to Giles Constable for introducing me many years ago to the theme of charity in the Middle Ages, and to my colleagues in AARHMS who encouraged my studies over the years: Rev. Robert I. Burns, S.J., Joseph O'Callaghan, James F. Powers, Bernard Reilly, and Jill Webster. Larry J. Simon of Western Michigan University graciously provided the cover illustration, and Jill Webster and Pilar Salmeron, an archivist at Barcelona's Hospital de Santa Creu i Sant Pau, helped to establish its provenance. A graduate student at the University of Central Arkansas, Rebecca Prestwood, diligently helped me to sort out the notes. I am grateful for the financial support given to this project by the Program for Cultural Cooperation between Spain's Ministry of Education and Culture and United States Universities. At the University of Pennsylvania Press, Jerome E. Singerman, Humanities Editor, and Ruth M. Karras, editor of the Middle Ages Series, helped me through the review process, and Ellen Fiskett and Mindy Brown through the various phases of production. All errors are, of course, mine. My children, James and Meg, tolerated my long hours on their computer. A special thanks is owed to my wife, Marian Masiuk Brodman, who, through a patient reading of the several versions of the manuscript, always provided sound advice and needed encouragement.

I

Hospitals and the Poor

THE BEGINNING POINT for all studies of medieval hospitals, institutional medical care, and relief starts with the notion of poverty, a complex theme as it pertains to the Middle Ages. For some poverty was an affliction; for others, it was a source of virtue. Poverty was never seen purely in economic terms, but rather viewed as a form of degradation that rendered the individual vulnerable or dependent. Thus the sources speak of the poor man, the poor knight, and the poor cleric. For some, such as monks and friars, this humiliation was voluntary and thus a source of virtue, but others were merely victims of economic need, old age, or disease that made life difficult to sustain and even caused a diminution in rank or status. For the latter group, the defining concept was less the absolute level of their subsistence — what we today call the poverty line — than their lack of power to sustain a particular status without some sort of assistance. Thus, as Michel Mollat notes, the word *poverty* was used in the Middle Ages first as an adjective. Its transformation into a collective and abstract noun, to designate the poor as a group distinct from the rest of society, dates only from the thirteenth and fourteenth centuries.[1]

Patristic writers, echoing both biblical injunctions as well as the sentiments of Roman stoic philosophers, acknowledged that Christians had an obligation to assist the poor. But, curiously, their focus was more on the spiritual needs of the wealthy than on the material concerns of the needy. Thus the *vita* of Saint Eligius states: "God could have made all men rich, but He wanted there to be poor people in His world, that the rich might be able to redeem their sins."[2] Inherent in the writings of John Chrysostom, Basil, Jerome, and Augustine of Hippo is a contempt for wealth, a sense that the individual could strive for God only by rejecting the material. Their injunctions to aid the poor thus reflected a spiritual motivation quite divorced from the economic and social realities of poverty. While a genuine concern for human suffering must have played some role in patristic

thought, nonetheless, this attitude lent a ritualistic character to charity in
the early Middle Ages. For example, cathedral churches and, later, monasteries would support poor persons, often called the *matricularii*, who frequently were fixed in number at the apostolic twelve.³ Monastic hospitality,
too, developed its own ritual in the form of the welcome, the washing of the
feet, the provision of hospitality (i.e., food and shelter), and the presenta-
tion of a farewell gift. Such folk were treated more as symbols than as real
people because the monks viewed themselves as the real "poor of Christ,"
having voluntarily laid aside the accoutrements of power for a life of humility. Those assisted did not represent any particular economic group or class
because this was a society of serfs and tenant farmers where most people by
any sort of objective standard could be labeled as poor. Instead, charity
focused on travelers, rich and poor alike, whose distress was of a temporary
and transient nature.⁴

During the eleventh and twelfth centuries, there emerged the concept
of the pauper as someone distinct from the great mass of society, as one who
derived his subsistence from alms and begging rather than from work.
Furthermore, such individuals came to be identified, along with monks and
other practitioners of voluntary poverty, as members of Christ's poor even
though their distress was not a matter of choice. The conclusion that paupers were thereby owed some form of material assistance is the result of the
convergence of several phenomena: among them are the Gregorian reform
movement, with its revival and redefinition of the canonical life, the articulation of canon law, which gave the pauper a specific legal identity, and an
economic transformation that stimulated the growth of towns, the mone-
tization of the economy, and the creation of a distinctive class of the eco-
nomically disadvantaged.

The development of a commercial economy in Europe, beginning in
the eleventh century, created new hierarchies and cleavages within society. While some individual entrepreneurs as well as organized groups of
traders and artisans prospered, others like unskilled workers and unat-
tached women became marginalized. The age, furthermore, exalted values
of acquisition and profit that were alien to a traditional morality that had
always scorned attachments to material possessions. This, Lester K. Little,
in his *Religious Economy and the Profit Economy in Medieval Europe*, has
argued, created a serious tension between morality and behavior, religion
and life, within the emerging urban centers. One product of this tension
was the creation of the *new orders*, which collectively espoused the ideal of
apostolic or voluntary poverty. Some, like the Cistercians, Carthusians, and

Premonstratensians, attempted to reform monasticism toward greater asceticism and isolation from the world of affairs. Perhaps this same notion of ascetic detachment is also tied to the popularity of pilgrimage, which permitted ordinary laypeople to escape temporarily from the cares of their everyday life. Others, however, revived the canonical movement, which was an effort to organize the secular clergy into communities that observed a vow of poverty while practicing an active apostolate within the world. Although first envisioned as a reform of the urban clergy, the initiative in the twelfth century spawned not only numbers of reformed cathedral and collegiate chapters but also several new religious orders (the Antonines, Victorines, Trinitarians, and so on) organized under the Rule of Saint Augustine. The monastic and canonical movements took radically different approaches to poverty and to the poor. The first is typified by Saint Bernard of Clairvaux who, in extolling voluntary poverty argued: "It is one thing to fill the belly of the hungry, and another to have a zeal for poverty. The one is the service of nature and the other the service of grace." The canonical movement, on the other hand, saw that its vocation lay precisely in service to the involuntary poor.[5]

Canonists, at the same time, began to define the legal status of poor persons; they concluded that, because poverty itself was not a moral evil, individuals so afflicted should not be deprived of their legal rights. Consequently, in ecclesiastical courts paupers were exempted from the payment of certain court fees and in some instances were to be provided with free counsel. Perhaps because the canonists attempted to reserve for ecclesiastical courts any case where justice might be threatened by a litigant's poverty, secular courts in the thirteenth and fourteenth centuries also responded by taking note of the indigent. Within Iberian communities, for example, the office of public defender emerged to protect the rights of the poor.[6] The Church, for its part, came to accept a special duty to protect *miserabiles personae*, or poor wretches — namely, widows, orphans, the blind, the mutilated, and those debilitated by long disease. Out of this developed in the early thirteenth century the theory that the poor had a right to help from the patrimony of the Church, which represented the common property of the community, as well as from the superfluities of individuals. Michel Mollat argues that the gift economy of the early Middle Ages had thus given way to an economy of moral restitution, according to which the poor, viewed in the image of the suffering Christ, had a right in both charity and justice to material assistance.[7]

While the twelfth century witnessed a significant expansion of support for the needy, particularly in the form of hospices, hostels, and hospitals in towns and along pilgrim routes, charity retained some of the ritualistic character of the early Middle Ages. To a degree aid remained indiscriminate, dispensed equally to all who happened by. This is especially apparent in the development of the network of hospices along the way of Saint James and other pilgrimage routes. Perhaps the best evidence that we have for the poor as a kind of religious abstraction is found in the wills of this era. These testaments often provide that, after all bequests have been paid out and claims against the estate resolved, the residue would go the "poor of Christ" as universal heirs.[8] Theologians in the twelfth century, however, began to distinguish between two types of poor: *pauperes cum Petro* and *pauperes cum Lazaro*. The former, like the Cistercians or Carthusians and, later, the mendicants, espoused a poverty that was voluntary and which imitated the vocation of the apostle Peter. The latter, however, like the biblical beggar Lazarus, were *miserabiles personae* who suffered some form of physical or material need.[9] Iberian literary sources tend to classify the *pauperes cum Lazaro* into three groups: those who could not work (invalids, widows, orphans), those who would not work (knaves, vagabonds), and those who experienced a temporary need (day laborers, refugees). Modern historians and social scientists distinguish among these with the terms endemic, epidemic, and episodic poverty. Regardless of his or her own individual situation, each is treated as belonging to a marginalized group which, to use the corporal metaphor employed by such medieval Catalan writers as Vicent Ferrer and Francesc Eiximenis, existed within but was not an intrinsic part of the body politic.[10]

So long as the numbers of the poor were manageable, the documents show little attempt to differentiate among the needy. All were the "poor of Christ" and in a quasi-ritualistic fashion equally due alms. Indeed, the concern of early-thirteenth-century observers like Jacques de Vitry was focused more on fraudulent hospitallers and collectors of alms who were able to deceive unwary donors than on unworthy paupers. But Gratian and later canonists, including the Catalan Dominican Ramon de Penyafort, argued that charity to all is possible only in times of abundance. In eras of scarcity, it is proper to discriminate among the poor by giving preference to family and friends over strangers. The *Glossa ordinaria* to the *Decretum*, furthermore, states that the Church should not give aid to able-bodied but idle beggars "for strong men, sure of their food without work, often do neglect justice." The writings of Thomas Aquinas and Castilian legislation of the mid-thirteenth century sounded a similar note.[11] By the fourteenth century, when economic hardship struck not only in Catalonia but throughout Europe, assistance to the poor became increasingly discriminate. From the early thirteenth century—as early as 1208 and 1214 in Barcelona and 1238 in Vic—a distinction between the *pauperes verecundi* (or *vergonzantes, vergonyants*) and the *pauperes matricularii*, or *pobres captaires*, begins to appear. The latter, the so-called public poor, were nonresidents, drifters, or foreigners.

In Barcelona, and elsewhere, individuals who lacked a place within society increasingly became subject to restrictions.[12] King Jaume II, for example, forbade pimps, prostitutes, the crippled and lame, the blind, those with foul diseases, and those who lacked a hand, arm, or foot to enter and loiter around the plaza of Santa Ana in Barcelona.[13] In 1322, furthermore, nonresident beggars were permitted to linger within the city for no more than a day, on penalty of expulsion and whipping; kindhearted residents were discouraged by severe penalties from helping outsiders to evade this regulation. Elsewhere in Iberia, Pedro I, at the Cortes of 1351, attempted to outlaw begging altogether within the Kingdom of Castile and ordered that all except the young, the old and the sick should work by the labor of their hands.[14] On the other hand, the honest poor, or those who were too ashamed to beg (*pauperes verecundi*), were friends and neighbors who had fallen on hard times through no fault of their own; they could no longer maintain their status within the community and were thus worthy of assistance. In 1311, the bishop of Ravenna differentiated between those who publicly accepted alms and those who had to be sought out at home to be helped. The neighborhood poor, as a distinct and separate group worthy of charity, emerges in the middle of the thirteenth century in Italian communes such as Modena, Arezzo, Cremona, and Piacenza, where confraternities and even a religious order, the *fratres verecundorum*, were established to tend to their needs.[15] Wills extant from Catalonia and the Kingdom of Valencia from the mid-thirteenth century single out the ashamed poor as an object of special attention, and court records from fourteenth-century Barcelona show that the idea of *pauperes Christi* was being interpreted to favor relatives and the working poor.[16]

Laws against vagrancy and the emergence of the notion that some paupers are more deserving than others indicate an evolution in attitudes toward the poor even as the older notions remained in force. In the thirteenth century, for example, such mendicant writers as Adam di Salimbene and Giordano di Rivalto and the Castilian historian Rodrigo Ximénez de Rada (d. 1247) continued to focus on charity's benefits for the giver by insisting that paupers had a reciprocal obligation to pray for their benefac-

tors and by emphasizing the redemptive nature of charity.[17] Into the fourteenth and fifteenth centuries, wealthy individuals continued the custom of
bequeathing funds to provide handouts of bread, meals, or money indiscriminately to whosoever of the poor should appear on the day of their
funeral or the anniversary of their death.[18] Alongside this tradition, however, developed forms of assistance like parochial alms funds that targeted
particular individuals or specific groups to the exclusion of others. Furthermore, commentators like the Franciscan Francesc Eiximenis issued stern
warnings against helping the false poor. Some see here a hardening of
attitudes toward the poor but, in light of charity's earlier focus on the
benefactor, this position is difficult to accept at face value.[19] Without a
doubt, however, society in the fourteenth century took a more conscious
account of the recipient's external circumstances than did the ritualistic
charity of earlier centuries and responded more directly to occasions of need
like plague, famine, and unemployment. Efforts to restrict begging or to
regulate wages are one side of this response; the reorganization and even
extension of caritative assistance are another.[20]

Medieval charity in its various forms, therefore, was intended to as-
suage the sins of the well-to-do and to ameliorate the condition of the
deserving poor. It was not until the sixteenth century, as Brian Pullan points
out, that society seriously attempted to assist and reform the lives of the
marginalized poor. Before then, prostitutes, criminals, and other street people lived only at society's fringe, exposed to the uncertainties of begging and
the law, and were blamed for their idleness and dissolute behavior.[21] How,
then, can we characterize medieval practices toward the poor? A useful
place to begin is with Gratian, the twelfth-century canonist, who distinguished between two forms of assistance: *hospitalitas* and *liberalitas*. The
former is the giving of alms gratuitously and is thus, properly speaking,
charity. As Gratian puts it, "In hospitality there is no regard for persons."
Liberalitas, however, discriminates between friends and strangers, the honest and the dishonest, and the humble and the arrogant. Gratian says, "In
this generosity due measure is to be applied both of things and of persons;
. . . of persons, that we give first to the just, then to sinners, to whom,
nevertheless, we are forbidden to give not as men but as sinners." Because
its purpose is to advantage particular groups, *liberalitas* is predicated on a
social policy and is thus a form of welfare.[22] Medieval assistance contains, as
the following chapters will demonstrate, elements of both ideas.

Because hospitals and other providers of aid had to rely substantially
on private offerings, bequests, and endowments, the issue of poor relief can

never be separated from personal motives and intentions. To the degree that these derived from religious and expiatory considerations, the economic and social needs of individual paupers were irrelevant. The poor were passive players in a larger drama that focused on the salvation of the giver rather than the improvement of the recipient. But this does not reflect the full reality because individuals, as well as corporate groups, increasingly began to discriminate in the disbursement of this charity, justified by the notion that resources were insufficient to succor all. Therefore, maidens, children, widows, relatives, and neighbors were preferred to vagrants, prostitutes, and able-bodied idlers. If these distinctions lack the rationally calculated engineering of a public welfare program, they do contain the kernel of a social policy.[23] This kind of assistance was not an early "War on Poverty" precisely because the medieval poor were not treated on an equal basis. To the degree, however, that private and public assistance attempted to sustain a particular social order, medieval charity reflects Gratian's notion of *liberalitas*. This concept of welfare, joined with its complementary and sometimes contradictory idea of charity, will form the context within which this study of public assistance in the Catalan lands will be framed.

2

Feeding the Poor in Medieval Catalonia

The Role of the Cathedral Almshouse

POPE URBAN II'S CALL AT CLERMONT at the end of the eleventh century that launched the Crusades took place during a period of economic hardship that explains some of the dynamic unleashed by popular preachers like Peter the Hermit. While most of Europe was spared the acts of violence associated with events like the People's Crusade, this era nonetheless inaugurated a period in Western medieval history in which the poor became an identifiable and permanent element within society. The crop failures of the late eleventh century were followed periodically by other catastrophes that cast many off the land. These events created a marginalized underclass of beggars who wandered the countryside seeking alms from monasteries or who sought out urban centers for work and sustenance. In addition to these victims of economic dislocation, the roads in the twelfth century became populated with pilgrims, crusaders, students, tinkers, merchants, and others. As a consequence of a more mobile and needy population, the old Christian and monastic tradition of hospitality would have to be substantially modified and expanded to cope with these new and harsh realities.[1]

One of the most basic forms of assistance to the needy is the provision of food. Monasteries had long offered meals to passersby, and at the beginning of the twelfth century this monastic tradition of hospitality was augmented by new forms of urban charity. Within the medieval Catalan lands, the most characteristic form was that of the *pia almoina*, an almshouse established at the cathedral church and administered typically by the bishop and chapter. At such places, the poor were fed in various ways — at certain seasons of the year or daily, with a meal or with only bread or even with cash in lieu of food. There is documentary evidence for such establishments in Catalonia, as well as in Aragon, as early as the eleventh century, at such sites as Barcelona, the Seu d'Urgell, Jaca, Roda, and Huesca.[2] But none seems to have been well organized or adequately funded before the later twelfth or early thirteenth century, when Barcelona and Catalonia emerged from a prolonged period of economic stagnation.[3] The gestation of these charities thus was slow. Records show that their economic and institutional development was incremental and that they did not emerge as fully formed, rationalized organizations until the fourteenth century.

The *Almoina* of Barcelona

The Pia Almoina of Barcelona is the best known of the Catalan establishments, due principally to the work of Josep Baucells i Reig. Here the earliest instance of ecclesiastical charity dates from the late tenth-century will of Bishop Vives, which directed that his estate be given to the cathedral, the poor, and pilgrims. After al-Mansūr's raids of 985 and the subsequent restoration of the chapter, Bishop Aeci, on March 9, 1009, donated property to feed the canons and the poor; Baucells notes that these two constituencies were closely associated with each other in the minds of eleventh-century donors, who had not yet made any clear distinction between voluntary and involuntary poverty.[4] By the twelfth century, there developed the *mandatum*, a custom of feeding a number of poor folk during Lent, which was associated with the liturgical practice of washing the feet of the poor on Holy Thursday. Before 1160, distributions of food were generally ritualistic and by nature only occasional.[5] In 1161, however, Pere de Claramunt, cathedral sacristan, established an endowment in land and money so that three poor persons, chosen by the chapter, could be fed a midday meal throughout the year. In 1210, another canon, Ramon d'Hostalric, willed money to endow a daily meal for one poor person, and between 1227 and 1241 the canon and academic Master Martí left property and rents for three additional paupers.[6] At the same time, the bishop of Barcelona, Berenguer de Palou, who may have fed as many as 120 per day during Lent, established his own permanent endowment. As early as 1217, he directed the beneficiary of the altar of Sant Miquel to feed the apostolic number of twelve poor; the bishop's will of 1241 provided a permanent grant of lands to endow these meals, although no number is explicitly mentioned.[7] Over the next few decades, new endowments were forthcoming from other canons as well as from such lay notables as Ramon de Plegamans; these gifts funded daily meals in the canonical dining room as well as other, special meals that were to be handed out on the anniversary date of the donor's death.[8] At first, the organization of this largesse was haphazard. Individual donors, like Bishop Berenguer and the layman Pere Grony (in 1264), nominated their own agents, while earlier and presumably smaller gifts were handled in some fashion by the chapter.[9] The scheme was finally rationalized by Bishop Arnau de Gurb in his constitutions of December 1275. All of these funds were now placed under the administration of two canons, who were appointed for a term of two years by the bishop and his chapter, and were subject to an audit at the termination of their service.[10] These proctors named two other clergy of the cathedral to supervise real estate, which amounted to thirty different parcels in 1317 and, a century later, forty others. Other minor officials, such as a key-holder, butcher, collector of rents, and distributor of portions, appear in the records. At the same time, the identification of the individual endowments with their original donors seems to have faded, as they all now were merged into this larger, well-organized cathedral soup kitchen.[11] The establishment, with its kitchen and dining room, continued to function until the 1420s when fears of fraud (namely, that some of the poor were selling, rather than consuming, their daily ration) and the exigencies of construction created a new regime. The old facilities were closed in 1421, and the daily meal was replaced with a payment in cash, four diners on meat days and three on those of abstinence, along with a pound and a half of bread. Even after the *almoina* had acquired new quarters, first in the new cloister, and then on a nearby site purchased from the Mercedarians, the meals were not resumed.[12] Although lesser known and yet to be studied, a second *almoina* existed at Barcelona, one that belonged to the Jewish community.[13]

The *Almoina* of Lleida

The beginnings of the Pia Almoina of Lleida compare chronologically to that of Barcelona's cathedral, although the circumstances were very different. Here the foundation is thought to have been directly episcopal and to have occurred between 1149 (the date of Count Ramon Berenguer IV's conquest of the city) and 1168 when Bishop Guillem Pérez de Ravidats organized the cathedral chapter. In the capitular constitutions, the bishop gave to the *almoina* (or *Limosna*), located in the cloister of the cathedral, a tenth of all tithes, first fruits, and death duties that emanated from three villages along the Segre, north of the city, and a tenth of other episcopal revenues. An almoner named Odon is a witness to the constitutions.[14] Agustín Prim Tarragó, however, argues that because these tithes are not found in the accounts of the *almoina* the initiative for its foundation lay with the chapter, which donated a portion of its daily meal to a proctor of alms.[15] It is not known what aid was initially offered the poor, but it is unlikely that they were fed at the table of the canons. By the late 1200s, however, the *almoina* had its own house, located in the cathedral cloister, from which it dispensed food or its equivalent in money.[16] Endowments similar to those at Barcelona began in 1277 when a canon willed money to feed three paupers; clerics and others, including Bishop Jaume de Roca, continued this tradition throughout the fourteenth century, but it seems to have ended after 1400. Thereafter, the old refectory was remodeled into a chapel where the poor would hear mass, and then be given three diners apiece. Before 1300, the *almoina* seems to have been the joint responsibility of the bishop and chapter, but thereafter of the chapter alone. The canons, in turn, delegated their authority to two senior almoners or proctors, who in turn appointed an administrator or *rector*. The latter was obliged to reside in Lleida, buy and distribute food, collect the rents, and dispense alms on Sundays to the poor, the sick, and pilgrims, to those who came to the *almoina*, and to the inmates of the city's hospitals and prisons. The administrator was assisted by lesser proctors, who collected rents within specific districts, and by a lawyer and a notary. In 1338, the cook was a woman named Na Gordana who had the assistance of two servants; supplies were purchased by one En Sijamo. In addition, two priests were paid three hundred sous per year to celebrate mass each day as the poor were being fed. In the hard times of the 1340s, in response to the increased pressure upon the *almoina* for assistance, the bishop and chapter limited admission to no more than fifty persons per day.[17]

The *Almoina* of Urgell

In the Seu d'Urgell, an *almoina* appears soon after the death of Bishop Ermengol (d. 1035) and may be a by-product of the spiritual renewal that he had begun in the diocese, but the early evidence is fragmentary. In 1048 a priest named Oriol was in charge of an almshouse; and Bishop Guillem Arnau de Montferrer's will of 1096 suggests that it, along with a small hospital, was located in a building near the church door. In 1161 canons were obligated to pay any fines levied against them to the "prior-almoner for use of the poor." At this time, it seems the poor were fed in the capitular refectory, a site renamed the *almoina* when the chapter abandoned its common life at the end of the twelfth century. In the thirteenth century, the *almoina* was relocated in the new Romanesque cloister. Unlike the *almoina* of Barcelona, this institution failed to attract private donations sufficient to underwrite its work and in 1279 had to be rescued with a grant of tithes from the bishop and chapter.[18] Despite occasional gifts from clerics and laics — in 1347, for example, one Jaume de Cava donated one hundred pounds — the institution's resources remained so meager that it had to suspend operations in years of famine and plague, like 1333 and 1348, precisely when its services were most needed. To compound this problem, after the plague the canons diverted the *almoina*'s revenues to their own support, until the bishop in 1352 ordered a restoration of the expropriated foodstuffs to the institution. When the chapter responded by declaring the almshouse abolished, protests from townspeople forced its restoration, albeit on a reduced basis.[19] The general lack of vigor exhibited by this institution throughout its history may perhaps be due to the relative abundance of grain in this region, which frequently exported its surplus to Barcelona, and a concomitant smaller incidence of hunger.[20]

The *Almoina* of Girona

The origins of organized food distributions in Girona are first detected in the year 1228, when laypeople bequeathed two endowments for this purpose. The smaller of the two, the *almoina* of Bernat de Subiranegas, provided only a ritualistic assistance to the poor in the form of distributions of bread on All Souls' Day (November 2) and Good Friday.[21] The second endowment established in 1228, while undoubtedly growing out of the same pious intentions, eventually became a local institution of some importance. While this institution belonged to the cathedral, it received its initial grant from Arnau Escala, in the form of houses that he had purchased from the chapter; after the French siege of 1285, a new building was constructed east of the Mercadell. During the fourteenth century, the Almoina del Pa, as it came to be called, became a popular charity among the citizens of Girona. Unlike institutions in other Catalan towns, however, Girona's almshouse distributed only bread, daily between Ash Wednesday and Pentecost. Hard times in the fourteenth century caused this term to be extended; by 1347 it began at Saint Martin's Day (November 11), and in 1355 at All Saints' Day

(November 1), with a terminal date of May 1. A will of 1324 names Pere Casadevall as "proctor of the bread alms" and he appears to be tied to the chapter.[22] By the mid-fourteenth century, the Pia Almoina had also acquired a sizable patrimony between the Ter and Fluvia rivers, from which it drew tithes and rents in kind and in coin, collected by bailiffs, or, after 1347, farmed out to others. Unlike the situation at Urgell, neither the plague nor periodic famine seems to have seriously affected its financial stability. Even in the difficult years after the plague, donations continued to expand the patrimony.[23] For example, 78 percent of rural wills, and 35 percent of those from Girona itself, bequeathed something to the *elemosina panis*, to use its Latin name.[24] The onset of the bad years caused complaints that the institution no longer adequately served the poor because its proctors and their bailiffs had become negligent. To remedy the problem, Bishop Arnau in 1346 appointed a commission to revise the original statutes of 1228. These were reported in 1347; in 1355 Bishop Berenguer added others. Their intent was to provide closer supervision of accounts, inventories, and the amount of bread actually given poor people.[25] According to these statutes, the *almoina* was to be operated by two clerics appointed by the sacristan, a doorkeeper, and a serving woman, but the accounts of 1376–77 list, in addition to this proctor, four serving women, a baker, a person to weigh bread, a carter, and a "scholar." Evidently either men or women could mix and knead the dough, but the baking was entirely a male occupation.[26]

Other *Almoinas* in Catalonia

In Tortosa, where the documents have yet to be closely studied, there is disagreement about the nature of the effort to feed the poor. Enrique Bayerri, on the one hand, argues that work of feeding and sheltering the poor was combined and directed by the Hospital of the See, or that of Santa Maria. Christian Guilleré, on the other hand, believes that a separate *almoina* existed for this task, although it does not yet seem to have been studied.[27] Tortosa, the entrepôt for the Ebro valley's grain exports to Barcelona, like Urgell, may also have experienced fewer difficulties with food shortages.[28] At Tarragona, there is no evidence for any food distribution; the chapter in 1171 included a hospitaller but not an almoner.[29] Likewise, there is no evidence that Vic possessed an almshouse before the fourteenth century when one finally emerged, but under the administration of the municipal councilors and not the canons of the cathedral.[30]

The *Almoina* of Majorca

Hunger, however, was an ever-present concern on Majorca after its conquest by King Jaume I in 1229. Here legacies to purchase *cuarteras* of wheat (about fifty kilos) were the most common caritative benefaction in the thirteenth and fourteenth centuries. Typically the testator would establish an endowment to underwrite the distribution of flour or bread on major feasts or during Lent. Particularly generous was Bernat Scala de Sóller who in 1269 left enough money to distribute to the poor some two hundred loaves of bread on each day of Lent; his motives, however, were as much personal as religious. The bread had to be dispensed at the site of his tomb outside the town of Sóller, on the northern part of the island, so that paupers would not only acknowledge the identity of their benefactor but also pray for his soul. Majorca, however, had no central agency responsible for distributing these alms of bread. Instead this duty fell to individual executors, municipal officials, and parish authorities; toward the end of the fourteenth century, however, municipal *almoinas* began to appear, administered by proctors selected by the local council. Under extraordinary circumstances, however, there could be collective action. In 1349, just after the outbreak of the plague, King Pere III agreed to the request of the island's outlying rural communities that the urban alms funds be consolidated, and their proceeds used to assist farm workers in need.[31]

The Ordinary and Extraordinary Poor

The evidence shows that by the later thirteenth century almshouses functioned in most if not all Catalan episcopal towns, especially the larger ones, and that they were endowed by the local clergy and laypeople to provide food to those in need. Now let us turn and examine their clientele and the nature of this alimentary assistance. In global terms, the numbers helped must have been small within populations where the poor may have comprised between 25 and 50 percent. Thus, for example, Barcelona, whose size ranged from about 25,000 to 40,000 in the thirteenth and fourteenth centuries, would have had between 6,000 and 20,000 poor people.[32] Such statistics would obviously be subject to fluctuation, increasing during periods of shortage, such as 1315–17 and 1340–50, and decreasing when the crisis had abated.[33] Baucells's studies at Barcelona, nonetheless, indicate that the cathedral *almoina* actually helped about two hundred individuals at any one time, or only between 1 and 3 percent of Barcelona's poor.[34] At the Seu d'Urgell, the almshouse tried to feed only fourteen persons a day before the plague years and the institution's decline.[35] At Lleida in 1338 there was enough income to feed 137 poor people each day, the so-called "ordinary poor," and 386 "extraordinary poor," namely those who were fed once a year, typically on an important feast or an individual's anniversary of death. While Pere Sanahuja sees this number rising throughout the rest of the century, Prim Bertrán i Roigé is skeptical, arguing that the income from endowments in 1338 was insufficient to feed so large a number.[36] The numbers he cites fluctuated greatly—90 per day in 1338, 50 in 1343, between 80 and 85 in 1358, growing to the range of 171 to 200 in 1409 and to 145 to 151 in 1415. Indeed, Sanahuja himself acknowledges that the chapter in 1341–43 attempted to limit assistance to no more than fifty per day, and accepts as valid a daily average of ninety, which ultimately suggests that several endowments eventually were eroded or dissipated.[37] At Girona, where the *almoina* just handed out bread and only for seven months of the year (from November through May), the numbers of those assisted were much larger. Fluctuations of distribution—for example, more bread was handed out in December and January than in other months, peaking on Christmas day—make it difficult to estimate the numbers of poor fed during the cold months of the year. Guilleré believes that during the difficult years of 1347 and 1348 some sixty-five hundred individuals were assisted; in 1376–77, out of a population smaller than eight thousand, eight hundred were fed.[38]

What was the major limitation of this aid? Apart from the growth of prejudice against those who were not members of the community, cost must have been a major constraint on a charitable scheme that relied on voluntary gifts. Evidence from fourteenth-century Lleida, for example, suggests that a hundred sous were required to feed one pauper for a year, or nearly three diners a day. Because much of this money derived from endowments, the capital that a donor had to provide was considerably larger. For example, in 1295 when the executors of Bishop Jaume de Roca purchased an annuity worth three hundred sous a year from the abbot of the monastery of Escarp to endow three places at Lleida's *almoina* the immediate cost to the estate was forty-two hundred sous, or thirteen times the annual aid to the poor.[39]

If only a minority of the urban poor were fed by these cathedral charities, who exactly was chosen? There appears to have been three categories of individuals assisted. First, among the "ordinary poor," that is, those who were fed a daily meal, there were those especially singled out for aid by either the donor or the chapter and those who had no special connections or claims. Then, there were the "extraordinary poor", those who were fed an occasional meal on a feast or anniversary. We know the most about the first group. It was common enough practice for benefactors to endow specific places at the *almoina*'s table, and frequently these were reserved for family members. Pere Grony, for example, a canon at Barcelona from 1291 to 1329, endowed three such places, one of which was given to a nun named Saurineta Gronya, and another to the man who lived with her. Likewise, the priest Ripoll de Cortades, in his will of 1302, directed the *almoina* of Barcelona to feed the poor of his own kindred, especially individuals who had moved from the family's home district of Ripoll to Barcelona to pursue studies or to serve as clerics — but for no more than eight years.[40] A year earlier, Gueran de Cervelló underwrote five places and asked that preference be given to students from his home town.[41] This practice of reserving places for family members is also found at Lleida and, given the evidence of Jaume de Cava's 1347 will, not unknown in Urgell.[42] At Barcelona, the *almoina*'s proctors, who were granted the right of presentment by many donors, reserved places for individuals in special circumstances, like students and teachers. In 1256, for example, the bishop accepted the petition of the nuns of Sant Damià that a legacy left by a ropemaker be used to support their chaplain. In 1369, a portion was allotted to Francesc de Mas, a poor student, as long as he studied science, and from the middle of the fourteenth century a portion of the *almoina*'s income was applied to the support of the cathedral boys and to the salary of a lecturer in theology, whose duties included delivering public talks in the cathedral to instruct the canons, curates, and the faithful. During the reign of Jaume II, the king also gained the right of presenting three paupers to the proctors of the Pia Almoina, a privilege that Alfons III invoked in 1330–31 to assign places there to Bartomeu Carbonell, the nephew of his chaplain and a poor student, and to two women, one a widow and the other left without support by her deceased father.[43]

But reservations were also made for the more typically needy, like Arnau de Sanç in 1327 who was old and not able to work, or to a poor youth with an injured arm. Baucells argues, however, that at Barcelona few places were available that had no strings attached, perhaps only the original, small group of twelfth-century endowments, those of the *mandatum*.[44] Maria Echániz Sans's study of Barcelona's *almoina* in 1283–84 concludes that the poor helped here were not the marginalized but rather the so-called deserving poor.[45] At Lleida, the story is much the same. Among those aided were twenty students, a beadle of the *Estudi General*, and two acolytes attached to the chapter. There were also handouts to a diverse group of individuals temporarily in need: abandoned children aided until they could be sent to the local orphan hospital, the father of two captives being held in Granada, an Italian bishop on pilgrimage, and the victim of a highway robbery.[46] Of the fifty or so paupers who received a daily meal, as few as eighteen (only those whose places were funded with tithes directly by the chapter itself) were without connection or claim.[47] At Lleida, however, the distinction between ordinary and extraordinary poor disappeared at the beginning of the fifteenth century, when food distributions were replaced with cash subsidies. During the difficult years of 1409 and 1415, the numbers that the *almoina* aided fluctuated between 145 and 200 individuals a day, for a total of 68,566 payments in 1409 and 59,219 in the 1415.[48]

Beggars, vagrants, and other marginalized people were more likely to receive handouts that were distributed at funerals and on the anniversaries of a benefactor's death. This custom, dating back to the twelfth century, had several variants. In its simplest form, baskets of bread would be left on or beside the tomb on the day of a funeral, and in subsequent years as well, to solicit prayers for the deceased from paupers who would congregate around church porches and cemeteries. In some instances, however, the bread would be given to the residents of convents and monasteries, and in other cases, particularly from the fourteenth century, small sums of money might be substituted for the loaves.[49] At Lleida, for instance, the bread offerings donated at funerals, usually enough to feed between ten and fifteen persons, were collected by the clergy and given to the Pia Almoina for use in its daily distribution of food.[50] In other places, such money was placed in endowments, whose income would be used to feed a given number of the "extraordinary poor" on the anniversary of the decedent's death.

Baucells's studies at Barcelona, the most complete on this account, enumerate the endowments of over three thousand such meals that were dispensed between 1200 and 1500. For various reasons, some endowments eventually lapsed, but in the year 1317, for example, 1,920 such meals were delivered to the poor.[51] Some generous individuals bequeathed money for full-time places in the *almoina* as well as smaller amounts for the commemoration of their anniversaries. We can cite the gifts of Bishop Berenguer de Palou that not only fed fourteen paupers a day but also another hundred on his anniversary, or that of Ramon de Riera who endowed two daily portions and a hundred special meals, fifty on his anniversary and another fifty on the first Friday of Lent. In 1250, Master Ramon made a kind of hybrid donation, twenty meals on the last Friday of each month.[52] At Lleida the numbers are smaller but the practices are similar: in the fourteenth century about 350 annual meals were given out on anniversaries and on the feasts of the Mother of God, the Holy Cross, and All Saints as well as during Holy Week.[53] At Girona, where the Pia Almoina distributed only bread — 130,000 loaves in 1347–48 and 44,000 somewhat larger ones in 1376–77 — there would not have been a distinction between the ordinary and extraordinary poor. Here, assuming that each person was given a quarter loaf, as many as 2,500 individuals were served on a daily basis in 1347–48, with an estimated distribution of 6,500 portions, or 1,625 loaves, on Christmas day. Thus, at Girona a wider category of poor was served, but in a lesser amount, than was assisted at either Barcelona or Lleida; it seems likely that they were not selected at all but rather served on demand.[54] At Urgell, there likewise were large-scale distributions of bread from the cloister, but seemingly on an irregular basis as funds became available.[55]

Apart from the cathedral almshouses, handouts of food were also made by wealthy households, of which the best known is that of the king. King Pere the Ceremonious in the midfourteenth century systematized royal alms in the form of the *Almoina reial*, and among its functions was the daily distribution of food to those who presented themselves at the royal residence, wherever it was at the moment. The *almoina*'s ordinances of 1344 specified that bread would be given daily to sixty paupers, that leftovers along with the bread, wine, fruit, and cheese that had grown stale or old should also be distributed each day, but to a different group of needy persons, and that, as a remembrance of Christ's humility, thirteen others should be given a meal every day, with the king himself serving it on Good Friday. Extra rations of bread would be provided on feast days, as well as on fast days when what was saved provisioning the royal table was to be given to paupers.[56] Like the recipients of bread distributions and anniversary meals, the poor served seem to have been not a special privileged group, especially given the itinerant nature of the royal court, but rather merely those who presented themselves at the king's back door.

Parochial Charity

Within the Crown of Aragon, the marginalized, itinerant, and criminal poor were the responsibility of the cathedral, while the local poor increasingly were entrusted to newly developing parish institutions.[57] In 1288, within the Kingdom of Valencia, for example, a "father of the poor" was elected in each parish. His duties were to dole out money each Saturday and meat and rice in addition on holidays. On All Saints' Day, warm clothing and blankets were distributed against the upcoming winter.[58] In Reus, there was a *bacinus pauperum* (or collector for the poor) in the fourteenth century.[59] On Majorca by 1300, the legacies left to benefit the poor were pooled into municipal alms funds administered by almoners appointed by the town council or in rural parishes by the local pastor.[60] In smaller towns, however, care for the deserving poor remained in the hands of some central agency. In Vic, it was the city council that took the responsibility for distributing alms. Here the city councilors administered not only the Almoina General but also a fund or *bací* to provide clothing to the poor. In Girona, the Vestuari, a charity established by the canon Bernat Vilafreser in 1245 and subsequently administered by the chapter, distributed shirts and breeches to the poor at Easter, and tunics on the feast of All Saints.[61] Castilian parishes in the fifteenth century developed an institution that, like Italian *montes de pietà*, distributed and loaned money at no interest to parishioners in need.[62] In Barcelona, relief funds were established in each of the seven urban parishes under the titles of *bací, colecta,* and *plat* for the deserving poor. The earliest was founded in the neighborhood of Vilanova del Mar, at its parish church of Santa Maria del Mar. Its existence is documented in 1320, but it may have been functioning as early as 1296 or even 1275.[63] Each fund was administered by elected lay parishioners, called *baciners,* who collected, managed, and distributed money as alms. In the parish of Sants Just i Pastor, for example, there were three such officials who oversaw collection boxes (*bacins*), one placed at the cathedral, another in the parish church, and the third midway between the houses of the Franciscans and Mercedarians. One *baciner* was an "honored citizen," the second a merchant or artisan, and the third a worker. Alms were to be distributed twice a year, a few days before Christmas and during Holy Week, and could be in the form of clothing, flour, and/or money. At Santa Maria del Mar, normally one or two *baciners* were elected, but there could be as many as five in difficult years. Most were merchants, but also chosen were notaries, apothecaries, artisans, and silversmiths.[64] At Santa Maria del Pi, detailed ordinances describe the election of the three *baciners* (on Candlemas, later on New Year's Day), their obligation to collect alms each Sunday at various locales throughout the city, and their distribution of alms to the poor. They were specifically forbidden to give anything to beggars, idlers, or the "depraved." As at Sant Just, meals were not given out because the needy had homes where they could presumably prepare their own food. Instead, flour was distributed at Christmas and on the feast of Saint John in June, bread on the feast of All Souls' (November 2), clothing once a year, and small amounts of money once a month. In 1423 and 1428, for example, each poor person was given two *canas* of cloth, enough for a suit of clothing; in 1423, most recipients received one or two *arrobas* of flour (or twenty-six to fifty-two pounds). Cash grants were evidently proportional to need with most, in the 1420s, ranging from one and a half to three sous. Statistically, more women were aided than men; the size of the cash grants was influenced both by gender and class, with males and those of prominent families getting more. In 1423, the largest dole went to an ailing widow, with other grants recorded for a sick lawyer, a bricklayer, a draper, a silversmith, and Jaume Rossell's widow who had a daughter. None of those assisted was a rural worker.[65]

Anecdotal evidence suggests that the "deserving" poor break down into two distinctive groups. The first, which included people like the lawyer Joan Albanell and his wife, consisted of those who could no longer support themselves due to some permanent disability. Sickness, old age, and widowhood are the most frequently cited justifications for assistance at Santa Maria del Pi.[66] Lacking the support of family or a corporate body like a guild, such individuals could fall back only on the assistance of their neighbors. Members of the second group were victims of the economic cycle, able to get by in good times but in need of help during periods of famine and unemployment. Catalonia, for example, suffered from food shortages in 1315–17 and from 1333 to the onset of the plague; the period 1380–1420 was an era of general economic crisis during which as much as 80 percent of the population was reduced to poverty.[67] A study of poor relief in Barcelona's parish of Santa Maria del Pi suggests that there was also some geographical basis to poverty. In the district of the Arrabal, located across the Ramblas from the parish church, needy families who received parochial assistance in the fifteenth century were found on practically every street. But the most needy, that is, those who received regular doles, tended to congregate in just six areas that seem to be the "poorer" neighborhoods. Handouts in other areas fluctuated a great deal, presumably following the cycle of the economy.[68]

The assistance to these two groups is revealed in the scattering of accounts that have survived from some of Barcelona's *bacís* from the early fifteenth century.[69] These records show that the actual solicitation of coins from parishioners had become largely symbolic and yielded only a small percentage of the revenue expended on the needy. Most of the money now came from legacies,[70] most often in small amounts between two and a half and ten sous, but which could include exceptional gifts like the 133 pounds, 6 sous, and 7 diners that Arnau Serra contributed to the alms fund of Santa Maria del Pi in 1400. All of these gifts were capitalized in the form of *censos* and *censales*, rents on pieces of property owned by the *plat* or income from public obligations issued by entities like the Kingdom of Majorca, the Generalitat of Catalonia, or the City of Barcelona. Government bonds and real estate investments generally paid a return on capital of between 5 and 10 percent.[71] The total income available for the poor varied considerably from parish to parish — at Sant Just, just over £13 a year, but rising to the range of £300–350 at Santa Maria del Pi and between £336 and £576 in the wealthy parish of Santa Maria del Mar.[72] In comparison to this investment income, revenue derived from direct alms collections was insignificant. At Santa Maria del Pi, collections averaged no more than £4 per month in 1423, less than a sixth of the *bací*'s total income.[73]

We know less about distributions from parochial alms funds than we do about their sources of income. The best study of alms distributions is that from Santa Maria del Pi for the years 1423 and 1428. It is difficult to quantify the reasons that underlie the need of these parishioners because, while permanent disability was the justification for assistance cited most frequently, in the majority of cases no reason whatsoever is recorded. One suspects, however, that cyclic economic hardship was an important, if unstated, cause because the second of the two years studied, 1428, was one of unusual hardship. The records of the *bací* reflect this, showing a greater number assisted in 1428 than in 1423, with the largest monthly disbursement occurring in March 1428. While in the typical month more women were aided than men, in October and November 1428, the gender ratio was reversed, suggesting a problem of unemployment. Furthermore, those who appeared on the dole list in 1428 for the most part did so only once, and this also suggests that their need was a temporary one.[74]

The Diet of the Poor

Now that we have discussed where, when, and to whom food and other assistance were distributed, let us examine the nature of the assistance and its delivery. Neighborhood charity, as we have seen, tended to be discreet. It provided the needy with clothing for the winter, flour, and monthly supplements to income, all of which were designed to permit the poor to continue living in a normal fashion within their neighborhood. Cathedral charity, on the other hand, was public; the poor had to appear daily at the *almoina* to receive food, a daily monetary dole, or a combination of the two. Today, the former would compare with various forms of public welfare, and the latter with the soup kitchen.

Detailed accounts permit us some insight into the character of the assistance distributed in the form of daily meals. Typically medieval Catalans took two meals a day, one around ten in the morning and the other near six in the evening.[75] The poor, however, were served only once, around midday.[76] The menus were dull and repetitious, except for the special meals that were served on religious holidays, or on the anniversary of some benefactor. For example, the leper hospital of Sant Llàtzer in Barcelona served its inmates special menus on fifteen holidays; Barcelona's Hospital of Sant Macià did the same on Christmas and on the feast of its patron saint.[77] The expenditure of Valencia's Hospital of En Clapers on various items of food consumed by inmates and the staff suggests the outline of a fairly typical medieval institutional diet. In 1388–89, of the over six thousand sous spent on consumables, 30.1 percent went for wheat, 25.7 percent for wine, 18.4 percent for mutton, 14.3 percent for condiments, 5.2 percent for oil, 4.5 percent for fish, and 1.8 percent for eggs.[78]

The staple of the diet was bread, for rich and poor alike; at Girona, as we have seen, this was the only item of food dispensed to the poor. According to the depictions in murals at the almshouse of Lleida, the bread could be large, round, and fluffy loaves of yeast bread or else the flat, hard, unleavened variety found elsewhere in the Mediterranean. At Barcelona, two sizes were common: the *dinal*, a small loaf used as offerings at funerals, and the *dobler*, the size commonly consumed and which cost two diners.[79] Bread could be made of rye, wheat, or a mixture of grains that could also include barley, millet, and even melon seeds. At Urgell, where rye predominated in the grain restored to the *almoina* in 1352, it would seem that the bread was rye; Bertrán supposes the same to have been true at Lleida.[80] But throughout the peninsula, rye was gradually supplanted with wheat bread.[81] Not only was rye bread disparaged as being the food for poor and rural folk, but it also carried the threat of ergotism.[82] At Girona, the pattern was slightly different. Here wheat bread was a special treat reserved for Christmas and Easter; on other days, the poor were served bread made from barley flour. At Barcelona in 1283–84, 61 percent of the grain received by the *almoina* as rents in kind is known to have been wheat and 9 percent barley and other grains; the remainder, which is not identified in the sources, may well have been wheat too.[83]

There have been various estimates of the amount of bread served to the poor. Estimates are a low at Girona, where large numbers of the poor were given quarter loaves, which amounted to about 200 grams of bread per day in 1347–48 and 250 in 1376–77. Pere Desvilar mandated that his hospital in Barcelona serve each inmate a loaf made from sifted wheat that weighed eighteen ounces. At the other end of the scale, Bertrán estimates that the poor of Lleida, for the week of June 19–25, 1338, received 715 grams of bread per day. In between the extremes would be the 560 grams per day served at Barcelona after 1421 when other food distributions were replaced with cash. At the Hospital of En Clapers, in Valencia, the daily ration ranged from 531 grams in 1374/75, a period of shortage, to 768 grams in 1388–89, a more normal year. Other studies suggest that the ration of the poor here was somewhat less than the general population elsewhere would consume.[84] The portion of bread amounted to, in Bertrán's calculations, 78.43 percent of the total caloric intake of the meal; Echániz Sans at Barcelona is less precise but still concludes that the combination of bread, wine, and meat amounted to over 75 percent of the food provided and consumed.[85] By way of comparison, the *Constitutio cibaria*, enacted at Lleida in 1168 by Bishop Guillem Pérez de Ravidats, provided that each canon was to be given a daily ration of bread amounting to about 750 grams, which means that the various charitable regimens provided the poor with less bread than typically consumed by the clergy.[86]

Besides bread, wine was the other principal staple served to the poor at Barcelona every day except Holy Thursday and Good Friday. [87] It was normally purchased at the local market to save cartage and because it could be purchased for less money than the higher quality vintages produced on the *almoina*'s own estates commanded. At Lleida, the wine came from both sources. There are no estimates of the ration provided at Barcelona's table, but the Hospital of Pere Desvilar dispensed a sixth of a quart per day. Bertrán has estimated that Lleida in 1338 gave each poor person .53 liters per day, amounting to 12.34 percent of the total calories provided by the *almoina*'s meal.[88] This is close to the fifteenth-century portions provided by Burgos's Hospital del Rey (.75 liters of poor, local wine) and Toledo's confraterntity of San Pedro (.84 liters), but only half what the average medieval person seems to have consumed. Even the residents of Valencia's Hospital of En Clapers imbibed between .77 and 1.25 liters per day in the later fourteenth century.[89]

Apart from bread and wine, meat was the most commonly served food; it was part of the diet of all social classes, albeit in small quantities.[90] At Girona in 1360, for example, there were some forty butchers to serve a population of ten thousand.[91] Meat, of course, could not be consumed on days of abstinence—Fridays, the eves of certain feasts, and certain days during Lent and Advent. Echániz counts 155 days of abstinence so observed in Barcelona in 1283–84, although Bertrán's work at Lleida for 1338 suggests that far fewer were meatless. In any case, the records show that meat was served on 253 days out of 365 at Lleida, and on 185 days out of 340 at Barcelona.[92] By contrast, the canonical constitutions of Lleida (1168) permitted meat on only 180 days a year to a clergy who presumably followed a stricter regimen.[93] Mutton was by far the meat eaten most often, representing 174 of the 185 meat portions given out in Barcelona in 1283–1284; beef was second, with twelve servings at Lleida and seven at Barcelona; the menus were rounded out at Lleida with one serving of pork and at Barcelona with four of veal. The mutton was presumably very mature lamb; in Castile the custom was to slaughter sheep only after they had reached forty to forty-five kilograms. Beef typically came from old milk cows or diseased animals; indeed, at Barcelona, Echániz speculates that much of the meat for the *almoina* was purchased from butchers who specialized in discarded animals and served, especially in the summer months, with salsa to hide the bad smells.[94] The records of the *almoina* show no poultry served—understandable because chicken was typically priced as high as pork, which next to lamb and veal was the most expensive meat and considered to be suitable only for the sick or for special occasions. In general, the cheapest meats predominated.[95] Neither Bertrán nor Echániz have estimated the size of meat portions, but that served to pilgrims at the Hospital del Rey in Burgos is thought to have been about 300 grams.[96] In Catalonia, however, the portion might have been as small as 100 grams. At Pere Desvilar's hospital, for example, inmates by statute were supposed to receive either 90 grams of mutton or 110 grams of veal or beef.[97]

Fish, salted, dried, or smoked, was served more rarely, only 14 times in Lleida in 1338, but 110 times in the seaport of Barcelona. At Lleida, conger eel, the only variety of fish consumed, appeared during Lent, especially on the Thursdays and Sundays between the feast of the Annunciation and Holy Thursday. It was completely absent from the rest of the year; instead, on other days of abstinence, the poor would be given wine, oil, dried beans, and salsa plus a half diner (or *òbol*) with which to purchase a main course.[98] At Barcelona, where a greater variety of seafood was available at the *pescateria del mar*, fish like mullet, sea bass, or dolphin were fairly common during the colder months, especially during Lent. Like meat, fish was purchased daily from local sellers, but as at Lleida the custom of paying out money in lieu of fish seems to have developed also.[99] At Lleida, Bertrán estimates the portion of eel served to have been 62.26 grams, which we can contrast to the pilgrim portion at Burgos of 83 grams plus one sardine.[100] The Church at this time also permitted cheese and eggs to be served on days of abstinence; for the poor, cheese was a staple, not a condiment. At both Lleida and Barcelona, cheese seems to have been served on Fridays, especially in the summer when fish was hard to come by, but never during Lent or Advent; in addition, eggs also appeared on the menu at Barcelona. Portions were small, estimated to be about ninety grams at both locales.[101]

In the *Book of True Love*, Juan Ruiz, the archpriest of Hita, assigns as a penance for the sins of greed, pride, avarice, lust, perjury, gluttony, and envy to the Lord of Flesh a diet of vegetables — chick peas, string beans, asparagus, spinach, lentils, and beans.[102] Arnau de Vilanova, in his widely read *Regimen sanitatis*, furthermore, argued that legumes were unsuitable for the healthy body, that vegetables should be eaten only after being cooked, and that fruit was suitable only as medicine.[103] While such foods were clearly less esteemed than bread, wine, and meat, they nevertheless formed a significant, and the least expensive, part of the diet of the poor. Echániz's study at Barcelona reveals a monotonous selection, limited almost exclusively to cabbage, spinach, and beans. Cabbage appeared on the menu 75 percent of the time, spinach 13 percent; beans appear to have been served along with flour, oil, and a little meat as cassoulets. At Lleida, there was more variety but fewer servings. Bertrán lists broad and kidney beans and other vegetables like spinach, swiss chard, lettuce, broccoli, and cabbage as major components of 109 meals and garlic and onions for 50 more. At Barcelona, spinach and cabbage were served in the cooler months, with salsa substituted in the summer as a condiment to improve the taste of meat. In Valencia, the garden of the fourteenth-century Hospital of En Clapers grew cabbage, garlic, spinach, onions, peas, beans, various kinds of melon, gourds, eggplant, lettuce, basil and other herbs, and leeks. At Lleida, beans were served in June, August, and November, and other vegetables were served as they were in season. Here too there was a *salsa de casa* that, according to a 1311 recipe, consisted of pepper, ginger, and saffron. Olive oil was used in small quantities with fish and in stews; salt was used in seemingly large amounts; but very little if any fruit was used, since it was regarded as a food for the sick or merely as a condiment to accompany other dishes.[104]

Estimates of the nutritional value of these free meals vary. Judging by

medieval standards, Echániz describes the diet as privileged, being more
secure and varied in content than the normal food of the working class.
Bertrán, judging it by modern norms, finds it woefully inadequate, unbal-
anced, monotonous, deficient in key minerals and vitamins, and in terms of
calories adequate for women but 20.9 percent too low for men. The 2,372.9
calories that he estimates were provided by his sample menu were certainly
far below the 4,700 to 6,882 calories that have been estimated as being
typical for medieval religious, or the 3,500 required by the average laborer.
Of course, almshouses with more limited aims, like that of Girona, which
distributed only bread, provided a far smaller proportion of nutritional
needs.[105]

The Iberian sources are silent on questions of gender and status, but
studies elsewhere reveal that these could influence the quality and amount
of food given the poor. The accounts of the English Hospital of Saint
Leonard from 1461 to 1462, for example, show that while all received the
same basic allotment of bread, meat, and beer, a woman received slightly
less (6.5 percent) fish, unless she had purchased and held a sacerdotal, that
is, a man's, place.[106]

*   *   *

The four centuries of charitable assistance to the hungry that have been
reviewed here demonstrate an evolution from the occasional and ritualistic
distribution of food to a few local poor into a complex and articulated
system of assistance. Many forces were responsible for this development—
the growth of towns, the differentiation of the poor into various groups
and classes, the maturation of ecclesiastical and then of municipal institutions, the gradual accumulation of permanent endowments. To a great
degree this charity was motivated by religious concerns, which might explain why many deferred making contributions until the end of their lives.
In such circumstances, because the identity of the poor themselves would
be irrelevant, the assistance would be open to any person of need.

In Catalonia, however, this was less and less the case. Eastern Spain,
like Italy, was a region of seaports and towns and, in addition, was on the
fringe of the frontier. More so than more predominately rural and agricultural regions, Catalonia attracted numbers of outsiders who, during difficult years, could easily overwhelm the mechanisms of assistance. Thus, no
later than 1250, as early as in Italy, contributors and others in Catalonia
began to distinguish between the deserving and undeserving poor and to

discriminate on that basis in the distribution of charity. After 1250, we see no new *almoinas* established, and those already in existence begin to reserve a considerable proportion of their places for the *pauperes verecundi*, that is, poor scholars, officials, or relatives. With the formation of new parishes in towns like Barcelona, most new caritative initiatives after 1250 took place within the neighborhood and focused exclusively on the local and deserving poor. In smaller towns like Girona and Urgell, where there were fewer parishes and perhaps a smaller marginalized population, cathedral or municipal assistance continued to dominate, but this assistance was seasonal and supplemental, being limited to basic staples. As a consequence, even in smaller locales, the bias toward local people temporarily in need is clear. While the older *almoinas* would continue to distribute some food to the marginalized, increasingly the task of dealing with those without a neighborhood fell to the public shelter, which in the medieval period bore the title of hospital.

3

The Origins of
Hospices and Hospitals

SHELTER FOR THE TEMPORARILY HOMELESS, whether or not they were needy in the modern sense, was as typical a charity in the towns and villages of medieval Europe as was providing food to the hungry. The Rule of Saint Benedict, as well as local Hispanic customs, imposed the obligation of hospitality upon monasteries.[1] Likewise, in the reviving towns of the eleventh and twelfth centuries, there was a need to provide beds for those who were not householders. Urban hospices served a diverse lot: pilgrims wending their way to a shrine like Santiago, clergy and others in town on business, wandering beggars, and the local poor. Increasingly, those with means seem to have secured their own accommodation in inns or residences, while paupers sought out the more public shelters operated by churches, monasteries, town government, and even private individuals. By the thirteenth century, every town of size in Europe, including Iberia, had several of these shelters. The texts describe these institutions as hospitals or, less frequently, by the old Byzantine term *xenodochium*. While they functioned primarily as shelters, these hospitals would at times offer other forms of care because their guests needed refreshment and might also require medical assistance.[2]

Hospitals Outside the Catalan Lands

The earliest known hospital in Christian Iberia was the *xenodochium* established by Bishop Masona at Mérida in 580, but, in post-Visigothic times, the stimulus of urban development and the pilgrim road to Santiago gave rise to many hospitals in the northern portion of the peninsula. This was a new development of the eleventh and twelfth centuries. Studies at León, for example, have demonstrated that older benefactions to its cathedral would form no part of the endowments of the caritative shelters that began to appear just before 1100.[3] These shelters served the local poor and sick, but especially pilgrims who were often in as much need of care as shelter, given the dangers of the journey and the preexisting illnesses that motivated many pilgrimages. Thus, in 1052 King García Sánchez III of Navarre established the hospice of Santa María de Nájera; at León, in 1084, Bishop Pelayo opened a place near the cathedral for the sick, lame, blind, deaf, and hungry, as well as for pilgrims, and, twelve years later, Bishop Pedro moved it to a larger site just outside of town; Archbishop Gelmírez of Santiago in the early twelfth century followed this precedent. Elsewhere along this pilgrim route, we find the Hospital de San Juan in Oviedo, where the feet of pilgrims were washed, the late tenth-century Hospital de la Trinidad de Arre, near Pamplona, the eleventh-century Hospital de San Esteban at Astorga, the Hospital de Santa Cristina at the pass of Somport, and the early twelfth-century hospices at Aubrac and Roncesvalles in the Pyrenees.[4] In Burgos, among some thirty known hospitals, were the Hospital del Rey, the Hospital del Emperador, and the Hospital de Santa María la Real, all of which specialized in sheltering pilgrims on the Santiago road, the Hospital de San Lucas that housed invalids, and a capitular hospice near the cathedral for the local paupers. Other, smaller institutions served the needs of specific parishes or those of individual confraternities.[5] Elsewhere, Astorga had twenty hospitals and Salamanca twenty-eight.[6] León's first hospital was the episcopal Hospital de San Juan (1084), and by 1250 it was joined by eight others. At Valladolid, the Hospital de Esgueva, which dated from the end of the eleventh century, was but one of twenty institutions in the fifteenth century. Seville, a Castilian town only after 1248, had five hospitals by 1300 that included pilgrim hospices established by King Alfonso X and another by Aragonese settlers in the region; five others were founded in the fourteenth century, including that of San Bernando for poor, elderly residents of the town.[7] Córdoba counted at least thirty-three hospital establishments founded in the thirteenth and fourteenth centuries.[8] Valencia, another "new" city, saw a half dozen hospitals established in the immediate decades after its conquest, most under ecclesiastical governance, and by the fifteenth century this number had risen to fourteen. Thirteenth-century Saragossa had eleven hospitals and Toulouse more than a dozen.[9] In Portugal, there were over forty-seven hospices just north of the Douro, and another twenty-five leprosaria; the town of Porto itself had eight hospitals.[10]

The Iberian phenomenon was typical of the situation elsewhere in Europe. In Paris, there was the large Hôtel-Dieu near Notre Dame Cathedral for transients and the sick, as well as other hospices for lepers, pilgrims, orphans, ex-prostitutes, and the blind. Paris itself had about sixty hospitals in all, and the smaller towns of Narbonne, and Arles had fifteen and sixteen.[11] The chronicler Giovanni Villani reports that Florence had about thirty hospitals at the beginning of the fourteenth century, and a century later there were ten more. In 1350 Rome counted twenty-five.[12] In the Low Countries, there is record of pilgrim hospices from 1137 and of urban hospitals from 1090 (at Louvain).[13] In 1154, England had 113 known hospitals, and more than 700 by 1300, not counting monastic infirmaries, establishments of the Hospitallers of Saint John, and the ubiquitous small, undocumented establishments.[14] Thus, the phenomenon of public shelters was one that Catalonia shared with the rest of Europe.

Catalan Hospitals

While the oldest hospital in Catalonia will likely never be identified, two of the earliest were the hospices for pilgrims and travelers located at the Benedictine monasteries of Sant Pere de Rodes, which dates from the late tenth century, and of Sant Pere de Casserres, which was founded in the eleventh century. Both were constructed outside the monastic walls as simple two-storied hostels. At around the same time, the count of Cerdanya in 965 established a hospice for travelers at the Coll de la Perxa, a deserted spot on the road from Cerdanya to the Conflent, which was served by a community of lay brothers and servants.[15] There were other refuges at the Hills of Puymorens and Arnés, and at Sentillà and Santa Cecília de Rella. In the valley of Clusa three other hospices for pilgrims depended on the monasteries of Sant Hilarde Rasez, Arlés, and Soreda. Instances of other such shelters, located in towns, villages, and rural locales, proliferate during the eleventh century. At Barcelona, Bishop Deodat donated to a hospital for the poor in 1024, and another named "En Guitard" was established circa 1045, the same year someone named Arnau opened a hospital for the poor next to the cathedral at Urgell; Girona possibly had a hospital within the old Roman fortifications in the tenth century. Another hospital was established at Cardona in 1083, and in 1068 Arsendis, the wife of Arnau Mir of Tost, asked her spouse to establish shelters for the infirm poor at Tost as well as at Algar, Montmagastre, and Artesa. In the eleventh century Vic had an *Albergueria,* located behind the cathedral, that served as a residence for clergy as well as a hospital. At the beginning of the next century, in 1101, the chapter of Ager established a shelter for travelers, and, in 1116, Count Arnau de Roselló instituted a shelter for Christ's poor at the Church of Sant Joan at Perpignan.[16] Throughout Catalonia, as indeed throughout Christian Iberia and western Europe,[17] bishops, chapters, confraternities, prosperous and perhaps pious individuals, and eventually even municipalities established a myriad of such shelters to house and, at times, offer various types of material assistance to an assortment of temporarily or permanently homeless persons: travelers and pilgrims, the old, the sick and the dying, and the destitute.[18] Here we shall endeavor not only to chronicle this hospitaller explosion, but also attempt to fathom the social forces that created the phenomenon.

The Hospitals of Barcelona

Barcelona possessed one of the earliest of the cathedral shelters in Catalonia,[19] but dating the Hospital of the See, sometimes called En Guitard, is difficult. One tradition connects its foundation to a legacy of land on Montjuic given in 938 to the sacristan of the cathedral; legacies from 995 and 1011 confirm the existence of a shelter for the poor and pilgrims. Another tradition argues that the hospital was founded by the chapter and Bishop Deodat in 1023, perhaps as part of the town's reconstruction after al-Mansūr's raid, or perhaps earlier in 1009 when the chapter itself was established. A third version attributes an early foundation to a viscount of Barcelona named Guitard, which was reendowed in 1045 by Count Ramon Berenguer I. Whatever the actual date of its foundation, the construction of a new Romanesque cathedral, consecrated in 1058, disrupted its operation and it is little mentioned in the sources until after a reconstruction in 1090. In the twelfth century, it acquired an endowment of lands in Sarrià, Las Cortes, and Reixac, and after 1133, at the behest of Archbishop Oleguer, received the beds and linen of all deceased clergy. The hospice was overseen directly by the bishop and chapter until 1175 when its supervision passed to the chaplain of the altar of Sant Nicolau, who was named *custos* of the *xenodochium*. Just as the bishop and chapter collectively attended to their obligation of feeding the poor in only a ritualistic fashion, as we have seen, so also they do not seem to have placed any great priority upon the operation of the cathedral hospital. It did not benefit from the considerable wealth of the bishop and canons, who were not only the largest landowners in Barcelona but also lords of a considerable rural patrimony. The hospice's lack of adequate endowment, in fact, led to its suppression and merger into a newly established hospital of En Colom.[20]

Joan Colom was an important member of the cathedral chapter; he oversaw capitular finances for the month of December, often served as a judge and arbitrator, and may have been a treasurer for King Jaume I. He was also a contemporary of Bishop Berenguer de Palou, whose benefaction was so essential for the cathedral's Pia Almoina. This hospital was established and endowed in 1229, just before the redaction of Colom's will. It was located on land abutting property of the Knights of Saint John, in the Raval, a yet undeveloped agricultural district across the modern Ramblas, near the future site of the Hospital of Santa Creu and on the modern Carrer de l'Hospital. This was the least desirable suburban district of the city, an area of poor drainage that was thought to be unhealthy.[21] The small establishment, with a house and a chapel, was placed under the administration not of the chapter or bishop but of a kinsman, Berenguer de Plan, and three nephews. In 1236, Berenguer agreed to its merger with the Hospital of the See, but because he retained the usufruct of Colom's goods, he acquired control over the unified hospital. But the bishop and chapter considered the new institution as a continuation of the cathedral hospice and thus diocesan property. The merger document of 1236 speaks of the hospital's mission to serve the poor, vagabonds, and pilgrims, which suggests that this served as a temporary shelter rather than an asylum.[22] But a census of inmates conducted in 1307 also reveals individuals whose term was likely more extended: ten sick persons, four abandoned children around the age of five, eight children still being nursed, and two poor boys being given academic instruction by the rector. All in all, in the early fourteenth century the hospital had a patient population of some twenty-seven persons and a staff of sixteen or more.[23]

Pere Desvilar was another canon of Barcelona's cathedral who founded a hospital in the thirteenth century. Under the patronage of Sant Macià, this institution was also located in the Raval district, close to that of En Colom and the leper hospice. Unlike Colom, Desvilar played no direct role in the establishment of the hospital, but instead left the task to his manumissors or executors. The will of August 1256 directed that Desvilar's goods be used to establish a hospice and chapel, to be directed at first by his executor, Pere de Sales, and thereafter by a rector nominated by the chapter. Desvilar instructed that any income derived from lease renewals and transfers, *laudesimos*, be dedicated to expanding the initial endowment; notices of additional gifts and bequests commence in 1269. The donor requested that the hospital provide care for the poor but specified a special preference for "men of the sea," sailors who were too old or sick to provide for themselves. (Valencia, another port town, would in the fourteenth century have a hospice for fishermen.)[24] In addition, he guaranteed lifetime support for his friend Pere de Sales, in sickness and in health, reserved a portion of the hospital's income to endow a memorial lamp for himself, and required support, until her death, for his maid Maria.[25] As illustrated in 1278 by Bishop Arnau's nomination of Bernat Ferrer to be administrator of Sant Macià, the overall responsibility for the hospital passed to the bishop. The terms of this particular appointment, however, because they required Bernat to transfer some eight parcels of land to the hospital, suggest that the diocese's commitment to its financial support was limited.[26]

The first important hospital established by a layman was that of Bernat Marcús, a rich resident of the parish of Santa Maria del Mar.[27] Endowed with urban houses and land on Montjuic, the hospital, chapel, and cemetery were located on the entry road into Barcelona from France. According to the donor's will of 1166, the hospital was meant to serve pilgrims, abandoned children, and the sick poor. The foundation's history illustrates the pitfalls of private foundations. While Bernat's sons, Bernat and Ramon, completed construction of the chapel and hospice that their father had begun, the family's patronage ceased in the next generation, whose only members were the three daughters of the younger Bernat. Future administrators, it seems, were nominated by the bishop of Barcelona, eventually with some participation by the Consell de Cent, Barcelona's municipal council, as well. By the end of the thirteenth century, the initial endowment provided by Bernat Marcús's family proved inadequate for the hospital's needs and presumably there was no new infusion of family funds. Consequently, Pere Bertran as administrator was forced in 1281 to borrow two hundred sous just to maintain the hospital's operation. The economic crisis of the later 1330s finally brought En Marcús to the verge of insolvency, and its administrators were forced to sell the hospital to the Consell de Cent for one hundred sous, making it the first hospital in Barcelona to be governed by the municipality.[28]

Pere Desvilar, not to be confused with the thirteenth-century canon, was another Barcelona layman who founded a hospital, but unlike Bernat Marcús, he conferred its governance directly upon the Consell de Cent, much the same way his contemporary in Valencia, the merchant Bernat dez Clapers, entrusted a hospital for infirm paupers to the "honored citizens" of Valencia.[29] While the origin of Pere's hospital may predate 1300, we know of it only from the document transferring it to city control in 1308. The property then consisted of a small building and chapel (dedicated to Sant Pere and Santa Marta) in the Ribera district, which is along the shore and near the modern Ciutadella Park. Desvilar's will of 1311 left an endowment sufficient to feed and shelter twelve paupers, but four of these places were reserved for his own kinsmen. Pere Desvilar oversaw his foundation until his death, and, perhaps because the needy here included his own relations, even specified the type and amount of food to be served. Afterward, his place was taken by a son, Jaume, but thereafter the administrator and chaplain were appointed by municipal authorities.[30]

Outside and to the east of Barcelona, near the modern Ciutadella, another hospital of the poor was established at the old monastery of Santa Eulàlia. Founded in the tenth century, the cloister was reformed by Bishop Oleguer in the 1120s as a community of Augustinian canons. By 1212, the date of a legacy, there existed a hospital on the site, located alongside the monastery. It seems that two laypeople, Berenguer Canet and his wife Pereta, perhaps as members of an unnamed confraternity, purchased this land in 1210 to build a hospital for the poor. Because it was located within the domain of Santa Eulàlia, Berenguer promised not to construct either a chapel or a cemetery, which would infringe upon the monastery's rights. What follows becomes somewhat convoluted. In 1213, in response to a series of disagreements between the canons and the hospital concerning the former's fiscal rights, the prior renounced any rights over the hospital. In 1221, however, when the hospital was definitely in operation along with a chaplain and oratory, and in what has the tenor of a testamentary bequest, Berenguer returned lordship over the hospital to the monastery. Presumably at some point in the preceding decade, Berenguer had obtained the right to build a chapel, whose chaplain was to be selected from among the canons of Santa Eulàlia. In return, Berenguer was made an oblate of the monastery with its attendant material and spiritual benefits. But, in 1237, his daughter, Berenguera de Rubí, hinting at serious scandal of some sort, complained that the monastery was unable to provide a fit chaplain.[31] Thereupon, she appointed a secular priest as chaplain, and eventually, presumably after Berenguera's death, Bishop Arnau de Gurb intervened and, at a date unknown, appointed two canons of the cathedral as the hospital's administrators. Episcopal supervision, however, could not have been strict, because the priest Bartomeu Descoll, who became rector in 1297, was able to destroy the hospital's reputation. A pastoral visit conducted by Bishop Ponç de Gualba in March 1305 found that Bartomeu had embezzled funds, raped a twelve-year-old female patient, and committed public scandal by bearing arms and playing musical instruments. There were no sheets on the beds (they had been pawned!), and the chaplain lacked food. Despite the bread alms from Barcelona sufficient to feed fifteen persons a day, and over one thousand sous in rental income and alms, patients and staff lacked adequate amounts of food. Furthermore, the rector evidently had refused admission to new patients since on the date of the visitation only six of the thirty places available were actually occupied. The lengthy suit that followed a second visitation in 1307 only reconfirmed the decadence into which the hospital had descended.[32]

Another hospital on the fringes of Barcelona was established at Olesa de Bonesvalls, near Vilafranca del Penedès, along a well-traveled route, to serve traveling Franciscan and Dominican friars and pilgrims. Its initial endowment came from the will of Guillem de Cervelló in 1262. Up until the seventeenth century, its rector was named by the pastor of the Church of Sant Pau and confirmed by the superiors of the two mendicant communities in Barcelona.[33] At Vilafranca del Penedès were the Hospital de Sant Valentí, in operation in 1141, and the Hospital de Santa Maria, which belonged to the Trinitarians in the fourteenth century.[34] Other hospitals in the diocese of Barcelona were located at Arraona-Sabadell, Piera, Cubelles, Vila-Rodona, Cornellà, Terrassa, Sant Celoni, Hospitalet, Subirats, Caldes d'Estrac, Sant Cugat del Vallès, and Cervelló. A hostel at La Garriga in 1287 had seventeen beds.[35] Manresa had two hospitals in the thirteenth century, and in 1300 Pere Salvatge added a chapel to serve the infirm of Sant Andreu, which was administered by the town council. At Granollers, Bertran de Seva established a hospital circa 1325, but this too was transferred to municipal authorities by his descendants.[36] And at Sitges, Bernat de Fonollar's will of June 9, 1306, endowed a shelter for poor pilgrims, orphans, the sick, and other needy.[37]

Public shelters were not confined to the Christian community of Barcelona. In 1277, Abraham of Alexandria and his son, Astruc, the founder of the *almoina* for the Jewish community of Barcelona, endowed a hospice for the poor and travelers in a house of the call (or Jewish quarter) that had been established earlier by Rabbi Samuel ben rabí Isaac Ha-Sardí, a native of Cerdanya. At the end of the fourteenth century it was known as the hospital of the poor Jews, and was governed by four hospitallers or proctors. A document of 1385 records the gift of a bed made from four boards, a mattress, a bolster, and associated bedding. Despite such gifts, however, this and other charities in Jewish *aljamas* were actually funded by an informal system of taxation, in which each man was expected to pay stated assessments and also make voluntary contributions. The destruction of the Jewish quarter in the riots of 1391, however, probably eliminated the hospital.[38]

An unusual association is revealed in the notarial records of fifteenth-century Barcelona: the confraternity of the Holy Spirit for the Lame, Blind, and Poor of the City of Barcelona, also called the confraternity of Sant Andreu. In 1442, Joan de Mayo, a blind man, and Jaume Blavi, a beggar, were its rectors, and its treasury included the cash amount of 139 sous. It also rented a modest house, received legacies and presumably alms. The record does not show how the confraternity helped its members, but one can assume that modest material assistance and burial would have been important priorities; there is no evidence that the confraternity was able to operate a shelter, although it does appear that Barcelona's blind beggars were confined to certain sections of the city.[39]

The Hospitals of Urgell

The hospitaller phenomenon that we have seen in the region of Barcelona was replicated, albeit on a smaller scale, throughout Catalonia. In the north of the principality, at the Seu d'Urgell, the earliest institutions of charity focused on the local poor, travelers who fell ill, and pilgrims to the Virgin of Urgell and its cathedral relics. Throughout the Pyrenean passes there were shelters for pilgrims, such as that at the Benedictine monastery of Sant Serni de Tavèrnoles, which guarded the bridge of Sant Esteve over the Valira River. Within Urgell itself, the first mention of a hospital for the poor, or *albergueria*, is found in a will of 1059.[40] Many parishes and locales in the diocese eventually followed the example of the cathedral, and similar hospitals were established at Organyà in 1156, Agramunt circa 1175, and Sanaüja before 1201. The will of Bishop Guillem Arnau de Montferrer in 1096 suggests that Urgell's hospital shared quarters with its *almoina*, both being dependencies of the chapter. Twelfth-century residents bequeathed the hospital gifts of money, clothing, blankets, and beds; as at Barcelona, it became the custom for local clergy to will their bedding to this institution. Eventually an endowment of lands and rents was assembled. While the bishop originally had the title of proctor of the house of charity, by the later twelfth century this position devolved upon the prior of the church of Sant Miquel, and in the thirteenth upon the precentor of the chapter. The proctor in turn appointed a hospitaller and the other staff of the institution.[41]

First mentioned in 1247 is a second or new hospital that seems to have been established by the municipality itself. It was located in the old church of Santa Eulàlia at the Cerdanya gate; the apse remained a chapel for its inmates, separated by two doors from the nave that in the fifteenth century contained five beds. The first hospitaller was a woman named Aledis, but the fourteenth-century hospitallers who are known were male. The hospital was primarily a place of shelter or residence; there is no evidence of any ties with Urgell's small medical community. Beds, along with mattresses and bed linen, were the most frequent material gifts; money donations in wills averaged a mere six diners. In most instances, the identities of the inmates and the duration of their stay is unknown, although its proximity to the local cemetery suggests that some individuals came here to die. In any case, the local and transient poor became the responsibility of the town. The property itself was transferred to the Dominicans in 1364, but it is unclear whether the Town Hospital, as it was now called, remained or was moved elsewhere.[42]

By 1258, the old hospital of Urgell had been renamed the Hospital of the Chapter or that of Poor Clerics, and it now served old or enfeebled clergy without means or those whose benefice was inadequate to support both a curate and a pension. This problem of impoverished clergy was universal, and Urgell, or Catalonia, was not unique in making such provision for retired clerics.[43] The custom of local clergy donating beds and linen to the older hospital continued to be mandated by the bishop until 1299, when it was replaced with a diocesan annuity of sixty sous, but some clerics continued the practice into the fourteenth century. Because the laity had transferred its charity to the municipal hospital, the clergy, and a few pious women, were now the only financial support for what had become a clerical old folks home.[44]

Then, during the early fifteenth century, both of these hospitals were consolidated into a single unit. While the chapter and bishop evidently continued their subsidy to the merged hospital, the burden of its support fell upon the town consuls; certainly the endowment of rents and land, along with private alms, provided a diminished proportion of the budget. The popular nature of the institution itself was reinforced by the new custom of electing two or three proctors as its governors at an annual assembly of all heads of household.[45]

At Solsona, south of Urgell, the custom of private hospitaller foundations continued into the fifteenth century. For example, Francesca, the daughter of a local merchant and the wife of a noble, endowed in her will of

1411 the Hospital of Llobera, a gothic structure, as a shelter for the poor. The charity remained a family enterprise for a century, since the position of administrator descended through several generations of male descendants.[46]

The Hospitals of Girona

The earliest known hospital in Girona is the Hospital of Sant Pere of the See, also known as the Old Hospital, the Hospital of the See, and the Hospital of the Capellans. It was located next to the church of Sant Nicolau, between the plaza and the monastery of Sant Pere de Galligans. Although the first reference to it dates only from 1228, it must be considerably older since a "new" hospital had been founded by the confraternity at the church of Sant Martí in 1211. In fact a legacy to a "hospice" for the poor is extant from 1095.[47] Documents of the late thirteenth and fourteenth centuries establish the old hospital as the responsibility of the bishop and chapter, who appointed the hospitaller and took at least some financial responsibility for its support. The ceremonial nature of the charity dispensed here is evidenced by the hospitaller's responsibility to attend not just the poor but also its benefactors.[48] The New Hospital, on the other hand, was a lay foundation that, according to reforms of 1317, was governed by a commander, selected by the *jurats* of the city, and by three consuls drawn from each of the town's social orders. Both hospitals had endowments of rural properties, but the municipal hospital was clearly favored by townspeople, if the evidence from testaments is representative.[49] In addition to these two hospitals, there was a hospice located on a bridge over the Rio Onyar for those on pilgrimage to Santiago. Evidence for its existence dates back to the twelfth century, and in 1386 it was governed by two "good men" selected in the same manner used for municipal and diocesan alms collectors.[50]

The Hospitals of Vic

At Vic, only a hospice to the rear of the cathedral predates the twelfth century. This *hospitaleria* for the poor and sick existed in 1133, when the bishop entrusted its care to the abbot of l'Estany; testamentary references to such a hospice, however, date from 1054 and 1063.[51] In the thirteenth century, with the construction of a chapel, this establishment became known as Sant Jaume dels Malalts or, in the fourteenth century, as Sant

Jaume's house of lepers, and was served by a small male confraternity. By this time, at least three additional hospitals were in operation: En Cloquer established in 1217 outside the walls and at the foot of the bridge into Vic; a shelter for travelers, vagrants, and the elderly at the church of Sant Bartomeu, which was founded in 1246 (but soon absorbed by En Cloquer); and the Hospital de la Santa Trinitat established by Ramon de Malla in 1275. These structures, however, were more than mere shelters for the poor, that is, the homeless, because they also served lepers (who elsewhere were usually more segregated) and victims of the plague. In the next century, the Hospital de la Santa Creu was established by a wealthy citizen, Ramon de Terrades, who bequeathed six hundred pounds in his will of 1338 to build a traditional shelter for pilgrims, the sick, and abandoned children. It began to function with twelve beds in 1384, and in 1441 gained a chapel.[52]

The Hospitals of Lleida

The roots of organized charity at Lleida are found in the Aragonese town of Roda, whose bishop was transferred to Lleida in 1149. He brought with him an almoner and infirmarian, whose offices at Roda have been documented in the late eleventh century.[53] Within the reconquered city itself, the care of needy clergy was an early and prominent concern (manifested here a century before Urgell) that gave rise to several foundations. One was an infirmary established in the cloister by Bishop Guillem Pérez de Ravidats, circa 1174, for invalid canons because the chapter at this stage was still living a community life. At around the same time, other clergy, presumably those who did not belong to the chapter, established a confraternity to support and shelter the needy within their ranks. These acquired their own hospice opposite the cathedral. The cathedral also maintained a shelter for outsiders, the Casa de la Caritat, first mentioned in a document of 1180. Initially it served as an inn for visiting canons from Lleida's sister see of Roda and their attendants, as well as a more general constituency of traveling clerics, pilgrims, almoners, and others. But by 1237, it functioned exclusively as a hostel for traveling ecclesiastics and their entourages.[54] The work of sheltering the nonclerical poor, which was elsewhere an episcopal or capitular responsibility, was initiated here by a lay couple, Guillem Nicolau and his wife Falerna. Shortly after the city's reconquest in 1149, but before 1156, the couple established a shelter for the sick, travelers, and pilgrims, along the banks of the Segre River and near the bridge into the town from

Barcelona and Bellpuig. The hospice was directed by Guillem as its proctor and master, and endowed with the tithes owed by his lands, which would otherwise have accrued to the bishop. Guillem and Falerna were also joined by others who formed a small community of brothers in service of the poor, assisted by a confraternity of townsmen. Because of the quasi-religious nature of the establishment and the application of episcopal tithes, the hospital itself was deeded to the diocese; a document of 1162, which records the relocation of the hospital from a flooded site to higher ground, notes Guillem's pledge of obedience to the bishop. The bishop in turn sanctioned a chapel with two bells in which the community and the poor could hear mass, providing that the bells, and presumably the masses, did not compete with those at the cathedral. There was also a cemetery for the hospitaller community and for inmates who died there.[55]

Pere Moliner, a knight who had profited from the conquest of Lleida, established a hospital for the sick. It was destroyed by flood, circa 1170; a document of 1179 notes its reestablishment in houses acquired from the Templars outside the walls near the monastery of Sant Antoni Abat, the municipal slaughterhouse, and the Gardeny gate. Unlike Guillem Nicolau, Pere Moliner did not deed his establishment to the bishop; as late as 1384 his heirs maintained the right to name the hospital's proctor. In the mid-fifteenth century, on the eve of its merger with five other hospitals to form the Hospital General de Santa Maria, its patrons numbered members of the cathedral chapter and municipal council.[56]

Several other of the original settlers of Lleida also established shelters or hospitals of some sort, although little is known of them. Among these are the Hospital of Pere Tarasco, first cited in 1225, and that of Pedro Belvis, which was donated to the bishop in 1201, and perhaps to the Trinitarians in 1204.[57] Other hospitals, like that of Santa Maria Magdalena, directed by the confraternity of weavers, a hospital of the furriers, the Hospital de la Vista, the parochial Hospital of Sant Martí, and that of Sant Tomàs, are little more than names that appear in the odd document.[58] Institutions like the Hospital of the Toulousains, which was destined to shelter travelers from that region, probably never functioned at all. In this case, the presumptive founder, Hugo of Toulouse, willed money for this purpose should he die without sons, but the birth of an heir made the bequest moot.[59]

Better known are the establishments founded by or for religious orders. There is the hospital of the Knights of Saint John, in existence by 1185. A canon, Gerald de Zacozola, may have established two hospitals, one in 1213 in service of the poor, the infirm, and Christian captives, and granted in his wills of 1216 and 1222 to the Trinitarians, and another in 1214 for the poor and sick granted to the Templars.[60] A will, redacted by Bernarda, the wife of Tomàs de Sant Climent, bequeathed fifty mazmodins to the "hospital of my father located on the other side of the Segre River (at Cap Pont) that is held by the Brothers of the Holy Trinity," but it is unclear whether this is the same or a second redemptionist hospice.[61] The Antonines, who were dedicated to the care of those with major skin disorders, especially ergotism, had a hospice in Lleida by 1271; a shelter for abandoned children may have been founded as early as 1166 but was eventually (by 1214) ceded to the Order of the Holy Spirit.[62]

The Hospitals of Cervera

In Cervera, on the road between Barcelona and Lleida, the first notices of hospitals date from the early thirteenth century. Besides the Hospital of Santa Magdalena, dedicated to the service of lepers, the will of Joan de l'Hospital and his wife Ermesinda in 1235 set aside two houses as support for a small shelter that could serve two paupers. In 1328, another couple, Domènech Aguilar and Guilleuma, established the Hospital de les Onze Mil Verges for the traveling poor, which prospered under the patronage of such prominent voyagers as Infante Joan d'Aragó, the archbishop of Tarragona. Financial problems in the difficult years of the early fifteenth century, however, forced its administration to turn to the town government for help. The municipality itself, in 1356, already supervised three hospitals and a leprosarium, all located within the city walls.[63]

The Hospitals of Tarragona and Its Region

In the archiepiscopal see of Tarragona, reconquered and resettled in the years after 1129, no reference is made to a cathedral hospice for the poor before the will of Archbishop Huc de Cervelló in 1171 that bequeathed a hundred morabetins for the construction of such a hospital at the gate of the cathedral near an ancient cemetery. A papal bull of 1184 notes that the income and tithes of two churches, Sant Miquel and Sant Lleonart, had been assigned by the chapter to the "Hospital of the Poor." Archbishop Ramon de Rocaberti made additional donations in 1214. In 1220, there was a hospitaller, a canon named Ramon. An interesting document from 1246 tells us that residents objected to the hospital's practice of appropriating the beds (and bed linen) belonging to all the deceased of the town. This was evidently done immediately after the body had been transferred from the bedstead, on which it had been conveyed to the cemetery, to the grave. In an effort to mediate between the sensibilities of heirs and relatives and the hospital's economic needs, Archbishop Joan of Aragon arranged a compromise by which the hospital forswore its claim to these beds in return for an annual cash subsidy from town residents. As at Girona and Lleida, the chapter had its own infirmary that was served by canons as hospitallers and infirmarians. César Martinell cites, but then discounts, an anonymous source which argued that the former hospital served town residents, while the latter was reserved for poor clergy and their family and servants. Tarragona's town council was established in 1255, but it was not until 1362 or 1370 that a municipal hospital, the *hospital nou*, was founded, with a priest as its first administrator. In 1372, it was given the quarters of an old leprosarium that had been built between 1174 and 1214. Given its poor state of repair, however, the city had to construct a new and larger structure in the 1390s. Hard times during the troubles of the early fifteenth century led to its merger in 1464 with the cathedral hospital as the Hospital of Sant Pau and Santa Tecla, but a new building was not provided until 1588.[64]

South of Tarragona, near the village of Cambrils, Queen Blanca's will of 1310 established the Hospital de l'Enfant, named for Jaume II's son, Pere, count of Prades. It was at first administered by the monks of Santes Creus, but later by the Hospitallers of Saint John.[65] The nearby monastery of Poblet, the necropolis of the count-kings, had its own hospices for monks, travelers, and pilgrims, and in the nearby village of l'Espluga del Francolí there was a hospital belonging to the Knights of Saint John.[66] Nearby, at the Cistercian monastery of Santes Creus the Hospital of Sant Pere dels Pobres was established in the early decades of the thirteenth century and is known from a series of endowments granted it in 1229 by aristocratic patrons.[67]

In the later thirteenth century places of shelter appeared at Montblanc, where a will of 1266 mentions the Hospital de Santa Magdalena and the Hospital de Sant Bartolomeu. The former was an extramural establishment on the Tarragona-Lleida road that belonged to the confraternity of the Poor of Jesus Christ. A fourteenth-century church was built on the site of what might have been an earlier twelfth-century hospital; and the Hospital de Santa Magdalena built alongside the river was a two-storied rectangle, surrounding a courtyard. Of the Hospital de Sant Bartolomeu virtually nothing is known except its association with the Franciscans. A third institution, the Hospital de Sant Marçal, was established for the poor in the midfourteenth century alongside the town wall with proceeds from the will of

Jaume Marçal who had died in 1339. In addition to a chapel with three altars, there was a simply constructed arched hall.[68] There was also a pilgrim hospice next to the sanctuary of La Serra that was served by two priests and two boys (acolytes); in 1397 the priests received protection as familiars of the royal household.[69]

The Hospital de Sant Joan at Reus, near Tarragona, was constructed in the mid-thirteenth century to serve the sick. The administrators were chosen annually at the final meeting of the town council and were given charge of the hospital and its patrimony, the poor, and the hospitaller church; thus, these officials were frequently called the sacristans of Sant Joan. By the fourteenth century, however, the terms of office were much longer and frequently were held by married couples. The hospital's receipts from its lands (which grew wheat, grapes, and olives) must have been substantial, since in 1379 it paid a tax assessment of 112 sous and 3 diners to the lord of Reus, the archbishop of Tarragona.[70] The hospital itself was situated in the new town, near the walls, and mostly likely was a two-storied structure built around a central patio. There is no evidence of any medical staff before the sixteenth century.[71]

The Hospitals of Tortosa

The first notice of the Hospital de Santa Maria, or the Hospital of the See, in Tortosa is in a document of 1172. As is typical, its function was the care of the poor and infirm, and its governance capitular. Tortosa's Code of Customs of 1279 mentions a municipal hospital, that of la Grassa, which functioned under a hospitaller who was also a cathedral canon, but one commentator suggests that this might just have been an inn or hostel. In the early fourteenth century, there was also a hospice for feeding the poor eight kilometers away in the hamlet of Hospitalet de l'Infant.[72]

The Hospitals of Majorca

At Palma on Majorca, soon after its conquest, three hospitals were quickly opened, perhaps spurred on by the outbreak of the plague in January 1230, just weeks after the capitulation of the city. Nunyo Sanç, the nephew of Ramon Berenguer IV and the count of Roussillon and Cerdagne, endowed the Hospital de Sant Andreu. Located in the moat of the citadel, the Almudaina, Sant Andreu contained twenty beds for the sick and poor and was served, under the supervision of the bishop and chapter, by a rector, priest, sacristan, serving woman, and seven laborers for fieldwork, some of whom were slaves. Provisions and freshly baked bread were supplied by farms located in the village of Santa Eulàlia.[73] During the same decade, and certainly before 1248, two other hospitals were also established. The first, Sant Antoni Abat, resulted from a land grant given by Jaume I to the Augustinian canons; the second, that of Santa Magdalena, was the gift of Pons Huc, the son of Count Huc of Empuriès who was the most prominent victim of the 1230 plague. The first hospital designated specifically for the poor did not appear until the foundation of Santa Catarina dels Pobres in 1345.[74]

The Jewish community of Majorca, like its counterpart in Barcelona, established a network of beneficial institutions. In addition to an *almoina* or house of alms, Moisés Cabrit established a shelter in Santa Coloma de Queralt for the unfortunate and Sayt Mill established a hospital in the Jewish quarter of Palma in 1377 with five beds and endowment for bread and clothing.[75]

The Hospitals of Valencia

The city of Valencia, like Majorca, only came under Christian lordship during the reign of Jaume I, who first entered the city on October 9, 1238. Over the next several years, its lands were given out to a myriad of Christian settlers, as recorded in the famous *Repartiment de València*, which meant that whatever hospitaller tradition that had existed under Muslim rule ceased and had to be rekindled by the city's new masters. Here the situation would be similar to that which we have already seen in Lleida and Majorca. With the bishop and his chapter preoccupied with establishing their own institutional apparatus, the initiative for establishing houses of charity fell to individuals who had profited from the conquest and to religious orders who were attracted into the new realm by grants of land and property. A case in point is the Hospital of Sant Guillem, founded in 1242 by the wealthy settler Guillem Escrivá, and entrusted to the care of the Order of the Trinity, a group recently founded in France to ransom captives and shelter the poor. The Hospitallers of Saint Mary of Roncesvalles, who were established in 1132 to provide shelter to pilgrims and the sick traversing the Navarrese pass, also operated a small shelter within the city, as did the Knights of Saint John. The important royal hospital, with its accompanying church and shrine, was that of Sant Vicent, which Jaume I established in 1238 to honor the patron saint of the new kingdom. It was entrusted to monks of the powerful Aragonese monastery of Saint Victorian, and briefly to the Catalan ransoming order of Santa Eulàlia (or Merced). All of these sheltered the poor, and Sant Vicent sheltered a group of royal corodians or pensioners.[76] There were several significant foundations in the fourteenth century. Queen Constance, the widow of King Pere II, left a bequest to establish a hospital, formally called Santa Llucia, but more commonly Hospital de la Reyna. The royal endowment, however, was inadequate because the Franciscans, to whom the hospital had been entrusted, were forced to seek a municipal subsidy in the famine year of 1333 and to cede all control to the city council in 1379. In 1311, the burgher Bernat dez Clapers established an eponymous hospital, formally dedicated to Santa Maria, that under municipal governance became the principal hospital within the city. Between 1333 and 1340, the Antonines established a shelter for victims of ergotism; and in 1334 Ramon Guillem Català founded a hospital for the Beguins, a lay penitential group, which shared its governance with municipal authorities. The clergy of the diocese organized a confraternity to support a shelter for poor priests in 1356. A hospice for poor migrants, particularly Castilians, was established in 1377 near the N'Avinyó gate by the confraternity of Sant Jaume, with the support of the municipal council. In the 1390s, an apothecary, Francesc Conill endowed a hospital for the sick, and a burgher, Pere Bou, a shelter for invalid fishermen.[77]

The *Llibre del Repartiment de València* mentions a hospital for the poor in Xàtiva in 1248 that served as the major hospital in the region until the fifteenth century. At first, it was entrusted by King Jaume I to the Friars of the Sack, and after their dissolution it was operated by the confraternity of the Mare de Deu de la Asunción. A second hospice seems to have been established by Pere Soler in 1265 with a grant of land from the king, and in the early fourteenth century Bernat de Bellvís, a friend of Valencian philanthropist Bernat dez Clapers, donated five hundred pounds toward the foundation of yet another.[78] In the northern part of the kingdom, Castelló de la Plana in the thirteenth century possessed only a small shelter for the sick. The first mention of this town hospital is in a will of 1290 that granted a vineyard to the institution. A century later, when Guillem de Trullols left an endowment of three hundred sous, the hospital contained ten beds.[79]

* * *

If the idea of the public shelter, whose purpose was to assist anyone who needed lodging, germinated shortly after the year 1000, it came to bloom and flourished in the twelfth and thirteenth centuries when towns, large and small, and rural locales as well, supported one or more of these establishments. The initiative for their creation was for the most part episcopal, but by the twelfth century wealthy individuals, clerical and laic, and religious communities also served as sponsors and patrons. A century later, municipal governments began to assume some responsibility for sheltering the poor. Those establishments in rural locales and in the smaller towns tended to retain more of their initial character as shelters for travelers and pilgrims, as well as the local poor. Urban hospices, on the other hand, seemed to have paid as much attention to needy residents as to transients. By the fourteenth century, the idea that the primary purpose of a hospital was the provision of bed and board would be on the wane, with the appearance of new institutions who saw their function in narrower terms, to treat disease and other physical ills. The earlier concept of serving all of the poor, however, was not entirely lost. This evolution of function can be seen in the admission policies of Valencia's Hospital of En Clapers. Founded by a merchant in 1311, it served various classes of the sick but refused entry to those whose disability was merely material. Nonetheless, the poor were not entirely ignored by En Clapers, because small alms, handfuls of pennies, were dispensed to those who came begging for food.[80] As for travelers with means, however, the provision of shelter increasingly became a commercial enterprise, as private homes, hostels, and taverns began to take in paying guests.[81]

4

Hospitals and Hospitallers

THE HOSPITALS THAT EMERGED in Catalonia and elsewhere in Europe in the centuries after 1000 grew out of a myriad of institutional and individual benefactions and were thus highly decentralized in character. Relatively few hospitals, in Catalonia or elsewhere, were connected to external institutions, such as religious orders, or operated according to any standard norms of governance. The majority were, as we have seen, independent foundations over which individual patrons often asserted various proprietal rights. In addition, most were of such modest size that the typical Catalan town was able to accommodate several hospitals and shelters of various sorts. What were the consequences of this institutional fragmentation? In order to answer this question, we must first investigate the personnel of the Catalan hospital, examine the motives and the character of their service, and sketch the physical space of the typical institution. A study of their administration reveals complaints in the fourteenth century that some hospitallers abused their autonomy, which led Church and municipal authorities to claim rights of supervision and oversight. In the fifteenth century, limitations of size, problems of governance, and economic disorders caused many of these small medieval institutions to be dissolved and consolidated into larger general hospitals.

Patronage and the Medieval Hospital

Virtually all Catalan hospitals were founded and endowed by individual or corporate benefactors who thereby claimed rights of patronage over their future administration. This power included the authority to appoint present and future administrators, to conduct visitations, to set rules of behavior, and to determine the types of individuals whom the hospital would assist. Illustrative of such a patron is Joan Colom, who established an eponymous hospital, En Colom, in Barcelona circa 1229. Even though Joan was an important officer in the cathedral chapter, he did not entrust this new foundation to the bishop or to his fellow canons; instead he turned to a trusted kinsman, Berenguer de Plan, to be both administrator of his hospital and the guardian of his two nephews and a "natural" son, Bernat. Significantly, Berenguer continued to govern even after En Colom had been consolidated with the capitular hospital in 1236.[1] In another example, the layman Pere Desvilar served as director of his own hospital in Barcelona, and then passed the responsibility on to his son. Pere, however, recognized the limitations of familial governance because in 1308 he directed that, once his family had relinquished control, the hospital would then pass into the jurisdiction of Barcelona's Consell de Cent.[2]

The case of the Hospital of Llobera at Solsona illustrates how difficult it was for a founding family to maintain its patronage over a hospital for more than one or two generations. This institution was established in 1411 by the will of Francesca, the daughter of a prosperous local merchant. Francesca nominated as its administrators three of her relatives, who were merchants in Barcelona. Future heads were also to be chosen from within the family, but by the local Dominican prior and the abbot of the Augustinian monastery. Subsequently in 1446 these two ecclesiastics nominated three younger kinsmen to take up the task, but unlike those of the earlier generation, they no longer wished to accept the responsibility. Thus, in 1447, the relatives hired a canon of Urgell, Bartomeu Travesset, to serve as rector.[3] Given difficulties such as these, many heirs, like those of Bertran de Seva of Granollers, simply relinquished their rights over a hospital to others, usually to the bishop or chapter, but also to municipal councils, religious orders, and confraternities.[4]

Long before the fifteenth century, therefore, most hospitals had come under some sort of external control. At first, this governance tended to be ecclesiastical, with the bishop and chapter being especially important; in the fourteenth century, town councils also assumed supervisory functions over hospitals.[5] As we have seen, virtually every episcopal town had its cathedral hospice; other shelters, if they were ecclesiastical in character, were also often subject to the bishop's oversight. In some instances, this authority was granted by the founding family to the bishop, and in others it fell by default. Even when the bishop lacked any formal powers, he still would claim the right to monitor how hospitals took care of the poor and to audit their accounts.[6]

Some, like Agustín Rubio Vela who has studied the hospitals in

fourteenth-century Valencia, argue that the appearance of municipal supervision of hospitals is a sign of their gradual secularization. Most Valencian
institutions founded in the thirteenth century, he observes, were entrusted
to various religious orders, while only two of seven fourteenth-century
foundations had an ecclesiastical administration.[7] Although Rubio Vela
sees this as a significant paradigmatic shift, hospitals at the end of the
Middle Ages continued to exhibit patterns of mixed and even shared governance. Girona's New Hospital, for instance, was a laic foundation of the
early thirteenth century that had come under municipal control; nonetheless, it possessed a chapel and priest and was placed under the invocation of
Santa Caterina. Even greater integration of religious and secular authority
can be seen in such fifteenth-century institutions as Barcelona's Hospital of
Santa Creu, which was established in 1401 through the merger of six older
hospitals. Governance was entrusted to a board of directors, two of whose
members were selected by the bishop and his chapter, and two by Barcelona's municipal government, the Consell de Cent.[8]

In addition to the indifference of later generations, the need for some
sort of financial oversight and assistance precipitated external interventions.
Reacting to complaints of malfeasance, Pope Clement V, in his decretal of
1311, *Quia contingit*, established a measure of episcopal control over most
hospitals in Europe by requiring that hospital administrators render an
annual financial accounting to the local bishop and by empowering the
bishop to correct any abuses that would thereby be uncovered.[9] Problems of
this sort, including a failure to attend properly to the poor, caused the bishop
of Barcelona in 1326 to relieve the rector of the leper hospital of Sant Llàtzer,
who had been jointly named by the bishop and the Plegamans family. The
rector's administrative functions were then turned over to a new officer
appointed by the bishop alone.[10] Similarly, in 1341 the municipal council
and bishop of Valencia appointed a joint committee to investigate charges
that the city's hospitals were turning away the sick, and in 1346 the council,
now acting alone, sent two men to each hospital to see whether "sick and
miserable persons were being received and housed and provided with the
necessities" by the various hospitaller administrators.[11] Finally, it is clear that
financial irregularities were a major reason that authorities in Barcelona
promulgated an elaborate set of ordinances for the Hospital de la Santa Creu
in 1417, some sixteen years after its foundation. Not only did the prologue of
this document complain about fraud, malfeasance, and a general confusion,
but the ordinances also elaborated a complex scheme that mandated regular
audits of everything from alms to supplies and bed linen.[12]

Rectors

Presumably, the individual whom the bishop, chapter, and/or municipal council would select to direct a hospital was a trusted and reputable member of the community. Various factors came into play in the making of this appointment: kinship, friendship, and even money. In 1278, for example, Bishop Arnau of Barcelona agreed to appoint a priest named Bernat Ferrer as administrator of the Hospital of Sant Macià, after Bernat had promised to give the hospital all of his property. This was a substantial endowment that included eight vineyards and personal property worth thirteen hundred sous. This was not a case of Bernat adopting the status of a religious, taking a vow of poverty as either a *frater* or *donat*, and entering some sort of community life. Instead, the new administrator was given a life's interest in his income and property, and thus his style and standard of living would seem not to have changed. Yet because this concession would ultimately benefit the hospital, the bishop tells us, Bernat was given his commission.[13] But there could be other considerations as well. For example, there is the case of Nadal, a convicted killer who was taken out of prison in 1348, in the middle of the plague, to tend the over eighty patients languishing in the hospital of the poor in the Minorcan town of Ciutadella. Evidently the regular attendants were already dead, and no volunteer could be found to work among the sick in the hospital. Under Nadal's solicitous care, however, some of the patients survived the plague. In 1349, as a reward, the municipal council of Ciutadella appointed Nadal as permanent administrator, and King Pere absolved him of his past crimes.[14]

The day-to-day operation of hospitals, nonetheless, fell to various administrators, usually called rectors, who were charged with the governance of the institution and the protection of its interests. Some served for life, while others were appointed for a fixed term.[15] Pere Desvilar, the founder of the Hospital of Sant Macià in Barcelona, demanded that all its future administrators swear to serve the poor, never to alienate its property but seek to expand it, and to preserve all its rights.[16] The letter of appointment that Berenguer de Molendinis received in 1347 as administrator of the Hospital of En Colom of Barcelona obligated him to render annual accounts and seek episcopal confirmation for any appointments to the hospital staff.[17] Bishop Ponç de Gualba's reform of the leper house at Barcelona in 1326 stipulated that the new administrator would collect offerings and alms, insure that donors of property renounce in writing all their rights to the property, make an annual accounting of all income before any official named by the bishop, and supervise all the hospital's leaseholds. The accounts of Girona's Pia Almoina suggest that after the plague a deliberate market strategy was developed that allowed the institution to purchase and stockpile grain when the price was lowest; one would assume that everywhere similar decisions were also the responsibility of the rector.[18]

In some instances, there could be more than one administrator. In smaller hospitals, like Girona's Hospital Nou, the functions were often performed by a married couple, although technically the husband held the title of *comendador*, while his wife was a mere *donata*. In large institutions there would have been a hierarchy of officials. At Barcelona's Hospital of Santa Creu, for example, there were four nonresident overseers, chosen for two-year terms, who represented the hospital's patrons, the municipal council and the bishop. Next in the hierarchy was a resident official, the president, who appointed all subordinate staff, and under him were the prior and infirmarian, who actually supervised the spiritual and material well-being of patients.[19]

Maintaining discipline among inmates and patients was an important component in the establishment of strong leadership within the hospital. In 1334, for example, the municipal council at Valencia explicitly placed the lepers of the Hospital of Sant Llàtzer under the *regla e disciplina* of the proctor, stipulating that he could impose penalties as harsh as confinement for any transgression of the rules.[20] A collapse of discipline, on the other hand, led the municipal council of Lleida in 1412 to petition the papacy to replace the rector of an orphanage that operated under the care of the Antonines.[21] Santa Creu's ordinances compelled each member of the staff to take a solemn oath to obey the administration and the ordinances. Singled out as particular behavioral problems were swearing, fighting, and rumoring; in addition, there was an evident concern that hospitallers might misappropriate food, medicine, linen, supplies, and alms. To control these illicit behaviors, the ordinances established regular procedures for accountability and placed in the hands of the administrators the power to withhold salaries, to impose fines, and to inflict corporal punishment.[22]

If they were clerics, rectors also had priestly obligations toward both inmates and the hospital's financial benefactors. In 1210, for example, Pere de Granollers, a priest of Barcelona's cathedral, left his bed, bedding, and various rental properties to the cathedral's shelter on the condition that its proctor celebrate an anniversary mass on his behalf in the cathedral.[23] Evidently such duties could become burdensome. In 1363, this led the rector of the Old Hospital at Girona, who was obliged to say anniversary masses for three priests of the diocese, to employ other clergy to serve the spiritual needs of those in the hospital. The temptation to do so must have been strong because the income from such anniversaries amounted to sixty sous, while the cost of substitute clergy was only seven sous.[24] Indeed, the conflict between these two allegiances, to benefactors and to inmates, was one of the reasons Bishop Ponç de Gualba intervened in the affairs of the leper hospital of Sant Llàtzer at Barcelona in 1326. A benefactor, Ramon de Plegamans, had in 1218 established a beneficed priest to serve the chapel; for the balance of the century, this prebend was held by the rector of the hospital. The bishop, in 1326, as the result of a visitation, concluded that this priest's obligations to the benefactor's family left him little time to attend to the spiritual needs of the resident lepers. Consequently, the bishop established and endowed with an income worth twenty-five pounds a year, a second chaplaincy whose sole function was to serve the lepers. At the same time, presumably because his duties to the Plegamans family detracted from his ability to serve as administrator, the chaplain was also relieved of these functions, which were then turned over to a lay appointee of the bishop and chapter.[25] In Valencia, conversely, the ability of an administrator to "provide the sacraments during the day as well at night" motivated the *jurats* of Valencia in 1400 to name as head of the leprosarium of Sant Llàtzer the priest, Matheu Agramunt, to replace Pere Roig, a notary who had grown too old to serve. Presumably, in this instance, the difficulty of procuring clergy for dying lepers outweighed other considerations.[26]

There are other instances of expanding bureaucracy. In 1375 the *jurats* of Valencia divided the office of En Claper's administrator among three appointees: a hospitaller (and his wife) to supervise care for the sick, a proctor to manage the endowment, and an administrator. The administrator, now a personage of high estate who was appointed for life, no longer resided at the hospital. Instead he served more as the hospital's patron or protector. Santa Creu in Barcelona had an entire staff of clergy. A prior, in addition to his responsibilities for the other clergy, the liturgy, and the preaching of "notable sermons," prayed for confraters and other benefactors at his daily mass in the chapel, visited the inmates, and recorded all instances of child abandonment. A rector administered the sacraments to inmates, and four other priests assisted the prior and rector in their duties.[27]

Ostensibly, in all of these instances, the decision to create one or more chaplains as distinct officials reflected the increasing complexity of the hospital, presumably rendering the duties of administration, consolation, and commemoration too onerous for a single individual. Rubio Vela, in addition, argues that the separation of religious and administrative functions was a by-product of the secularization of hospitals in the fourteenth century. The office of administrator, he believes, was no longer regarded by many incumbents as a religious vocation, but was seen as a secular office that required specific skills.[28]

The economic status of hospitaller administrators varied immensely. Some, one suspects, were only marginally better off than the poor they assisted. For example, Bonanat d'Arques, administrator of the New Hospital of Urgell in the fourteenth century, had to sell off his blanket to buy wheat.[29] Not nearly so desperate was the administrator at Sant Llàtzer in Barcelona whose salary was fixed in 1326 at fifty sous (increased in 1343 to one hundred sous), plus bread, wine, and a daily stipend of two diners for food. This was not a princely sum at all, in light of the fact that other employees were paid nearly as much, nor atypical, because in 1347 Berenguer de Molendinis, administrator of En Colom, was paid the same amount.[30] But the priest Bernat Domenge, named administrator of the Hospital of Bonesvalls in 1349, and the rector of the *almoina* of Barcelona received three hundred sous each, and the rector of Lleida's *almoina* four hundred sous; still higher were the stipends of Antoni dez Clapers and Berenguer de Plan. The former, as hospitaller-administrator of the hospital established by his forebear, Bernat, in Valencia, was paid a salary of one thousand sous. The latter was the kinsman whom Joan Colom had named as procurator of his hospital. Berenguer, along with several of Colom's relatives, were housed in the deceased canon's house, and had rights of usufruct to a large assortment of the hospital's original endowment.[31] His successors, like Berenguer de Molendinis, who lacked any tie of relationship to the founder, did not fare nearly as well. Nonetheless, some hospitaller leaders were surprisingly prosperous, as an inventory of Girona's Old Hospital, done in 1362 upon the death of its hospitaller, Berenguer Verdaguer, demonstrates. Berenguer's quarters were well-furnished with a bed, chest, armoire, chair, stool, and storage closet. Among his personal effects were a saddle, sword, silver reliquary, a large supply of clothing that included sixteen overcoats, a gold altar cloth, two silver cups, a library of some twenty-five paper and parchment books, about two hundred sous in cash, and an account book showing receivables of over fourteen hundred sous. Interestingly enough, Berenguer's intellectual interests ran toward the theological; his library contained only one book of medicine and this seems to have been a legacy from a previous incumbent. The inventory also shows that rectors were responsible for the hospital's accounts and property records, since a chest containing these documents was found in Berenguer's room.[32]

Hospital Personnel

Jacques de Vitry, in his *Historia occidentalis*, tells us that hospitals were served by communities of men and women, who "lived according to the Rule of Saint Augustine, without property of their own, and in common under obedience to a single superior, and, having accepted the habit of the regular life, promised perpetual continence to the Lord."[33] But, in reality, the *hospitalarii*, the *fratres et sorores*, who served the poor, conformed to no fixed pattern. Some were religious, either in the formal sense of being subject to an established *regula*, or else in the practice of some form of community life. Other institutions were served by a mixed group, that might include those under some form of dedication, like *donats*, but also retainers who served for a salary, who themselves might have been reared in the house as foundlings, or who were even slaves.[34]

The clearest examples of religious communities are found in hospitals affiliated with the Antonines, the Trinitarians, Mercedarians, or with the Orders of the Holy Spirit, Roncesvalles, and Saint John. While greatly outnumbered by locally controlled institutions, these collectively represented a significant number of hospitals, and perhaps more importantly were models of organization and practice for local institutions.[35] For example, the Rule of the Hospitallers of Saint John, which evolved between 1125 and 1153, exerted a degree of influence over other orders and hospitals. The Order of the Holy Spirit, as a case in point, derived approximately a third of its statutes from the Hospitaller Rule.[36] Developed initially between 1204 and 1208, over time this rule grew into an elaborate code of 105 *capitula* that dealt with matters of governance, conduct, religious observance, and recruitment. The serving brothers and sisters were subject to the authority of an externally appointed superior, were bound by the vows of poverty, chastity, and obedience, and were compelled to follow a specific dietary, liturgical, and disciplinary routine. These impositions gave a shape and rhythm to their daily existence that would set them apart from hospitallers who served for pay. But even within religious communities, however, there were nuances of observance. In addition to serving brothers and sisters, who were bound by the rule, there were also lay affiliates, or oblates, who shared in the community's life but who were not fully bound by its discipline.[37]

Some hospitals not affiliated with an order also possessed the semblance of a religious life, although Carme Batlle argues that such observance in Catalonia had disappeared by the fourteenth century.[38] These independent communities generally saw themselves as Augustinian (*ordo s.*

Augustini); that is, they professed some version of the Rule of Saint Augustine, which in the twelfth century had come to be adopted by most nonmonastic religious communities.[39] An example of this would be the hospice for the poor and sick established by Ramon in 1156 upon his election as prior of a group of Augustinian canons at Organyà, a town in the Segre valley twenty-seven kilometers south of Urgell. A brother canon, Joan, was placed in charge, and the small establishment was endowed with a portion of the chapter's own resources.[40] This was similar to the regime at the English Hospital of Saint Leonard in York, where the staff consisted of thirteen chaplain-brothers who lived under the Augustinian Rule.[41] However, because this rule was no more than an outline, or prologue, derived from Augustine's 211th letter, there was in fact a diversity of custom that grew out of local experiences and circumstances. For the larger orders, these usages began to coalesce in the twelfth century; those of independent houses, however, did not emerge until the beginning of the thirteenth century. In France, for example, statutes for municipal hospitals began to appear around 1200, first at Angers, then at Montdidier (1207), Paris (1220), and Cambrai (1220). Indeed, church councils held at Paris (1212) and at Rouen (1214), under the presidency of the papal legate Robert de Courson, attempted to impose such norms of conduct on all those who served in hospitals and leprosaria. As a consequence, by the end of the thirteenth century, most important *Maisons-Dieu* in France had written statutes.[42]

Another version of religious observance would be found in communities of Beguins, individuals who imitated Franciscan spirituality but who did not always follow the order's spiritual direction. In the first third of the fourteenth century such a community was established in Valencia, by a layman named Ramon Guillem Català, to operate a hospital for the sick, variously entitled the Hospital de Santa Maria or Hospital de Jesuchrist or Hospital de Beguins. The founder, presumably himself a Beguin, manifested the movement's suspicion of ecclesiastical authority by placing the hospital under the dominion of Valencia's municipal council and by explicitly declaring that neither the bishop nor any other ecclesiastical person could interfere in its administration. Eventually, a dozen or so sick people were attended by a religious community, *homes de penitència*, led initially by a *frare,* Jacme Just. While strictly speaking they did not follow the Third Rule of Saint Francis, their regimen, influenced by the writings of Arnau de Vilanova and Ramon Llull, reflected mendicant spirituality. Indeed there is evidence that, in addition to sheltering the sick poor, the house of Valencia welcomed itinerant preachers as they passed through the city. Because they sheltered religious noncomformists alongside the traditional needy, Beguin hospitals were not a widespread phenomena.[43]

For most of Iberia, however, religious customs were less articulated. For example, there was no written rule until 1535 for the community that served the Hospital del Rey in Burgos.[44] The Aragonese hospital at Somport and the more ephemeral Order of Santa Cristina associated with it have left no written constitutions even though Innocent III in 1216 had explicitly recognized the community as Augustinian.[45] At Lleida, the hospital established circa 1150 by Guillem Nicolau and his wife was served by a small religious community for which no written customs are known.[46] Thus, in many hospitals the norm seems to have been an unwritten practice. Why? The hospitals were small; there is no known conciliar mandate, as in France, for formal constitutions; perhaps, as Batlle suggests, many municipal and even episcopal hospitals were served by salaried personnel. One of the few examples of written constitutions that we do have are those that emanated from the eponymous hospital established by the Barcelonan layman Bernat Marcús, in the late twelfth century. Its rector, appointed by the bishop of Barcelona until 1339, supervised a small community of *fratres et sorores* that in 1306 consisted of only three members. In 1307, after a pastoral visit made by Bishop Ponç de Gualba, the community adopted a rule entitled *Constitutiones fratrum et sororum hospitalis Bernardi Marcucii*. Because this hospital was in desperate condition and would be sold off in 1339 to the city, however, the appearance of a written customs in 1307 was more a sign of decadence than strength, perhaps a vain attempt on the part of the bishop to breathe new life into a dying congregation.[47]

Most Catalan hospitals, however, were not served by any sort of formal religious community. The Hospital of En Colom in 1306–9, for example, numbered among its staff an assortment of personages: a rector, two chaplains, two lay sisters or *donatas*, four female servants, who tended to the sick, three alms collectors who begged bread, two gardeners, and five wet nurses. The staff of the nearby hospital of Bernat Marcús, while smaller, reflects the same diversity; in 1306 there was a rector, one serving brother and two sisters, and several hired maids.[48] Barcelona's leper hospital in the fourteenth century had on its resident staff an administrator, several priests, a serving sister, a female porter, several messengers, and a male slave; in addition, the hospital paid salaries to nonresident alms collectors (*baciners*) and "informers" who seem to have been neighbors delegated to keep the bishop apprised of the hospital's situation.[49] At the beginning of the fifteenth century, Barcelona's Hospital of Santa Creu had a large staff of administrators and attendants, all of whom were salaried. Valencia's Hospital of En Clapers also had a staff of mostly hired retainers: a male hospitaller, his wife, and two female and one male servant, but occasionally the records show one of these serving for no pay. Staff at the nearby Hospital de la Reyna included an administrator, a proctor, a resident concierge, medical personnel, and attendants.

The ratio between inmates and staff, where it can be determined, was surprisingly small: one to seven at the Hospital of En Colom; one to five at Sant Llàtzer; and one to three at the Hospital de la Reyna.[50] But this did not translate into intensive care for patients since the majority of the staff was charged with other tasks, such as serving the chapel, collecting alms, and tending to the garden, building, and the endowment. This can be seen in the 1388/89 budget for Valencia's Hospital of En Clapers, where salaries for those who tended to the sick consumed only 3.8 percent of the total, about the same amount that was paid to the single collector of the hospital's rents, and less than the 6.6 percent paid to various priests. The only exception involved the care of infants, because in the same budget wet nurses received 18 percent of the total, which after food (47 percent) was the largest item.[51] Thus, in modern terms, each of these shelters seems to have borne a large overhead, both because such institutions were responsible for their own financial support, but also because they were used to house poor relations, dependents, and students.

Donats

Of particular interest among hospitaller personnel are the *donats*, whose relationship to the hospital was quite complex in its combination of personal and religious motivation.[52] Typically, a *donat* or *donata* conferred all or most of his/her personal property upon the institution, and promised to serve it for life. The hospital, in return, promised full support and lifelong care. The founder of a hospital, for example, could become a *donat*, like Roger de Uncastillo, a resident of Huesca and seemingly a widower, who built a bridge over the Rio Guatizalema and with it a hospice to shelter the poor. In 1199, he relinquished control of the hospital to the bishop of Huesca, but the bishop in turn recognized "Brother" Roger as its rector, and obligating him to provide a chaplain to attend to the hospital's religious needs. In a somewhat different vein, Huesca's bishop in 1196 conferred a

hospital already in his domain on Salvador Pescador and two brothers and
their wives, so that in return for material support they would serve the poor
there. In this instance, Salvador lacks the appellation "brother," but he and
the others may still have been *donats* since there is no compensation mentioned beyond their personal sustenance.[53] Much the same situation prevailed in Lleida where Guillem Nicolau and Falerna, his wife, presided over
their hospice with the assistance of a small community of lay brothers.[54]
Individuals could become *donats* in a variety of ways. Most directly, one
could enter into a contractual relationship with a hospital, in which one
would exchange service for support. An example is the contract signed on
June 7, 1336, by Bernat Albió with the Hospital of Sant Joan in Reus.
Bernat, a resident of Reus, offered himself "to the service of God and of his
poor" and granted his "person as a *donat* of the hospital of Reus," promising
the town councilors and the hospital administrator to serve the poor there
for his whole life and to procure the alms, rents, and legacies that belong
to the hospital. Furthermore, he granted the hospital thirty Barcelonan
pounds, in return for which he was to be given food, drink, clothing, and
whatever else he was accustomed to have. If future administrators wished
to terminate this arrangement, then Bernat was to have his money returned; but if Bernat decided to leave of his own volition, then he was not
owed any refund. A similar arrangement, but one involving a married couple, Bernat Vidal and his wife Ramona, was signed with Reus in 1323.[55]

The practice was also common in Barcelona. For example, Pere Desvilar, in endowing his hospital, required that support be provided for his
maid, Maria; En Colom's administrator, Berenguer de Plan, guaranteed
support to two nieces, Sancha and Borracia, Bernat, who was probably his
son, and to Bernat's mother. We can assume that the women lived as *donatas*, especially Sancha and Borracia because they were guaranteed transfer
to a house of religion should their places ever be eliminated. In Lleida, a
charter of 1220 contains the names of three *ministers* of the Hospital of Sant
Martí — Pere Rubio and his wife Maria, and Ermesenda de Canals, who
seem to have been *donats* of the house. In 1288, Pere Portolés, evidently an
elderly man, became a *donat* of the same hospital in return for a payment of
a hundred and fifty sous, but one wonders whether Pere was merely purchasing nursing home care rather than embarking upon a career of service.[56] In Vic, the hospitals of Sant Jaume and Santa Trinitat were served by
communities of *donats*. The Rule of the Order of the Holy Spirit hints that
serving sisters, at least, were recruited from among the orphans and other
young girls reared within its hospitals.[57]

Thus, the institution of the *donat* was multifaceted. On the one hand, it provided a vehicle for those who wished to live a quasi-religious life of service, without vows and outside the confines of a formally established religious community. But, in some instances, it is scarcely distinguishable from a corody, a type of medieval annuity that had nothing to do with service to the poor. Instead it was a vehicle for the elderly who lacked the support of a spouse and/or children to guarantee for themselves a modicum of care and perhaps spiritual comfort in return for a fixed payment.[58] Unlike other regions of the continent where shelters specifically for the elderly began to appear in the late Middle Ages, Iberia and Catalonia do not seem to have had such institutions. Thus, the elderly here are to be found dispersed throughout the hospitaller population as long-term residents (*donats* or corodians), or in the shorter term as *malalts* (invalids), or as indigents about to die. The Iberian evidence permits no insight into the age at which the elderly would enter such a shelter or the length of their stay. Patricia Cullum's study of Saint Leonard's in England, however, suggests that those who purchased places did so before the onset of serious disability, and that on average their care lasted about eight years for a man and ten for a woman.[59]

Nurses

Because surviving documents generally concern matters of finance, property, or governance, there is little information about the tasks performed by the men and women who served the poor in hospitals. The linkage of names and titles, however, does suggest that such tasks were assigned according to gender. Administrators, alms collectors, and medical practitioners, for example, were generally, although not exclusively, male. Those who tended to the ordinary needs of inmates, on the other hand, were generally female. The Rule of the Hospitaller Order of the Holy Spirit, for example, specifically assigned to sisters the tasks of washing the sick and their bedding, but for the sake of modesty spared the sisters from performing similar duties for the serving brothers. Nonetheless, the rule makes clear that sisters were dependents of and subject to the order's male leadership.[60] Women at the English Hospital of Saint Leonard (York), according to a visitation held in 1364, also acted as nurses, tending to the sick, feeding and washing them, and alerting the priest if any needed confession or the last rites.[61] Valencia's Hospital of En Clapers in 1375 had a male hospitaller, Rodrigo Serrano, who directed the other servants and oversaw the distribution of food and drink; his wife took charge of female patients. Under this couple served two other women and a man, all of humble estate. The man purchased and transported combustibles to the hospital, did some gardening, and washed the male patients, while the women tended to female patients, did the laundry, made bread, and prepared the meals.[62] While no narratives of hospital life have survived, Jacques de Vitry describes the life of medieval hospital attendants as a kind of living martyrdom:

> For the sake of Christ, however, they endure such an overwhelmingly pervasive foulness of the sick and illnesses of almost intolerable stench, taking upon themselves such violence because I believe that no other kind of penance can be compared to this holy and precious martyrdom in the eyes of God. Therefore those pieces of squalid excrement, upon which, like a fertilizer, their souls stumble in order to bring forth fruit, the Lord will change into precious stones, and the odor of the stench will become sweet.[63]

Other Members of the Staff

In addition to *donats*, the *familia* of the medieval hospital included individuals who served in a variety of capacities. Among them were the *acaptadores* (or *baciners*, or *bacinadores*), the alms collectors who stood at church doors on Sundays and feasts and at other likely spots in town during the rest of the week.[64] These were regulated by the bishop through the issuance of licenses. The three *baciners* who served the Hospital of En Colom, for example, wandered the streets of Barcelona six days a week to beg bread and on Sundays took up their station at the entrances to churches. Those of Sant Macià even brought abandoned children with them to arouse the pity of the faithful; on Good Fridays, they asked for mattresses and bedding. In the mid-fourteenth century the vicar general wrote to all the rectors, vicars, and chaplains in the diocese to remind them that these almoners had the right to collect alms inside or outside of churches whenever they wished.[65] At Barcelona's Santa Creu, the collectors were under the supervision of the infirmarian, to whom they were to deliver their proceeds each afternoon. Indeed, the rivalry among competing collectors produced the inevitable litigation. For example, in 1409, the Antonines of Lleida, claiming an exclusive right gained from King Pere III to seek alms in the streets of the city while ringing bells, obtained an injunction from King Martí that demanded that members of the Order of the Holy Spirit silence their hand bells.[66]

Because hospitals depended on the charity of others, the collection of funds was important. At large institutions like Santa Creu, collecting money became quite complex and spawned additional personnel. In addition to the donations collected by almoners or deposited in boxes placed in Barcelona's churches, gifts of clothing, money, or other goods might be given to any staff member, who was obligated to turn them in within twenty-four hours. Legacies were an important source of revenue, but it was difficult for the hospital to discover the existence of such gifts, or to enforce them once the testator died. As one remedy to the problem, the hospital's *reebedor,* or receiver of accounts, was obligated to visit each notary in Barcelona at least once a month, in order to examine the notarial manuals for the records of new bequests and wills currently being executed. In 1401, the year of its foundation, King Martí had also entrusted to Santa Creu the property of those who had neither a will nor children; in order to claim these goods the *reebedor* presumably also had to maintain contact with parish priests.[67]

Besides almoners, the receiver, and the administrators already discussed, the ordinances of Santa Creu list a wide variety of other employees. In charge of patient care were the infirmarian, two women who served as his assistants in wards that served women and children, a woman in charge of bed linen, a baker, a person in charge of beverages (*boteller*), a pantryman, a storage room supervisor, a transporter, a cook, a barber, several other physicians and barbers on call, an apothecary, and an unspecified number of attendants who served meals and cared for patients. The clergy included the prior, rector, and four other priests. The physical plant was entrusted to the porter, who maintained regular visiting hours, and a janitor in charge of maintenance. Administrators were assisted by a scribe or secretary, a purchasing agent, and an auditor of accounts. In the mid-sixteenth century, this amounted to a staff of thirty-one.[68]

At the other end of the spectrum, but probably not all that unusual in smaller establishments, was the Hospital of Sant Llàtzer in Valencia where inmates, while under the direction of a municipally appointed proctor, seem to have fended for themselves. A brief series of statutes issued in 1334 mention no staff, apart from the administrator. The inmates, female and male, are advised to select the dish that they wish to eat each day, implying that its preparation was their own responsibility.[69]

Hospital Space

While early hospitals and shelters were located in or near the cathedral cloister, later constructions tended to be located elsewhere. During the twelfth and thirteenth centuries, the cost of land and access to clients seem to have guided the choice of locale more than any fear of contagion. Thus, several of Lleida's early shelters, such as the Hospitals of Guillem Nicolau on the flood-prone banks of the Segre and Pere Moliner next to the municipal slaughterhouse, were sited on otherwise undesirable plots. Bernat Marcús placed his pilgrim shelter near the northern exit road from Barcelona; and other twelfth-century hospitals here were placed across the Ramblas in a still undeveloped area whose poor drainage rendered it unhealthy. At Valencia, several hospitals were clustered in the outlying suburb of Sant Julià. The fear of contagion could be an issue with leprosaria, which in northern French towns like Bourges, Paris, and Limoges were usually positioned downwind, on the north or east side of town. The leprosaria of Barcelona and Valencia, on the other hand, were established outside of the walls, but intermingled with other types of hospitals. The outbreak of the Black Death and its demographic catastrophe finally coalesced attitudes on the subject of quarantine; thereafter hospitals as a matter of course were relegated to peripheral areas. For example, the petition of the confraternity of Sant Jaume to King Pere III in 1377 to establish a new hospital in central Valencia was denied on the grounds that the locale was too populated; the monarch instead suggested a site on the edge of town.[70]

Medieval hospitals were generally small, consisting of a handful of wards or rooms with only a dozen or so beds.[71] It has been estimated, for example, that the entire city of Valencia in the fourteenth century, with its ten hospitals, had space for only forty-five to eighty sick people. Here, during the fifteenth century, an important hospital like La Reyna housed an average of 12.8 inmates. The largest, En Clapers, could shelter thirty-four, but rarely did so. Between 1384 and 1395, its average daily inmate population ranged from a low of 8 to a maximum of 18.4.[72] In Catalonia, before the fifteenth century, few could match in size the eighty-seven beds available at the Hospital del Rey in Burgos, and none came close to the great Hospital of Saint John in Jerusalem, or to Saint Leonard's in the English town of York, which could accommodate several hundred. No other town could match Paris, which had over a thousand beds for resident paupers and as many others for transients and pilgrims.[73] Instead, Catalan hospices rarely held more than a score of beds, and of these more were set aside for men than for women.[74] For example, the hospital founded by the noble Ramon de Montros in his village outside of Lleida in 1324 had only seven beds, which with accompanying linen cost seventy sous each; at Urgell, the New Hospital had but five beds; and Vic's Hospital de la Santa Creu contained twelve beds.[75] At Barcelona, in 1306, the Hospital of En Marcús had a total population of nineteen persons, staff and inmates together; in 1307, the Hospital of En Colom housed ten sick, four abandoned children near the age of five, and eight children being nursed.[76] Santa Eulàlia, despite a capacity of thirty, served just six inmates in 1305.[77] The Hospital of Sant Macià circa 1400, as one of Barcelona's larger hospitals, counted twenty-two beds for men and another six for women.[78]

With time medieval hospitals grew in size and function. The earliest were mere shelters that provided little else than a secure place in which to sleep. An example of this would be the small hospital established by the canonical community of Organyà in 1156. Here the poor and sick had the benefit of a space right at the entrance to the church of Santa Maria and within the church in the chapel of Sant Joan. Any further care was of a symbolic and ritualistic nature. For example, guests in the shelter were fed a meal of bread, wine, and meat only on four important days of the year: two that inaugurated seasons of penance (the first Sunday of Advent and Septuagesima Sunday) and the two most important feasts of the liturgical calendar, Christmas and Easter.[79] Later hospitals, particularly those in urban locales, not only sheltered larger numbers, but also afforded them various forms of extended care. The best evidence that we have for the size, configuration, and functioning of these shelters comes from a scattering of inventories that have been made of their contents. The four such examples to be examined here run the gamut from the larger to the smaller, and include representatives of those in a variety of town settings.[80] The impression is that none of the buildings was grand, but consisted rather of a warren of small rooms contained in one or two stories.

Of the four, the Old Hospital at Girona was the largest, with ten rooms and a porch. There were two sleeping rooms, one with eighteen beds for men and another with seven beds for women. In addition, there was a kitchen, with other rooms for making bread, storage, milling grain, and storing wine, a chapel, a sitting room, and private rooms for the hospitaller and female attendants. Sant Macià in Barcelona had nine rooms, five of which were dormitories that had the capacity for housing thirty men and six women, but this seems to include its permanent personnel. In addition, it had a kitchen, storage hall, and two dining rooms. The Hospital of Pere Desvilar in Barcelona had two small dormitories, each with six beds, and one with two smaller beds, probably for children. At Reus, there is no breakdown by room, but the inventory shows accommodations for nineteen and a modest amount of kitchen equipment. While we do not know the size of the beds, or whether they accommodated more than a single patient, the inventories show that each bed was equipped with a mattress, a pair of sheets, a cushion, a blanket (or two), and, less frequently, a coverlet.[81]

The inventories also give details about other facilities. At Girona, the kitchen was well-equipped and provisioned and must certainly have provided its clients with food and drink; Sant Macià, with a larger population, had two upstairs dining rooms but far less in terms of cooking space or equipment. Reus, with but one cauldron and fireplace iron, and Pere Desvilar, with its paella pan and fireplace iron (and despite the good intentions of a founder who had mandated an ample menu), were even less prepared to provide meals. Thus, there must have been considerable variation in the regularity and amounts of food served the poor. The impression is that space was cramped, because extra beds and mattresses were placed in every nook and cranny. Girona had four mattresses in the sitting room and another in the storage room; Sant Macià had an extra bed in each of the dining rooms and in the kitchen, although some of these beds may have belonged to the staff. At Girona, the attendant's room contained one bed; but surely more helpers were needed to do the cleaning and cooking. At Sant Macià where no separate accommodation for the staff is mentioned, the bedding provided in the dining halls and kitchen appears to have been of somewhat better quality. Of the four hospitals, religious services were possible only at the Old Hospital of Girona, which had a chapel equipped with various hangings, crosses, altar cloths, vestments, and liturgical books. Presumably the other hospitals followed the custom of En Clapers in Valencia, which was to pay the rector of the local parish a fixed annual fee to provide inmates with the sacraments (communion and confession) and burial.[82] Girona and Reus both had axes for cutting wood and swords for protection; Reus also had a pair of hoes for a garden, which Rubio Vela argues was an essential adjunct of every medieval hospital.[83]

The Patient Population

While most, if not all, medieval hospitals were dedicated to the service of the poor, the tendency to differentiate among classes of the poor is evident by the fourteenth century. There were those whose condition, age, or status required services beyond mere asylum; some hospitals were reserved for specific classes of individuals, like aged fishermen, impoverished priests, or abandoned children. Valencia's Hospital of En Clapers served the sick, but not lepers, the mentally disturbed, or the merely hungry, all of whom were refused admission.[84] A distinction was made between the deserving and undeserving poor, motivated by a fear that society's charity might be abused by the lazy and shiftless. Thus, the *limosnero* at the Hospital del Rey in Burgos was admonished to admit only genuine pilgrims and the true poor, and his colleague at the nearby Hospital de Santa María la Real was forbidden to admit knaves, scoundrels, vagabonds, and vile women. By statute, the Hospital of Jesucristo in Córdoba could not admit those who begged at the town gates or at the entrances to its churches.[85] On the other hand, some shelters, even in the fourteenth century, targeted the dispossessed. During the 1370s, several citizens of Valencia, assisted in 1377 with a municipal grant of two hundred sous, provided a house near the portal of N'Avinyó for the destitute who had fled from famine in Castile. Data from Barcelona's large general hospital of Santa Creu indicates that in the fifteenth century a majority of patients were transients, not only from the peninsular realms but also from all around the Mediterranean (France, Naples, Genoa, Greece, and even Rhodes).[86]

There were other criteria that could influence admission to hospitals and shelters. There is the distinction, studied by Patricia Cullum at medieval York, between those who were able to pay for their care and those whose poverty forced them to rely on the resources of the house, in English usage, a cremett versus a corodian. The institution of the corody has not been adequately studied in Iberia, although Robert I. Burns has noted it in his survey of Valencian institutions. Here the monastery of Sant Vicent, alternately monastic and Mercedarian, was required to maintain twenty corodians, nominated by the king from among his household and familiars, as a type of crown pensioner. What Burns describes, however, is a somewhat different institution, since at Sant Vicent neither the pensioner nor the crown, at least directly, handed over any cash; the expense was charged against the monastery's endowment. Hospitals, generally less well endowed than this royal monastery, could not afford such largesse and thus, insofar as we can see, demanded payments from those seeking lifetime care.[87]

Another factor influencing the admission policy is similar to the phenomenon at Sant Vicent, namely the reservation by the founder or by an important patron of the right to nominate the holders of a certain number of places in the hospital. We have already seen this at work in the hospitals of Barcelona, where Pere Desvilar in 1311 reserved four spots in his eponymous hospital for his own kinsmen.[88] The canon Pere Desvilar, in endowing the Hospital of Sant Macià, gave one place to his maid, Maria; Berenguer de Plan, as administrator of the Hospital of En Colom, provided for his two nieces, son, and mistress.[89] Some founders, however, like Bernat dez Clapers in Valencia, gave administrators no instruction at all concerning admissions and left these decisions entirely in their hands. In these circumstances, the primary factors used in granting entrance would be the number of beds available and the availability of economic resources.[90]

The nature and duration of services afforded the poor naturally varied with the type of institution. Many monasteries, for example, like the Cistercian monastery at Poblet, provided just hospitality, but in separate facilities for rich and poor guests.[91] At pilgrim hospices, stays were expected to be of short duration, and at the smaller and poor hospices meals were provided only on special occasions. In Burgos, for example, the Hospital del Emperador limited accommodations to one or two nights, except in case of illness or inclement weather. Guests were given bed, charcoal and firewood for cooking, but no food, except on Fridays and the days of Lent. The larger and better endowed Hospital del Rey was more generous. Those who came in the morning were given a meal; evening arrivals got bed and board; the sick received better food and a bed for the duration of their illness.[92] Only the sick could stay beyond the night. The Pyrenean hospital at Roncesvalles also limited hospitality to one night for travelers but up to three nights for genuine pilgrims.[93]

Within Catalonia, this same sort of discrimination is evident. The Hospital of Girona would provide shelter to the poor for up to three days but denied admission to "lunatics," the "wicked," or the type of vagrant who merely wandered from hospice to hospice. Sick people would be accepted, presumably for longer terms, but, to protect itself from excessive burdens, the hospital acknowledged an obligation to serve only the inhabitants of the castle of Palagret, where the hospital held lands and whose people were thus its responsibility. Completely excluded, for lack of proper facilities, were abandoned infants. But older children like Joan Bartholomeu of Esterria, near Banyoles, were helped. Joan's father was a poor widower, presumably unable to care for his son. Thus the hospital accepted Joan into its care, promising him sustenance, food, shoes, and all his needs.[94]

Inmate populations evidently fluctuated a great deal in size, if statistics for the Hospital of En Clapers in Valencia are at all typical. During the last quarter of the fourteenth century, the patient load was highest during the plague at the beginning of April 1375 when twenty-eight were housed. But in October 1384 the daily average had fallen to 4.8 inmates, slightly smaller than the hospital's staff of five. In 1394–95, because of an improvement in income, the average had risen to 18.4, still far below the hospital's nominal capacity of thirty-four.[95]

It is difficult to profile the exact character of the inmate population of medieval hospitals because hospitallers, except in the cases of abandoned infants, were generally not required to keep a record of admissions. The prologue to the ordinances developed in 1417 for Barcelona's new Hospital of Santa Creu contains this description of a hospital's population: "poor men and women, the crippled, paralytics, the mentally disturbed, the wounded, and others suffering from diverse human miseries."[96] As for earlier hospitals, what we know of medieval patients can only be derived from snippets of anecdotal information. For example, the record of deaths at Valencia's En Clapers in 1374–75 lists an infant, a youth, as well as an old woman, demonstrating a diversity of age. But here inmates were always Christians, never Muslims or Jews despite their significant representation within Valencia's population. Most patients were from the city itself, while some were residents of the realm and a few were foreigners. Despite the mention of a squire, a merchant, and a young fisherman, indications of social status are rare; most inmates were undoubtedly humble. At Barcelona's Santa Creu, on the other hand, where a larger number of patients were outsiders, records reveal a variety of professions: priests, pilgrims, tailors, farmers, fishermen, students, laborers, and, in 1481, even an Italian physician.[97]

Among Catalan hospitals predating Santa Creu is the hospital of En Colom in Barcelona, which had the charge to serve pilgrims, vagabonds, and the poor, individuals who would likely be transients. Yet in 1307 its inmate population also contained those whose stays must have been extended — ten sick people, four abandoned children around the age of five, and eight children still being nursed.[98] Some hospitals, as we have seen, also housed corodians like Bernarda, whose father, Ramon Cadena, had paid the New Hospital of Urgell three hundred sous in 1290 to care for his daughter from his death until hers.[99] The Hospital of Sant Macià in Barcelona was perhaps typical in the diversity of its clientele, which included those of diverse station who came to the hospital to die — the slave woman Margarita Baciners, a woman from the village of Llobregat named Na Bacona, an unnamed Beguin. For these the hospital had to provide care until their death, but the seriousness of their illnesses is indicated by the brevity of the stays — three days for Na Bacona and eight for the slave Margarita. Sant Macià then became responsible for the cost of their burial shroud and service, for which special collections seem to have been taken up. Statistics from Barcelona's Hospital of Santa Creu in the late fifteenth century show forty-nine percent of all patients admitted were terminal,

confirming the anecdotal evidence from Sant Macià.[100] Sant Macià also
provided shelter for travelers and/or pilgrims who had fallen ill. In one
instance, two individuals too ill to beg their own alms in the city were fed
and sheltered for six days at a cost of two sous. In 1390, shelter was given
here and at other hospitals in Barcelona to the casualties of the battle of
Bascara, at which Catalan forces led by Bernard de Cabrera had halted an
invasion by the count of Armagnac. There were also infants like the child of
four or five months who was found at the hospital's door on Monday
morning, August 30, 1389. This child was given to a woman named Alfonsa
who nursed it until its death in October. While most such abandoned
children were similarly given out to wet nurses, some were housed at least
temporarily at the hospital when a wet nurse was on staff or when goat's
milk was available. In 1386, for example, the administrator, Guillem Rossell, rented a slave to serve as a wet nurse for seven months. Finally, Sant
Macià dispensed charity to those who were not inmates, giving, for example, two sous to Eulalia to purchase medicine for her child.[101]

If hospitals were "sacred" and protected places within the medieval
town, with certain of their personnel protected by canon law, did inmates
also benefit from any form of special immunity? The only indication that
this was so is a charter of King Jaume II, dated October 31, 1314, that
exempted the patients of En Clapers in Valencia from any action resulting
from a crime, debt, reprisal, or any other cause.[102] Other charters generally
privileged only hospitallers. Staff members at Barcelona's Santa Creu, for
example, were granted various safeguards (*guidatica*) by the king in the
early fifteenth century, including the right to carry otherwise prohibited
weapons.[103]

The General Hospital

The end of the medieval era also marks a profound change in the character
of hospitaller services. Too small to provide much beyond shelter and custo-
dial services, and with endowments that, because of the economic crisis of
the late fourteenth century, had diminished in real value, many of the small
hospitals were consolidated into larger, general municipal institutions. In
addition to the inadequacy of funds, the usual justifications for reform —
improper diversion of funds, dishonest administrators, lack of adequate
supervision — are uniformly cited as motivating factors. Brian Pullan believes that preaching by Observant Franciscans, who feared that the poor
suffered from fraud and corruption within the older institutions, was im-

portant in encouraging the development of general hospitals.[104] For the most part, the initiative to reorganize hospitaller institutions in order to improve their efficiency would come from secular authorities, principally municipal councils and other local authorities, who had become the patrons of last resort. The exception to the pattern is England, where Henry V in 1414 proposed a general reformation of hospitals; but his motives were different — the diversion of "wasted" monies into the royal treasury.[105] In Italy, general hospitals were founded in Brescia (1447) and Milan (1448) and in Venetian towns like Bergamo (1457). In France, the *parlement* of Toulouse reformed the hospitaller structure in 1505, establishing five major institutions to treat specific problems like syphilis, orphans, and pilgrims.[106] In Portugal, Prince Duarte in 1430 requested and in 1437, as king, received the assent of Pope Eugenius IV to consolidate various small hospices throughout his kingdom. Subsequently, general hospitals were established in Lisbon and Coimbra. Within the Crown of Castile, general hospitals came later. The first was established only in 1499, when Queen Isabel and her husband Ferdinand endowed the Hospital del los Reyes Católicos in the pilgrim town of Santiago de Compostela. With its separate wards for men and women and for rich and poor, this institution became a model for later hospitals in Castile: Toledo (1504), Granada (1511), and Seville (1546).

This movement of consolidation came much earlier to the Aragonese Crown than to the other regions of Iberia and seems even to have foreshadowed developments in Italy. Within Crown lands, the first Aragonese general hospital, Nuestra Señora de la Gracia, was established in Saragossa in 1425 and another was founded in Majorca in 1456–58. In Valencia, municipal authorities in 1409 created the Hospital de Ignoscents, Folls e Orats for abandoned children and the mentally disturbed, and in 1495 a general hospital.[107] Within Catalonia, consolidation is seen in Lleida in 1453 when six of the medieval hospitals were joined together to form the Hospital General de Santa Maria.[108] Around the same time, the municipal and capitular hospitals of Urgell were joined in response to the economic difficulties of the era.[109] In 1464, the city and cathedral hospitals at Tarragona were merged and, later in the century, Archbishop Pere d'Urrea of Tarragona, acting in response to the wishes of King Ferdinand II, merged other hospitals throughout his archdiocese.[110]

Barcelona's consolidation was the earliest of all. On February 1, 1401, the Consell de Cent appointed a civil commission to study the condition of the city's hospitals; Bishop Joan Ermengol of Barcelona and the chapter subsequently did the same. On March 15, the two commissions agreed to consolidate the hospitals of En Marcús and Pere Desvilar, both of which were under municipal administration, with the capitular hospitals of En Colom and Sant Macià into the Hospital of Santa Creu, to be governed by a board composed of two citizens and two canons. On June 27, the leprosarium of Sant Llàtzer was added, and on July 23 the prior of Santa Eulàlia del Camp petitioned that the small hospital there also be included because "it does nothing useful." Subsequently and because the consolidation involved the alienation of church property, the approval of the Avignonese pope, Benedict XIII, was sought and received. The newly constructed Hospital of Santa Creu was dedicated to the service of the infirm poor and others who were accustomed to being sheltered in the city's hospitals. It endured as a medical facility until 1926, after which its functions were assumed by a new Hospital de Santa Creu i Sant Paul in the Eixample district. One of its last patients was the famed Catalan architect Antoni Gaudí, who died there on June 7, 1926. Today the medieval structure serves as the Biblioteca de Catalunya.[111]

The fifteenth-century structure, begun by the architect Guillem Abrill, is the largest example in Catalonia of the monumental style of hospital architecture, characterized by large halls surmounted by a beamed roof supported on diafragmes arches. Its chapel, however, utilized the nave of the older Hospital of En Colom. A painting of 1410 shows that the first of the great halls, ten by sixty meters in size, and half of another had been completed. Records in 1457 speak of five wards, including one for women. A second ward for women was built in 1472, and additional space was added at the end of the century. An inventory of 1564 indicates that Santa Creu had a capacity of between 120 and 200 patients.[112]

The actual operation of Santa Creu is described at great length in ordinances that were promulgated in 1417, which are reflective of the hospital's first decade of operation. Most valuable for our purposes here is their outline of routine patient care. While its size and resources certainly enabled Santa Creu to provide more comprehensive treatment to inmates than its smaller counterparts, its customs seem typical of late medieval usage. A lengthy section of the ordinances deals with the reception of patients, a duty performed by the infirmarian. According to our earliest statistics, from 1473 to 1491, Santa Creu during this period admitted an average of 264.5 patients each year, 191.8 male and 72.8 female. According to the ordinances, each one of these, after having his or her feet washed and "thoroughly cleansed," was to be provided with a bed and a meal. Then the rector, who as the hospital's chaplain had charge of the religious needs of patients, would arrive for confession, and perhaps communion and last rites. Meanwhile, the infirmarian was to summon medical personnel and then see that prescribed food and medicine were properly delivered. At some convenient time, the infirmarian and hospital scribe were required to interview the patient formally and ask "with gentle words" his name and geographical origins, compile an inventory of his money, clothing, personal and real property, and debts, and request the name of the individual to be notified in case of death. The emphasis on money and property was designed to protect the patient as much as to benefit the hospital. After verifying the accuracy of the patient's inventory, his property was to be kept safe, and returned in its entirety should the individual live. There is no indication that the cost of care would in any way be deducted from this amount. If, on the other hand, the patient died, then the hospital claimed all of his property and rights. In addition, clothing would be collected, cleaned, and sold off for the hospital's benefit. All of this indicates that inmates were indeed poor, that whatever money they carried would be meager in amount, and that residual property, if any, would not likely be claimed by heirs.[113]

The routine care outlined is one of bed rest, with a therapy of food and medicine. The condition of the patients was to be regularly checked by various personnel. The prior, in five daily visits, was to give spiritual consolation and summon the rector should the patient require confession and the last rites. The infirmarian was to make seven daily rounds to check on the quality of the food, patient hygiene, and the administration of medicine. In addition, barbers and physicians under retainer were to make morning and afternoon rounds, during which they were to provide medical care and report terminal cases to the prior so that the appropriate sacraments could be administered. There were separate wards for men, women, and children, each with its chief attendant and subordinates. Dinner was served at midday; attendants provided medicine and refreshments at other hours and cleaned up after patients. For those patients who did not die, the hospital realized the risks of premature discharge. The infirmarian was instructed not to release any patient until the cure was complete. To do otherwise, the ordinances argued, would make little financial sense because the person would undoubtedly relapse, be readmitted, and cost the hospital for additional care. The only exception to this rule was the case in which an individual would discharge himself by signing a release absolving the hospital of any future responsibility for his care and treatment.[114]

* * *

The specialization and diversity of purpose that mark the evolution of the hospital in medieval Catalonia parallel an internal development as well.

Just as these hospitals grew in number and size, their internal governance became more complex, as we have seen in this elaboration of the administrators, nurses and functionaries who staffed the hospital. With regard to institutions like the *donat* and the corody, or the effort of ecclesiastical and municipal authorities to exercise a measure of oversight, the experience of Catalonia is reflective of the rest of Europe. Eastern Spain, however, stands apart in other respects. For the most part, its caritative institutions were smaller than those found in larger urban areas, like Paris or northern Italy, or in even more rural areas like Burgos that lay astride major pilgrimage routes. Despite their modest proportions, however, Catalan establishments were at the forefront of institutional development, pioneering the concept of the general hospital. For reasons that remain to be studied, however, Catalan hospitals lacked some of the religious character of their French counterparts. Few were operated by formally, or informally, organized communities of religious; certainly by the fourteenth century, salaried staffs, which must have increased operating expenses, had become the norm throughout Catalonia and the Crown of Aragon. Finally, it is perplexing, in light of the relatively few number of available beds, that so many hospitals should have operated below their capacity. We have seen a number of instances in which financial hardships caused administrators to limit admissions, but such efforts also brought public rebuke from authorities. Attempts were also made to bar vagrants, the insane, and other undesirables from free bed and board. Nonetheless, given the level of poverty and disease during these centuries, it is hard to believe that there would be any lack of demand for these unoccupied beds. Perhaps this tells us that medieval communities had far lower expectations of public assistance than modern societies and that, for most, family and friends functioned as the principal providers of shelter and care in times of need.

5

Hospitals and Disease
in the Medieval City

UNTIL THE FOURTEENTH CENTURY, Catalan hospitals emphasized care over cure. As a consequence, most shelters did not discriminate in any fundamental way between the sick and the homeless; and, when the term *infirmi* was used to designate certain inmates, it is unclear whether the malady in question was chronic or acute. The condition that qualified an individual for assistance was poverty, and it did not matter directly if its cause was an affliction, such as blindness, old age, or disease, or the homelessness of the traveler and vagrant.[1] Even after 1300, this sort of hospital, which sheltered pilgrims, invalids, and paupers, continued to function; indeed, there were even a scattering of new foundations.[2] Alongside these shelters, however, new categories of hospitals began to appear. In the mid-twelfth century, there were those dedicated to particular groups of the needy, like lepers, the victims of ergotism, and orphans. In the fourteenth century, with its recurrence of plague and other diseases, new facilities, as well as older shelters, began to add medical treatment as a regular component of patient care. This culminated in the fifteenth century with the establishment of large general hospitals that offered, in addition to food and shelter, a broad array of medical and social services. Of these new and specialized institutions, the earliest and most numerous were the leprosaria.

Lepers and Leprosy

Instances of leprosy increased in Europe after 1000.[3] In the twelfth century the first leper colonies appeared, organized not too differently from the contemporary communities of Augustinian canons and frequently headed by the oldest surviving leper. Gradually a process of institutionalization and definition unfolded, as the leper settlements acquired a legal status and the right to own and receive property and alms. Ultimately, just as in religious communities, various statutes were drawn up to govern life within the leper colony. A significant ecclesiastical acknowledgment of their existence came in Canon 23 of the Third Lateran Council (1179), which gave leper communities an official status within the Church by stating: "When these men are gathered in a number sufficient to lead a common life, we enact that they can have a church and a cemetery, and the benefit of a priest among them." The establishment of a chapel, or the conferral of donations in property or cash, brought such communities to notice as a leper hospice or hospital, often under the invocation of a saint.[4]

Leprosy is caused by *Mycobacterium leprae*, which is related to the bacteria that produce tuberculosis, and which has existed, like the plague, as one of mankind's chronic diseases. G. H. A. Hansen first isolated the bacterium in 1874, but even today there is disagreement about whether it is transmitted by contact or through the respiratory or gastrointestinal systems. Five variants of the disease have been identified, the most serious of which is the lepromatous leprosy, which produces the extreme disfiguration that most associate with this malady. Today, we know its incubation period averages between three and five years, and that 90 percent of those infected with leprosy bacteria never show external signs of the disease. But most of this was unknown in the Middle Ages; the disease itself did not begin to be medicalized until the fourteenth century.[5] Before that time, its identification was the responsibility of priests, and then of barbers, who probably detected the malady only in its later stages, when victims began to show large lumps or patches on the skin, which eventually disintegrated into discharging sores. The disease was regarded by medieval physicians and other authorities as difficult to diagnose. Nonetheless, excavations of leper cemeteries have revealed signs of the disease in 77 percent of the skeletons, showing a relative accuracy in the medieval process of identification.[6]

Medieval thinkers regarded leprosy as degrading in both a physical and a moral sense. The disfiguring symptoms were viewed as marks of sin, from which prudent Christians should flee. It was commonly believed that the innocent could become infected by touching a leper, or breathing in his exhalation, or by having sexual relations, particularly during periods of menstruation. Consequently, it was a serious matter to label anyone as a leper; false accusations were regarded as slanderous, akin to calling someone a whore, traitor, or Saracen. Standards of diagnosis, moreover, did not coalesce until the fourteenth century when leprosy began to fall under the purview of physicians. In Catalonia, an important turning point was the great lepers' plot of 1321 when French lepers were widely accused of poisoning the water supply so as to infect others with their malady. As a consequence, in June 1321, King Philip V of France ordered their arrest and execution, causing many lepers to flee for safety into Catalonia, where Jaume II ordered them to be detained, questioned, and, if found guilty of some crime, executed. Perhaps as a reaction to the hysteria of false arrest, the following years saw greater physician involvement in the diagnosis of leprosy, clearer descriptions of the disease (like Arnau de Vilanova's *De signis leprosorum* and Jordanus de Turre's *De lepra nota*), and the development, particularly among those trained at the medical school in Montpellier, of a more clinical, and less moralizing, attitude toward the disease.[7]

The primary reaction of society to lepers was to house them far from populated areas. Some date these efforts at segregation to the *acta* of the Third Lateran Council (1179), but realistically such a policy is apparent only from the fourteenth century. The first French ordinance, for example, that called for the strict seclusion of lepers dates from 1321, the year of the alleged plot; in Italy, Florence ordered their expulsion from the city only in 1325. The most influential medical treatise to set down criteria and procedures for the seclusion of individuals suspected of leprosy, that of Guy de Chauliac, did not appear until 1363.[8] Earlier, such quarantine was relative. Towns, for example, usually located leprosaria, as well as other shelters for the poor, away from populated areas. Paris's Saint Lazare, for example, was two kilometers from the city, and Narbonne's hospice a kilometer away. In northern France, near Bourges, Paris, and Limoges, as we have already noted, leper hospitals were positioned downwind, usually on the north or east side of town, and only rarely to the south or southwest. But there was always some contact between the leper and the rest of society, if for no other reason than lepers begged as a principal means of their support. The law, for the most part, did not forbid lepers to interact with others, although it could restrict the nature of this contact. The Rule of the Hospitaller Order of the Holy Spirit, for example, insisted that members who had contracted leprosy be permitted to remain in and be treated as a part of the community. Lille in 1239, on the other hand, permitted lepers in town only with permission, but otherwise allowed them free passage through the countryside as long as they entered no houses. The Asturian town of Oviedo, perhaps because it had to cope with many northern Europeans traveling the pilgrim route to Santiago, enacted an ordinance in 1274 that was more severe, although it treated lepers and vagabonds alike. Because these unfortunates lacked any local roots, the ordinance forbade them entry to the town on penalty of expulsion for the first offense, whipping for the second, and burning for the third. In France, however, at Coutances lepers were merely barred from crowded places, like markets, and in the province of Auch, lepers were required only to wear distinctive dress as a warning to others. Ironically, in the fourteenth century, as leprosy itself began to diminish, restrictions upon lepers multiplied. Clickers and other noisemakers, for example, became common as a warning of approaching lepers. Because some believed that leprosy could be contracted by eating tainted food, lepers were forbidden to touch food or to enter kitchens and pantries. At Périgueux, they could not sell their cattle, poultry, or eggs to others. Towns like Amiens and Chartres barred lepers from municipal wells and cisterns; and at Chartres lepers were forbidden to wash their laundry with that of others. But, on the other hand, lepers were expected to carry with them a wooden goblet, into which others could place gifts of food, drink, and money without touching the leper. In France, these regulations culminate with the *Ordonnance cabochienne* of 1413 that forbade lepers to enter Paris or any other town.[9]

Leper Houses

If leprosaria began to appear at the onset of the twelfth century, the numbers of new foundations peaked between 1150 and 1250, and then fell off rapidly.[10] New establishments in the fourteenth and fifteenth centuries were usually just reorganizations of older institutions. It is impossible to estimate the numbers of these hospices, because most were small, with perhaps a half dozen inmates and few, if any, documentary traces. Furthermore, leprosaria were generally local institutions because this work never was taken up in any consistent way by the religious orders. Even the Order of Saint Lazarus, itself a society of lepers whose work was the care of lepers, remained small. While there were a large number of hospitals under the patronage of this saint, most had no connection to the order.[11] Thus, Louis VIII of France, in the early thirteenth century, bequeathed money to some two thousand leper shelters in his kingdom, but there must have been more than these in France since major regions at that date were still outside royal control.[12] It has been estimated that in medieval Yorkshire, in England, a quarter of all hospitals were leprosaria. All of these were established before 1300, with most in the twelfth or early thirteenth century. The most important shelters were of aristocratic foundation, but in 1200 at least half of all towns also had a hospice for lepers.[13]

In Spain, leper hospitals multiplied in the twelfth century, and their appearance might well coincide with the development of the Santiago pilgrimage route, which likely introduced numbers of lepers into the peninsula. One estimate argues that there were twenty thousand lepers in medieval Spain and approximately two hundred leper shelters. While we do not know the relative size of these Hispanic institutions, in nearby Toulouse, John H. Mundy's study shows an average of ten inmates per house.[14] One of the earliest Hispanic houses, established at Palencia in 1067, is attributed to the Cid who is said to have met and cared for a leper pilgrim to Santiago, later revealed to be San Lázaro himself.[15] In the province of Asturias, through which a branch of the Santiago road ran, there were over twenty leprosaria, established between the mid-twelfth and late thirteenth centuries.[16] At Burgos, there were two houses, both under the invocation of San Lázaro, one just outside the walls on the Santiago road, and the other in a more rural locale.[17] León had its own shelter in 1171, and Seville and Córdoba not long after the Christian conquest in the mid-thirteenth century.[18]

Lepers in Barcelona

The leprosarium of Barcelona, variously called the Casa del Malalts or Masells or Mesells, the Hospital of Sant Llàtzer, or the Domus Infirmorum, has no known act of foundation. Despite traditions that date its origins to the mid-ninth century, it is likely that its foundation, like those of so many others, took place in the second half of the twelfth century. One tradition credits its establishment to Bishop Guillem de Torroja (1144–71); the earliest direct reference to the leper hospital is dated 1200. The institution was located across the modern Ramblas from the twelfth-century city, in the plaza Pedró, a garden district that only became fully urbanized in the fourteenth century. Its chapel in the thirteenth century was under the invocation of Santa Maria dels Malalts, but later it became dedicated to Sant Llàtzer al Pedró. The hospice was supervised by the bishop and the chapter who appointed its proctor. The rector was the chaplain, who served at the altar of Santa Margarita, which was endowed in 1218 by the powerful Ramon de Plegamans, and later in 1295 by his grandson Marimon de Plegamans. Sant Llàtzer endured as an independent institution until 1401, when it was joined, first to the Hospital of Santa Eulàlia, and then to the new general hospital of Santa Creu. Subsequently, due to a rise in the incidence of leprosy in Catalonia during the fifteenth century, there was an attempt by the city council to establish a new and larger leper hospital outside the Porto Nou. This effort, however, floundered, not only because of its projected cost of six thousand florins, but also because of a fear that such a structure would only stimulate the immigration of lepers into Barcelona. Ultimately, the council decided to make due with the current facilities by barring their use to lepers who originated from outside of Barcelona itself.

Bishop Ponç de Gualba carried out a pastoral inspection on February 24, 1307, that reveals to us the personnel of the leprosarium: Bernat d'Orts, the rector; Jaume de Rocafort, a cleric and a leper who disliked the rector; Berenguer de Canal, the chaplain; and three male attendants. In 1379, the staff had grown to include an administrator, several chaplains, six full-time attendants, and several part-time alms collectors and neighborhood retainers. Statutes concerning its operation are extant from a reform by Bishop Ponç de Gualba in 1326, instituted to correct problems in the hospital's administration. Evidently, the rector, reacting to charges that the leper inmates were not receiving proper care, had responded by proposing a reduction in the number of admissions. The bishop's solution was to overhaul the hospital's administration in order to correct fiscal irregularities and to improve the inmates' access to daily mass and the sacraments.[19]

Financial accounts for Sant Llàtzer survive for the eleven-month period from May 1379 to April 1380, and these give us a brief glimpse of its economic status, the sources of its support, and some indication of its internal operation. The overall figures suggest that the hospital was prospering, with a budgetary surplus of over twelve hundred sous from revenues of almost forty-six hundred sous; yet this conclusion would be somewhat precipitous given the source of most of this income. Approximately one-half came from short-term giving: the sale of bread alms (30 percent), alms collected in town (11 percent), legacies (6 percent), and chapel offerings (3 percent). Only a quarter came from permanent endowment: investments, rentals and endowments established for anniversaries. The remainder derived from the sale of wine and other agricultural products (20 percent) and money contributed by leper inmates (5 percent). Thus, half of Sant Llàtzer's revenue was subject to the vagaries of Barcelona's economy and could be expected to fluctuate with the times. Lacking comparative figures, it is impossible to determine whether 1379 was a typical year, or an unusually good one.[20]

The largest expenditure of Sant Llàtzer was for food (38 percent), followed by wine (31 percent). While almost the entire expense of the latter was recovered through the sale of surplus vintage to others, all of the former went to feed both staff and inmates. While fragmentary to be sure, this evidence suggests something of the configuration of the house and the treatment of its residents. Because more was budgeted per capita to feed the staff, we can assume that they ate better than the lepers.[21] In 1379, furthermore, we know that the staff included an administrator, two or three chaplains, five staff members, and a slave. That being so, the food budget would seem to have allowed for the support of fourteen or fifteen lepers, a modest population indeed given a staff of approximately ten. This ratio, however, evidently did not translate into a high level of care for the leper residents, because of the ten paid personnel only one female attendant was directly charged with patient care.[22]

Lepers Elsewhere in Catalonia

Outside of Barcelona, one of the earliest leprosaria was founded at Lleida, where a hospital of Sant Llàtzer is cited in Berenguer de Boixadors's will of 1185. The hospice was located on inexpensive land on the left bank of the Segre, near the Hospital of Guillem Nicolau, on which there was an old mosque and a half dozen buildings. In the next century, a confraternity that enrolled men, women, and clergy was established to provide support; King Jaume II is said to have belonged. Another hospice on the road to Gardeny was established early in the thirteenth century.[23] At Girona, the Hospital of Sant Jaume de Pedreto, or Le Pedret, was located outside the walls.[24] The Hospital of Santa Maria Magdalena was probably a mid-thirteenth-century foundation at Urgell, with 1284 being its first citation. Like others, its location was extramural. It was a popular charity, with over a third of the wills extant for 1287 to 1291 remembering it with small legacies. Leprosy, however, must have soon declined at Urgell since the property in the early part of the next century was made into a residence for hermits.[25] At Vic, lepers were not segregated but rather included within the patient population of several public shelters. These include the hospice operated by the church of Sant Bartomeu, the Hospital of Sant Jaume and its confraternity, and the annex of the hospital for the poor that Ramon de Malla founded in 1275.[26] At Cervera, Santa Magdelena is first mentioned in a will of 1235 but the leprosarium's origins were in the twelfth century. The hospital and church must have existed under some manner of municipal jurisdiction because in 1246 town officers ousted the hospital's administrators in a dispute over its expansion.[27]

The lepers' plot of 1321, during which native as well as foreign lepers were accused of poisoning wells, led to scattered violence against lepers and the suppression of some houses by the Crown. King Jaume II gave leper property at Cervera and Tàrrega to the Franciscans, while Minorite nuns received the goods confiscated at Vilafranca del Penedès in Catalonia and at Morella in northern Valencia. Other lands at Tarazona and Borja were retained by royal agents. At Tàrrega, the Franciscans were given permission in 1322 to sell the leper house and use its proceeds toward construction of a new residence on the condition that they would care for all present and future lepers born in the town; but without the need for a separate leprosarium, their numbers must have been few. At Cervera there is no indication that the friars cared for lepers at all. Indeed, responding to protests from municipal officials that lepers were being driven to starvation, King Alfons III in 1331 forced the friars to restore the confiscated property to the lepers. Whether or not the loss of leper houses suggests any decline of the disease during the fourteenth century, as some have argued, the aftermath of the lepers' plot demonstrates not only the precariousness of the leper's place in society but also the increasing role the king was playing in the formulation of public policy.[28]

Lepers on Majorca

In Christian Majorca, the oldest known citation concerning leprosy is in the constitutions of the Monastery of Santa Margarida (circa 1330), which address the problem of leper monks. In the fifteenth century, Majorca had an officer called the *morbería* who was charged with keeping those carrying infectious diseases, which included the plague, tuberculosis, and leprosy, from disembarking on the island. Under him were various officials who dealt specifically with leprosy. The *vesador i instigador dels massells* was charged with identifying cases of leprosy; however, the disease here, as elsewhere, was evidently in decline because in 1468 this position was consolidated with that of a second official, the examiner of lepers. The Hospital dels Massells was functioning in 1440 with a physician to oversee the care of lepers. This was located outside the walls, near the gate of Santa Catalina, where lepers could beg alms at a safe distance from town residents. Frequently in the fifteenth century, the *instigador dels massells* also served as governor of the leper hospice.[29]

Lepers in Valencia

Sant Llàtzer in Valencia, located just outside the city on the road to Murviedro, is cited in wills as early as 1251 and must have been established shortly after Jaume I's conquest of the city in 1238. It is unclear under whose authority this asylum was first established, but it was the first of the city's charitable institutions to become the responsibility of the municipal *consell*. In 1319, the *jurats* and *consellers* decreed that the hospital be governed by a proctor, who was to be a citizen of Valencia, and who would serve a term of two years. In 1334, the councilors issued a brief handbook to govern the conduct of inmates and the administration of the house, and in 1474 they discharged Philip de Vezach as administrator after inmates had complained of his failure to provide sufficient food and fuel.[30] The hospital evidently used a panel of doctors to screen prospective inmates for actual signs of the disease. An instance in 1318 reveals that one such individual, Bernat Cubelles, who had been expelled as a leper from the Valencian village of Ontinyent, was declared to be free of the disease by these physicians and permitted to return home.[31]

The Care of Lepers

Were all lepers treated alike? All of these unfortunates were marginalized to the extent of being segregated from society and, whether or not they actually underwent the ritual of civil death, they were regarded as terminal patients, not as apt candidates for any sort of medical treatment.[32] Yet various studies — for example, in the Asturias region and in Catalonia — suggest that rich and poor lepers received different levels of care. Unlike cases of the sick, where the affluent were tended at home and the indigent in public shelters, wealthy lepers tended to reside in endowed hospitals where they were provided decent accommodations, a bed, and even some recreation, while paupers were more likely to end up as members of rural communities supported by begging. Hospital admission, in addition to being influenced by factors of family and wealth, also could be conditioned by geography, in that local residents were usually given preference over outsiders in the competition for a limited number of places.[33] At Barcelona, after 1326, a committee composed of the bishop's almoners and two upstanding citizens of the city decided whom to admit to Sant Llàtzer. First priority was to be given to lepers from the city itself, followed by those from the diocese, then other Catalan lepers, and finally transients.[34]

Perhaps the most important concern in deciding matters of admission was the cost of care, since anyone admitted might well remain in residence for several years. In France, and perhaps elsewhere, the presumption was that the property of the perspective inmate would belong to the leprosarium.[35] By the end of the thirteenth century, notarial manuals record contracts between lepers and shelters concerning the disposal of the former's property.[36] But many lepers were too poor to make any contribution toward their care. In some instances, the poor were expected to provide, as a minimum, their own clothing and bedding; in other instances, alms from the community supported the indigent. At Barcelona, lepers or their families in theory were required to pay nothing, but in fact those with means were expected to defray, in whole or in part, the cost of their care. Most if not all of Sant Llàtzer's inmates must have been indigent, however, since the records of 1379, for example, show that lepers contributed just over 5 percent of the house's total income. At Manresa, however, Guillem de Pujol was admitted into the leper house in 1326 only after paying his fellow inmates seventy sous, for which he was to receive bed, board, and a share of any alms received. Françoise Bériac's study of French leprosaria, indeed, reveals no consistent pattern of admission. Biases existed against the poor and against strangers (Sant Llàtzer's in Valencia, for instance, barred the admission of wandering minstrels), but these were not absolute. Likewise, the ability to pay was also no guarantee of admission. The leper community itself and its leader had a great deal of discretion in deciding these matters.[37]

Canon law imposed no particular form of governance upon leper communities, and the chaplains appointed by bishops did not always serve as rectors or administrators. At Toulouse, for example, the leper houses seem to have had no single head, but instead appear to have been governed by a council or chapter composed of hospitallers and/or the lepers themselves. In the thirteenth century, some bishops promulgated statutes for leprosaria that placed lepers and/or their healthy aides under a kind of religious observance.[38] In France, lepers at Meaux in 1300, for example, had to promise to live without property, observing chastity, obedience, and silence. At Saint-Lazare of Montpellier, inmates were forbidden to fornicate, quarrel, sell the house's property to outsiders, or steal, and were enjoined to pray together silently in church at the appointed hours. The English hospital at Sherburn required inmates to recite 161 paternosters a day, and another at Dover demanded 200 paternosters and Ave Marias during the day, and an additional set at night. At Sant Llàtzer's in Valencia, men and women evidently ate apart (but could not eat alone without good cause) and were forbidden to talk to each other "continuously."[39] But the archdeacon of Paris argued that lepers should not be treated like religious because many were married and had purchased their place in the asylum. For similar reasons, Bishop Ponç de Gualba of Barcelona in 1326 eliminated the requirement that inmates at Sant Llàtzer take vows of chastity and obedience, although he did express the wish that the lepers would live chastely and avoid sin. In the interests of maintaining order, however, even secular authorities attempted to impose a quasi-religious regimen upon lepers, but simultaneous promulgation of statutes against theft, assault, and battery and the threats of imprisonment also demonstrate that this ideal was rarely attained.[40]

Leprosy was a terminal disease from which no recovery was expected, and consequently leprosaria were, like most medieval hospitals, places of residence rather than centers of treatment.[41] Lepers would be fed and clothed; at Barcelona's hospital of Sant Llàtzer they were also given a small amount of spending money, one diner on each of the fifteen major feasts celebrated in the house. While those who became too ill to share the communal meal were given a special diet, the hospital's *Libre dels Comptes* reveals that only minor provisions were made for medical care. Regulations did permit a portion of the twelve diners that were set aside each week for an inmate's food to be used for lancets and bandages, but there is only a single reference to a physician being called to visit an inmate. Furthermore, the accounts indicate that virtually nothing was spent on any products of a therapeutic nature.[42]

Ergotism

In addition to leprosy, medieval people suffered from various other forms of painful and disfiguring maladies, the chief of which was ergotism. This is a disease caused when ergot, a wind-borne fungus, invades the ovaries of edible rye, producing a dark purplish-black mass called a *sclerotium*. Cold winters, warm and wet weather in spring and summer, or poor field drainage promoted the spread of ergot. The resulting ergotism recurred in epidemic proportions in Europe between the ninth and nineteenth centuries, where the descriptive terms holy fire (*ignis sacer*) and Saint Anthony's fire, for the intolerable burning pains felt in the limbs, came into use. There are two forms of the disease, although these were not distinguished until the seventeenth century. The first and most common is gangrenous ergotism, characterized by a sense of lassitude, painful contractures, alternating sensations of severe heat and icy cold, followed by the loss of all sensation and the onset of dry gangrene. The affected parts of the body became dry and mummified and eventually dropped off. Convulsive ergotism was more common in Germany than in France and was characterized by severe itch, sensations akin to ants crawling over one's body, and powerful spasms that could contort individual limbs or the whole body. The victim could also be subject to hallucination since ergot contains compounds related to LSD (lysergic acid diethylamide). Impairment of hearing and sight, glaucoma, paralysis, and epilepsy are other complications of the convulsive form.[43]

Because the victims of ergotism were at times viewed with suspicion and, like lepers, marginalized,[44] their care and cure came to be the work of the brothers of the Order of Saint Anthony, or the Antonines. This laic hospitaller community was established in France at Bourg-Saint-Antoine, near Vienne, the site of a Benedictine priory that preserved a reliquary of Saint Anthony. Here, around the dawn of the twelfth century, a noble named Gaston asked the saint's intercession to cure the ergotism of his son Guérin. While modern scientists speculate that "cures" in this region resulted from the local rye being free of the ergot fungus, Gaston attributed the remedy to the saint and vowed to establish a hospitaller community to serve other sufferers. The religious order that resulted was headed by a clerical master, but was composed for the most part of serving brothers, *donati* or *conversi*, whose habit was adorned by a Greek *tau*, and who lived according to the Rule of Saint Augustine. Shelters or *domus eleemosynaria* were established in France, Germany, England, Tuscany, Bohemia, Palestine, Constantinople, and Spain to serve the victims of skin disease of all sorts, and even travelers and pilgrims.[45]

There is no study of the history of the Antonines in Iberia, but a few notices testify to their existence in Catalonia and eastern Spain. Their first Iberian center may have been at Cervera, where a church and hospital dedicated to Sant Antoni functioned from the thirteenth until the early fifteenth century. Agustí Duran argues that this house possessed a royal *guiatge*, a form of protection, and sheltered the king and queen when they passed through the town. The Order abandoned the hospital circa 1401 because ergotism had disappeared from the region, and most of the brothers moved to a new hospital in Barcelona, taking with them the house's liturgical treasures and endowment, much to the consternation of the residents of Cervera.[46] But the Antonines have left few traces at Barcelona and Tàrrega and none at all at Girona, Tarragona, or anywhere else in Catalonia, where a hot, dry climate would not favor the development of ergotism. Lleida, on the other hand, where the order was established, controlled the grain produced on the plain of Urgell, Catalonia's principal granary.[47] At the beginning of the thirteenth century, the order functioned in Lleida, where it possessed a hospital and residence, called Pere de Deu, located outside the walls on the Gardeny highway, but near enough to town to be incorporated into the new wall constructed by Pere III in 1357. Income from the royal chapel in the castle of Zuda was donated by Jaume I.[48] Apart from Lleida, the Antonines were established in the Kingdom of Valencia, where in 1276 Geoffrey of Casca was identified as commander of the order in the dioceses of Valencia and Tortosa. The evidence suggests that he oversaw hospitals at Fortaleny and at other sites in the Kingdom of Valencia. A hospital opened in Valencia City itself sometime between 1333 and 1340, and there was another in Alicante; in 1353 the bishop acceded to the order's request to beg alms throughout his diocese for the support of those cared for in this hospital.[49]

Mental Disorders

People whose behavior we would now characterize as disturbed were not differentiated from the run of beggars until the fourteenth century when society began to sort the poor into various categories. Arnau de Vilanova, for instance, in his *De parte operativa*, attempted a differentiation of various types of mental impairment and distortion. But before the late fourteenth and early fifteenth centuries, the insane were considered to be primarily the responsibility of relatives. Those without family were generally housed alongside other needy individuals because their malady was not considered to be contagious. For most communities, the issue raised by insanity was not one of health, but one of public order — those whose behavior was violent and disruptive had to be kept under some restraint.

In regions like Germany, the response to mental illness was to flog and expel anyone who was not a resident. Locals so afflicted would be encouraged and paid to go on pilgrimage to a religious shrine to seek a cure. But for many others, for whom recovery seemed unlikely, institutionalization became necessary. Because their condition was chronic and their care would be of long duration, many ordinary hospitals, like Saint John's in Oxford, refused to admit the insane. Consequently, special shelters slowly began to appear in the fourteenth century to provide extended care, although these

institutions would not become common until the sixteenth century. Among
the earliest mental institutions were those located in Hamburg (1375) and
in London (1403). In Spain, the first such asylum is contemporaneous to its
northern European counterparts, the *casa dels orats*, which appeared in Barcelona during the 1370s as a division of the Hospital of En Colom. Here the
mentally disturbed were restrained at times by chains and shackles, or confined in closed cells, in the so-called house of lunatics. In the fifteenth
century, En Colom was absorbed into a general hospital of Santa Creu,
which continued to admit demented priests. Other general hospitals, in
Córdoba and Saragossa, included the disturbed in their inmate population.
In Valencia, the Hospital de Ignoscents, Folls e Orats, which Rubio Vela
argues was the first completely independent mental asylum to be established
in Europe, began to function in 1409. Another soon followed in Seville.[50]

Medical Practitioners

The association between hospitals and medicine, so axiomatic in the modern world, was not common in Europe until the fourteenth century. In
Spain, Catalonia, but not Castile, conforms to this general pattern.[51] The
necessary precondition to this conjunction of shelter and care was the pro-
fessionalization of medicine itself, that is, the articulation of recognized
standards for medical education and the licensing of its practitioners.
Among medical providers, there were four officially recognized categories
of personnel: the physician (*phisicus, fisicus*), the surgeon (*cirurgicus*), the
apothecary (*apothecarius, speciarius, herbolarius*), and the barber (*barberius,
barbitonsor*). The term *medicus* or *metge*, which is common in Catalan documents, is best translated as healer, and could apply to either a physician or
surgeon.[52] The first official notice of medical personnel within the Crown of
Aragon occurred when Jaume I in 1272, as lord of Montpellier, which was
one of the continent's premier centers of medical education, attacked practitioners who had no university degree or who had taken no examination.[53]
The Cortes that met under Alfons II at Monzón in 1289 was the first to
address medical issues. Section 18 of its *acta* placed physicians and surgeons
under the same regulations that applied to lawyers, which meant that prior
to being admitted to practice they had to be examined by the councilors of
their town and by members of their profession. This regulation was mod-
eled on the customs that had been established by Roger II in 1140 within the
Kingdom of Sicily, a territory that in 1282 had become part of the Crown of

Aragon. Similar practices had already been instituted by 1220 in Paris, by 1239 in Montpellier, and would follow in 1306 in Toulouse. The first Catalan towns to require practitioners to possess an academic knowledge of medicine were Cervera (in 1291) and Valls (in 1299).[54]

While such enactments did not specifically mandate any particular course of medical studies, the implicit expectation of competence became impossible to separate from some sort of educational regimen. The *Furs* or law code of Valencia in 1329, for example, demanded four years of study at a *studium generale* and successful examination before a panel of two municipally appointed physicians as preconditions of licensing for physicians, surgeons, and barbers. The physicians of Barcelona, undoubtedly influenced by the Valencian model, complained to Prince Pere about unqualified practitioners in the city. He responded in 1334 by mandating formal examination for any who had not attained the degree of master or bachelor of medicine. As king, Pere reacted to complaints from the Aragonese town of Teruel in 1348 that incompetent individuals were taking advantage of the emergency brought on by the plague and causing great damage. Whether or not the blame for these casualties was medical malpractice, the king forbade any man or woman from practicing medicine or surgery in Teruel who had not been examined before municipal officials by the magistrates of the confraternity of Saints Cosmas and Damian. The Cortes of Cervera in 1359, perhaps responding to other complaints of malpractice, legislated that all Catalan physicians were to have at least three years of university training.[55]

In 1300, King Jaume II, in recognition of the realm's loss of Montpellier and its university, established a new university at Lleida that also included a medical faculty, upon which the monarch then attempted to confer a monopoly over medical education.[56] But demands of the plague and the resistance of Barcelona's physicians to Lleida's privileged status led to the establishment of additional schools at Perpignan (1350), Huesca (1354), Valencia (1373), and Barcelona (1400), and a surgeon's school at Valencia (1462). The king evidently played some role in their governance, for in 1401 he granted licenses to Pere de Coll, a future physician at Barcelona's Hospital of Santa Creu, and to six others so that they could commence their study of medicine at Barcelona.[57]

How effective were these requirements for university study, licensing, and examination in uplifting the quality of medical care? Studies of enrollment patterns at the medical schools of Montpellier and Lleida suggest that only a few academically trained physicians were actually graduated; and

Michael McVaugh has been able to discover the names of only seven physicians within the entire Crown of Aragon in the 1340s who claimed any sort
of academic title.[58] The evidence from medical licensing is more abundant,
but the verdict from this source is decidedly mixed. On the one hand, the
level of medical knowledge required from those who underwent examination in Valencia, and seemingly elsewhere, was high; applicants were expected to demonstrate both theoretical and clinical experience. Conditional
licenses, which required a physician to consult with more experienced colleagues, were granted to those who failed a portion of the examination.
Because "these things pertain more to experience and manual activity than
to scientific understanding," would-be surgeons were examined about actual techniques, and the less competent were restricted to "minor surgery"
that avoided the three great cavities: the head, chest, and abdomen. But, on
the other hand, the vast majority of medical personnel, both within the
Crown of Aragon and elsewhere in Europe, never underwent the examination and licensing procedure. For example, even though some eighty-seven
physicians and surgeons have been identified as being in practice in Valencia
between 1376 and 1400, during that period only twenty-eight licenses were
actually awarded. And of these, only one was granted to an individual who
had the requisite university schooling, an Italian named Tommaso de
Maestre Tone. Indications are that licenses were not routinely sought by
new medical "graduates," but rather obtained only after an individual had
already been in practice, and then only if that person were coerced for some
reason to submit to examination. In the main, formal academic training was
regarded more as an ideal than as the sine qua non for practice. Furthermore, not all health professionals were subject to formal scrutiny. While the
barbers of Valencia were licensed, their counterparts in Catalonia were not.
The municipal council of Valencia did not begin to regulate apothecaries
until 1350, after the outbreak of the plague; and self-scrutiny by this profession did not begin until 1441 when a guild of apothecaries was finally
established.[59]

Communities of physicians, surgeons, barbers, and apothecaries,
nevertheless, became distinguishable in the fourteenth century.[60] Valencia,
for example, in 1347 had a dozen physicians and thirty-one barber-surgeons.
By 1283 the barbers had achieved a corporate identity through the establishment of a religious confraternity.[61] Along with the surgeons, they formed a
college in 1433 that by 1462 had evolved into a full school of surgery. By 1480
it had a full-time instructional staff, and in 1486 inaugurated a mandatory
five-year course of study. The apothecaries founded their own college in

1441, which acquired the right to appoint two of their number to serve the city's public institutions each year. In fourteenth-century Barcelona, apothecaries must have shared some common culture since all lived in the same district, on the *carraria apothecariorum* (the modern Carrer de la Llibreteria). Evidence from fourteenth-century Girona shows that barbers and apothecaries were trained through an apprenticeship system that required between five and seven years of service for the former, and between two and eight years for the latter. Physicians, on the other hand, were slower to develop a corporate existence, but they became visible in private practice and as providers of health care under contract to various municipalities, guilds, and confraternities.[62] Despite their lack of formal organization, physicians were capable of mounting collective action against unlicensed practitioners, as they did in Barcelona in 1334 and in Valencia in 1356. In 1356, for example, the physicians of Valencia declared that no one could practice in the kingdom without four years of university training and an examination of their fitness. Specifically, they convinced King Pere III to revoke the license that he had earlier granted to Guillem Carner, an apothecary, on the grounds that Guillem had served the poor without fee. Competence, or more likely privilege, here won out over charity. [63]

Recent studies permit us to reconstruct the configuration of medical communities in several towns. In the middle decades of the fourteenth century, Girona's medical population ranged from twenty-nine during 1320–30 to fifty-four during 1341–48 and included physicians, surgeons, barbers, and apothecaries, who served an urban constituency that ranged between eight and ten thousand. Apothecaries, in the years between the two outbreaks of plague, that is, 1348 and 1362, formed the largest group with twenty-nine practitioners, followed by twelve barbers, six surgeons, and six physicians. In 1366 twenty-seven of these organized themselves into the confraternity of the Ten Thousand Martyrs, or that of Physicians, Apothecaries, and Barbers, which met annually on the feast of Saint John the Baptist in the dining hall of the Carmelite convent. Girona's medical community was comparable to Perpignan, which just prior to the plague had nine physicians and eighteen barbers and surgeons, and Montpellier.[64] In 1334, Barcelona had fifty-five health professionals (ten physicians, eight surgeons, twenty-five apothecaries, and twelve barbers), while the statistics for Valencia show fifty-seven (respectively ten, nine, twenty, and eighteen).[65]

Among medical personnel, however, physicians were fewest in number, perhaps only four or five physicians and/or surgeons per ten thousand of population in Catalonia and Valencia, rising only to six or seven in towns

like Valencia, Barcelona, Lleida, or Tortosa. The figure rises to twenty practitioners if apothecaries and barbers are added.[66] Girona, according to Guilleré's count, had in 1360 one physician or surgeon for each eleven hundred
of population, dropping to one to about six hundred when barbers are
included among the medical personnel. Yet, statistics compiled by Luis
García Ballester and Michael McVaugh show that Catalonia and the Crown
of Aragon were much better served by medical personnel than the neighboring Crown of Castile.[67] The experience of eastern Spain was closer to that of
Toulouse, which in 1405 had as many as thirty-five practitioners in a population of twenty thousand, or Italy, where fourteenth-century statistics for
Venice and Florence show similar ratios. In both instances, where the ratios
rise to twenty per ten thousand of population, barbers and even apothecaries are included in the statistics. In the first half of the fourteenth century,
in contrast, Paris had approximately a third fewer physicians as a proportion
of the population.[68] In modern terms, however, no community was amply
served, and the relatively small size of the medical community meant that
villages, rural areas, and the poor in general were not well provided for at all.
In Catalonia, for example, the rate of twenty medical personnel per ten
thousand drops to 1.7 outside of the five largest urban areas.[69]

In the decades before the plague, the size of the medical community
increased. In Barcelona and Valencia, for example, the numbers, especially
of apothecaries and surgeons, grew by 50 percent between 1310 and 1335. A
decline set in, however, during the famine years of the 1330s and 1340s.
Barcelona's medical community peaked at fifty-eight in 1333; by 1340 its
size was down to forty-five, and in 1345 to thirty-two. Valencia also reached
its apogee of sixty-six in 1333, and this declined to twenty-eight in 1345.
Even more dramatic are the figures from Saragossa, which show a reduction from thirty-one (1330) to three (1345). The bad times, which began
in 1333, the introduction of licensing, and competition, particularly among
barbers and surgeons, have all been given as reasons for this decline. Nota-
bly, this shrinkage did not occur in smaller towns like Girona and Manresa
until the advent of the plague.[70]

The plague is another factor in the contraction of the medical community at midcentury, because medical personnel would experience relatively
higher mortality rates due to their exposure to infected individuals. Girona,
for example, which suffered a relatively modest mortality rate of about 15
percent during the first siege of the plague in the summer of 1348, still lost
40 percent of its physicians, 25 percent of the barbers, and a fifth of the
apothecaries. At Perpignan, where the plague is estimated to have taken

over half of the adult male population, only two of nine physicians and two of eighteen barbers and surgeons are known to have survived the pestilence. At Xàtiva in the Kingdom of Valencia, the king, acknowledging that after the plague scarcely a single surgeon was to be found in the town, reduced the legal requirement that two surgeons attend anyone found to be seriously wounded.[71] Yet, towns, as centers of culture and possessed with a population that could afford medical care, were able to recover from such losses by attracting practitioners from other venues. Florence, whose population had declined by half on account of the plague, nonetheless had as many medical practitioners in 1399 as in 1338.[72]

Medieval communities, like their modern rural counterparts, were concerned about the shortage of medical personnel, particularly after the devastation of the plague. Several stratagems were thus pursued to augment the supply of legally licensed medical personnel. The first was to petition the king for an exception, as did the lord of the town of Nules in Valencia in 1332; he asked the king to permit an apothecary (Ramon Sa Lena from Borriana) who could not meet the educational standards of the licensing statute to continue his practice. Such royally sanctioned exceptions became commonplace in the fourteenth century. A second stratagem was to utilize the services of non-Christians, despite the concerns of the Church, which, having little faith in the curative powers of medicine, saw as the prime duty of physicians the obligation to encourage patients to confess their sins.[73] Thus, the Cortes of Monzón in 1363 provided an alternative licensing procedure for Muslim and Jewish physicians who would not have access to Christian universities, and the registers of the bishop of Barcelona contain instances of licenses being granted to Jewish physicians to treat Christian patients. At the end of the century, after the persecutions of 1391 and 1392, some of these Jewish physicians changed their names and converted to Christianity.[74] On the other hand, few Muslim physicians practiced among Christians in Valencia; most of their numbers seem to have followed other members of the Islamic elite into exile in Granada or Africa. Among Muslims or *mudéjars*, medical practice continued to be carried on by *metgesses*, female practitioners who served not only as midwives, but also as general physicians and surgeons.[75] Such Muslim women were used not only by their own coreligionists, but by Christians as well. In 1332, for example, one such practitioner named Çahud resided within the royal household; and in 1338, when another, who practiced surgery in Barcelona, was accused of malpractice, the king did not automatically ban her from practice. Instead, he ruled that she be subjected to an examination by competent surgeons. Indeed, it may well be that the prohibition contained in Valencia's *Furs* in 1329 that "no woman may practice medicine or give potions" may have been aimed specifically against these Muslim *metgesses* and not against women in general. Nonetheless, given the scarcity of Christian physicians, especially in Valencia, both *metgesses* and Jewish physicians continued to practice well into the fifteenth century.[76]

Given such shortages, medical care was limited to private clients able to afford its cost, or to larger groups who would contract with medical personnel to provide services to their members. The inability of the poor to afford medical services undoubtedly was the motivating force behind the petition of the councilors of the Kingdom of Majorca to King Alfons the Magnanimous in 1420 that medical practitioners provide care at no cost to those unable to pay.[77] Among the early "health care alliances" were cathedral chapters. At Girona in 1296, the physician Ramon Cornellà was paid an annual retainer of one hundred sous to care for members of the cathedral chapter, and in 1305 the physician Albert received six hundred sous.[78] In the fourteenth century, increasingly detailed contracts were signed between the chapter and both physicians and surgeons. The Pia Almoina of Girona, operated under the direction of the chapter, evidently provided similar care for its *familia*, paying one Caravit three *mitgeras* of wheat in 1338–39 for his services. Beginning around 1300, towns would also make arrangements with medical personnel.[79] The earliest contract survives from the small town of Castelló d'Empúries, which paid two hundred sous in 1307 to the physician Bernat de Cremis, but it appears that this and other small communities like Manresa, Puigcerdà, and Cervera had difficulties retaining physicians, despite their payment of increasingly larger stipends. Larger communities, which could provide physicians more attractive conditions of practice and income, felt little need to enter into such contracts until after the onset of bad times and the plague. Tortosa, for example, had a physician and surgeon under contract in 1339, and Girona paid Guillem Colteiler twenty pounds in 1357, a substantial amount, but one which paled against the one hundred pounds or more that the count-king would lavish on his own doctors. Other towns, like Murcia in 1432, appointed a local physician to serve as surgeon of the poor, charged with providing free care to the needy of the town. The Kingdom of Majorca in 1372 paid a retainer of one hundred pounds to a physician and another hundred and fifty pounds to a surgeon to serve the poor, although the latter stipend was eliminated when the royal auditor discovered that no town then had a surgeon in residence. Perhaps the decree of King Alfons noted above had some result, because by the late fifteenth century the Crown was able to reduce the physician's allotment to forty pounds and the surgeon's to a mere ten pounds.[80] Before and after the plague, communities in the Kingdom of Valencia like Morella, Borriana, Xàtiva, and Alzira complained of a shortage of medical workers. Outlying villages, on the other hand, could at best support the services of a resident barber, but even he would have to be trained in a larger town.[81] Thus, these smaller municipalities might contract with physicians from the larger towns to visit periodically, but there were frequent complaints that such doctors failed to appear.[82]

Medical Care and Hospitals

Because of such shortages and their own lack of economic resources, the vast majority of small shelters that called themselves hospitals lacked any sort of medical personnel. Yet, by the thirteenth century, there are signs that medical care was being introduced into a few institutions. Timothy Miller argues that the European houses of the Hospitaller Order of Saint John were particularly influential in this development because, as early as its statutes of 1182, the order maintained four physicians at its large hospital in Jerusalem to diagnose disease and prescribe medicine. Within Europe, Roger I of Sicily tells us in 1137 that the Knights of Saint John were treating the sick within their houses, and in the thirteenth century several French Hôtels-Dieu, including that of Paris (1217), wrote statutes that mirror the provisions for care in the Hospitaller statutes.[83] The Knights of Saint John, however, do not seem to have practiced the healing arts in the realms of Aragon.[84] Indeed, evidence of medical care in Iberian hospitals does not emerge until the end of the thirteenth century or later.[85] In Valencia, the earliest example of the formal provision for medical personnel is the Hospital of En Clapers, where in 1311 the founder provided fifty sous as an annual stipend for a medical doctor. By midcentury, however, the administrators had difficulty locating physicians who would accept such "a small amount" and in 1379 were forced to pay four times that salary, or two hundred sous, to Jacme d'Avinyó for his services as a physician and surgeon. In return, Jacme was obligated to make the journey from town every day to visit the hospital's inmates. Jacme's expertise in both medicine and surgery was evidently not common because, when he was ultimately replaced in 1383, the hospital was forced to engage the services of Jacme Maderes, a physician, and Francesc Riera, a surgeon.[86]

Medical care was introduced into Catalan hospitals around the middle of the fourteenth century. Tortosa, which had been contracting with medical personnel since at least 1339, demanded in 1345 that the town physician also visit and treat the sick in the municipal hospital. Likewise, by the later fourteenth century, the Hospital of the Poor in Girona and the Hospital of San Feliu de Guixols had contracts with physicians.[87] At Barcelona's Hospital of Sant Macià, physicians like Berenguer Banyeres and Francesc Pedralbes were placed on an annual retainer of ten florins at the end of the fourteenth century; other physicians could also be consulted, but not frivolously because the fee was one sou per visit. In addition, the hospital would utilize as necessary the services of certain apothecaries. Instead it seems that Barcelona hospitals counted on an amount of gratuitous service from local medical personnel who had been commanded by King Pere in 1336 to visit all who were lying ill in the city's hospitals free of charge. In the early fifteenth century, the new Hospital of Santa Creu in Barcelona had a barber and an apothecary in residence, and there were additional barbers and physicians under retainer, who were expected to make their rounds in the hospital every morning and afternoon.[88]

Thus, by the end of the fourteenth century, hospitals like En Clapers would have a physician, a surgeon, plus a barber, an apothecary, and several *metgesses*, or female practitioners, to serve a patient population that ranged from between one and two dozen. It is difficult to gauge the level of care actually provided to patients, but, derived from the accounts of 1388 which show that 9 percent of the budget was expended on medicine and the salaries of medical personnel, the sense is that care was consistent if modest. Despite the requirement of the *Furs de València* that the physician was "obligated to treat the infirm poor without demanding any payment," the hospitals were forced to pay for these services and did so by placing medical personnel under some form of term contract or retainer.[89] Accordingly, at another Valencian hospital, that of Santa Llucia or La Reyna, the town council paid physicians two hundred sous a year, surgeons one hundred sous, and wet nurses fifteen sous a month. The *dides* or wet nurses were in residence, but others, such as apothecaries and barbers, came at regular intervals or as needed. The Hospital of Santa Creu in Barcelona, for instance, had a number of physicians and surgeons on retainer, sometimes at substantial sums. In 1409, for example, the surgeon Pere Garbí received 990 sous, but his payment evidently was variable because in later years the stipend was considerably less. Other medical personnel were paid about three hundred sous a year, a part-time salary that reflects the consultative nature of their employment.[90] Santa Creu accordingly worried that medical personnel might extort additional payments from individual patients, and so in its *Ordinacions* of 1417 banned this practice and stated that "they [that is, the barbers and physicians] should be content with the stipend or salary that the said honorable administrators will assign to them."[91] Unlike barbers and physicians, apothecaries were generally paid no salary, but derived compensation from the price of the medicine they provided. Nonetheless, hospitals like En Clapers, did give certain individuals exclusive rights to supply the institution with medicine. Barbers, according to the accounts of En Clapers for 1382–83, were paid per service, generally three or four diners for bleeding or shaving patients. Similarly, *metgesses* were summoned as needed, like the Muslim woman who was paid three sous in 1396 for curing a female servant at En Clapers of an inflamed spleen that the hospital's own physician was unable to treat.[92]

Records of late medieval hospitals show that the sick comprised substantial proportions of the inmate population, indicating that the transformation of these institutions from mere shelters to facilities dispensing medical care was indeed well underway. Among the inmate population in late medieval Valencia, for example, were individuals of various ages; many of these were awaiting some form of surgery, others had advanced cases of typhus, malaria, tuberculosis, cachexia (a wasting away due to chronic disease), dropsy, pustules, consumption, scrofula, and lesions of major organs and vessels. But, the largest number of recorded diagnoses were for those suffering from some sort of wound. There are also instances of the plague, both among inmates as well as the staff, and of the admission of children whose mothers had died from the pestilence. General hospitals like En Clapers refused entry to lepers, who were instead conducted to the leprosarium of Sant Llàtzer; and those who suffered from mental disorders would be held only until they could be returned to relatives.[93] At Barcelona's Santa Creu, the earliest *Llibre de entrades des malalts* dates from the period February 10 to November 23, 1457, and records the facts of some 346 admissions. Of these, 171, almost half, had some sort of fever and another 18 percent suffered from symptoms of the plague. An eighth of the patients came from vessels in the harbor, presumably sick but with no diagnosis specified; another three patients, described as *del mar*, presumably came from outside the harbor area. The remaining 20 percent of patients had a wide variety of ailments: dropsy (eight), apoplexy (two), ulcers (six), pains (four), leg and feet problems (five), fractures (two), old age (one), itching (one), and stomach problems (one). Fewer than 10 percent of the admissions (thirty-two) carried no diagnosis. Of all those who were admitted, only 26 percent (ninety-one) died, a much smaller statistic than the 49 percent recorded for the years 1473 to 1491; the rate was almost twice as high for women (47.8 percent) than it was for men (24.7 percent). Not surprisingly, the highest death rate, two-thirds, was experienced by victims of the plague. In contrast, only three of the eight patients with dropsy died, and 17 percent of those with fever. Unfortunately, data for other patients is too meager to be statistically significant, but it does indicate that those who entered the hospital did have a realistic expectation of recovery and discharge. Perhaps the reason for this is that, to judge by our meager information regarding admissions, there was a bias in favor of admitting the acutely over the chronically ill, individuals who would either be cured or die without the necessity of extended care. In terms of gender, higher mortality rates indicate that elderly women were more likely to receive admission and extended care than men.[94]

Late medieval physicians felt that their main task was to keep patients alive and comfortable and so generally shunned aggressive treatment.[95] Thus, besides prayer, the major forms of treatment within medieval hospitals involved diet, medication, and surgery. By all accounts, diet mimicked that of public shelters, and of the population at large, with its reliance on bread and wine, with small quantities of meats and vegetables, for the bulk of calories. This can be seen in the food accounts of En Clapers for 1388–89 that show an expenditure of 30 percent on wheat, 26 percent on wine, and 24 percent on meat and fish. Despite the fact that poultry was regarded as a proper food for the sick, most of the meat purchased was mutton, only 5 percent was chicken.[96] Thus, it seems in matters of diet the emphasis was on ensuring that the sick had food to eat, rather than on providing any kind of therapeutic diet. For example, when one individual arrived at Barcelona's Hospital of Sant Macià with fever, he was confined to the hospital and provided with a diet of chicken, raisins, and sweets, at a cost of nine diners; only if necessary would a physician be called because of the sou that the visit would cost. The ordinances of Santa Creu, which outline the general regimen of care, speak of foods, as well as medicines, being prescribed for various patients.[97]

The form of actual therapy that is easiest to document is the pharmaceutical, because herbal remedies, ointments, syrups, and other preparations had to be purchased from an apothecary. While drugs, most often elaborate recipes compounded from as many as a dozen ingredients, were available in Catalonia, they do not seem to have been widely prescribed for patients in hospitals, perhaps because of their cost.[98] The invoices of Valencia's Hospital of En Clapers, for example, show that the products most prescribed by physicians and other personnel were syrups (made, for example, from roses, sugar, vinegar, endive, maidenhair, fumitory, julep, a mixture of honey and vinegar, or violets), enemas, plasters, powders of various sorts, and ointments (made from roses, gold, camphor or sandalwood). Also purchased, but much less frequently, were pills of various sizes, confections, and eyewashes. There were also various potions, called variously waters (e.g. of the dog rose), oils (bitter almond, dill, quince, spinach, blue lily, mastic, myrtle, scorpions, or roses), conserves, juices, boiled wine, and concentrated syrups. The accounts also show quantities of tragacanth (a gum), musk, plaster, incense, small crustaceans, lemon juice, melon seeds, honey, black pepper, saffron, salsa, and sugar. Taking into account all the perils of medieval accounting, all of this represented between 5 and 10 percent of the hospital's total expenditure.[99]

Santa Creu, according to its ordinances, was as careful as modern hospitals in the distribution of medicine. Nothing could be dispensed to patients unless it were prescribed by a physician or barber. As a safeguard, these individuals were supposed to order the medication "in their own hand in the book of the apothecary of the hospital." The apothecary, for his part, was forbidden to compound or dispense any medications not prescribed for patients by medical personal; additionally, if the prescription were for a member of the hospital staff, it required the authorization of the upper administration.[100]

Positive medical interventions included bleeding and purging, although not to the extent that was once believed, and surgery. Given the lack of anesthesia and a means for preventing infection, surgeons were reluctant to open the body cavity. Their ministrations more commonly were confined to setting fractures, binding and suturing wounds, fixing dislocations, and dressing sores and rashes. One has the sense from the ordinances of Barcelona's Santa Creu in 1417 that the hospital functioned as a kind of emergency room. While most medical personnel were merely on call, one barber, who was to be expert in the art of surgery, was to be present day and night to serve patients who suffered some sort of emergency and the poor who might arrive at any hour and require immediate treatment.[101]

The final services that the hospital provided to inmates were comfort in death and a burial. A sworn deposition of 1335, for example, reveals that an attendant at Valencia's Hospital of En Clapers, Guillem Busquet, stood beside the dying Pero López d'Arbull, holding a candle and reciting various prayers. After a person died, the hospital had to prepare the corpse for burial, wrap it in a shroud, and if necessary inter the body in the hospital's own cemetery. Rubio Vela estimates, based on the amount of money spent on shrouds, that En Clapers buried an average of thirty or forty individuals per year, rising to almost ninety during the months of plague and famine between April and October 1375. It is difficult to estimate the hospital's mortality rate, even though we can estimate the average daily population, because there is no information concerning length of hospitalization. Nonetheless, given a daily population that ranged between eight and eighteen, the number of deaths suggests that many patients were seriously ill, and perhaps also reflects the hazards of medieval medicine.[102] Katherine Park and others have argued that hospitals served the economic function of protecting the urban work force from infection by providing a place for sick people, particularly victims of the plague, to die. These institutions might heal individuals and restore them to employment, but more importantly they served to quarantine those who might infect the healthy population.[103]

*   *   *

In the twelfth century, hospitals, even those that sheltered individuals suffering from a specific disease like leprosy or ergotism, served fundamentally as shelters. Their purpose was to provide a decent place in which the individual patient would die or, less likely, recover; care itself emphasized the welfare of the soul more than it did of the body. By the early fifteenth century, however, the outlines of the modern general hospital had emerged, staffed with physicians and nurses, who made rounds, prescribed medicine, and undertook other forms of treatment. While mortality rates remained high, a majority of patients recovered and returned as healthy members of the community. What forces are responsible for this transformation? Among the most important is the development of medicine as a profession, not only as an academic discipline taught in universities but also as a practical craft pursued and handed on by experienced physicians, barbers, and surgeons. Advances in pharmacology and diagnosis made their contribution. Essential as well was the evolution of municipal government, which could apply collective resources to procuring medical services for the less affluent, within hospitals and within the community. Efforts to inspire or compel medical personnel to serve the poor without charge met with indifferent success, and one suspects that limitations in society's ability to afford medical care is a significant reason for the concern, one with decidedly modern overtones, over a shortage of adequate medical services, particularly in smaller towns and rural areas. Catalonia, which had commercial and political ties to Italy and the rest of the Mediterranean and its own medical school, had an advantage over the rest of Iberia and much of northern Europe. With proportionately greater numbers of medical personnel and with some of Europe's first general hospitals, medieval Catalans and Valencians had gained some access to medical care, which was now considered to be part of the routine of hospitalization.

6

The Care of
Women and Children

THE MEDIEVAL EFFORT TO FEED AND SHELTER the poor and even to care
for the sick showed little regard for age or gender. In all but the smallest of
shelters, men and women generally slept in separate chambers, but few
differences are to be noted in the routine of their care.[1] Among the few
hospices specifically set aside for women and children were those operated
by the Order of the Holy Spirit, but not many of these existed in the Iberian
realms. Likewise the sort of shelters reserved for widows, reformed prostitutes, and other women that could be found in the Italian communes or in
Paris were mostly an urban phenomenon and, in the Crown of Aragon,
would be echoed only in places like Barcelona and Valencia. Indeed, among
the medieval needy, whatever privilege or precedence that was accorded to
gender most often benefited males. This can be seen most easily in the
allocation of space. Almost everywhere, more beds were reserved for men,
even though the material needs of males were not necessarily greater. For
example, statistics from Barcelona's general hospital between 1473 and
1491, the earliest that we have, show that women accounted for only 27.5
percent of the admissions, but 58 percent of all deaths.[2] There were two
areas, however, in which women were singled out for special consideration:
marriage and childbirth.

Marriage and Dowries

For poor women, the chief barrier to respectability, which was acquired
through an honorable marriage, was the almost absolute necessity of providing a dowry to the prospective husband.[3] In towns like Barcelona and
Girona, the dowry was paid in money and goods and tended to be quite
high. During the fourteenth century, for example, the almost five hundred

dowries recorded in Girona average 995s. In Barcelona, women of the lowest estate, for example, the offspring of slaves, were expected to provide four hundred sous, while the daughters of artisans and sailors were dowered with amounts between three hundred and seven hundred sous in the twelfth and thirteenth centuries, rising to eight hundred and twelve hundred sous in later Middle Ages. Even in a poor, rural town like Urgell, dowries in working-class families averaged between two hundred and three hundred sous, while affluent families paid out as much as two thousand sous. Such expectations precipitated a crisis not only for the very poor, who of course had nothing to give their daughters, but also for families of modest means. The pay of honest, but unskilled workers was barely adequate to feed a family, and often left little if anything available to daughters of marriageable age. Even those workers with some skill often had great difficulty managing the dower payment. Consequently, and perhaps precisely because the need extended upward from the ranks of the miserable poor into those of working classes, the provision of assistance to young girls seeking marriage became a favorite charity in Catalonia and elsewhere.[4]

Subventions or subsidies for dowries, as the alms list of Barcelona's parish of Santa Maria del Mar reveals, were extended both to honest young girls of marriageable age and to prostitutes in the hope of their reformation. Confraternities, at Vic and elsewhere, would subsidize at any one time dowries for as many as twelve daughters of members. Everywhere this was an important parochial charity; normally money for this assistance came from pious bequests contained in the wills of parishioners. Often, the amounts are but a few sous, but sometimes they were more substantial.[5] In general, it seems that the dimensions of this charity grew with time. Carme Batlle and Montserrat Casas's study of wills of the thirteenth century from Barcelona and Urgell, for example, shows that such bequests were few in number but large in amount, often ranging into the hundreds of sous, and frequently intended for the daughter of some poor relation. Teresa-María Vinyoles's study, on the other hand, shows a remarkably different result for the period 1375–1415, an era that had already experienced depopulation on account of famine, war, and plague and that was especially concerned with the promotion of marriage and families. Here a half of all wills contained alms for dowries. These were true charitable benefactions because only a fifth of the testators specified who was to receive the gift. Likewise, Batlle's own study of fifteenth-century wills in the parish of Sants Just i Pastor confirms that the charity to undowered girls had become the most common benefaction among Barcelona's parishioners.[6]

The Catalan experience is replicated in Italy, where Steven Epstein's survey of Genoese wills between 1150 and 1314 also depicts this to be a charity of the affluent, with only seven testators bequeathing enough money to dower over one hundred women. At Siena, like Barcelona, there was little popular interest in this charity until after the bubonic plague, when the bequests for dowries proliferated and soon became the largest category of pious bequests.[7]

Barcelona, unlike Lleida or Valencia, created no institutions specifically to distribute these legacies and other alms to needy women. Traditionally, the responsibility for their disbursement belonged to the clergy or to individual manumissors. In the fourteenth and fifteenth centuries, as parochial charity became organized into *plats* and *bacís*, female parishioners could receive assistance in amassing a dowry from these institutions. For example, in 1428, the alms fund of the parish of Santa Maria del Pi gave the grocer Lluis Batlle thirty-nine sous, in six installments, and Arnau forty-one sous, nine diners, in eleven installments, toward the dowries of their daughters. In 1423, this parish contributed approximately 2 percent of its total alms toward the payment of dowries.[8] While most parishioners, who left only a few sous in their wills for dowries, were content to let the parish or its alms fund decide on the recipient, other benefactors continued to entrust the responsibly to their executors, who seemed to have exercised a great deal of discretion in allotting those funds. Legal records, however, indicate that relatives of the deceased felt that they had some special claim on such legacies. For example, circa 1350, a man from Vilafranca petitioned the bishop of Barcelona's vicar to be given the dowry money left by a deceased relative and he was given one hundred sous. But the system was also open to abuse, as is attested by the vicar's decision to allocate three hundred sous from this alms fund to two notaries, Bernat Moyhoni and Guillem Vilella, who were regularly employed by the diocese and thus not among the *pauperes Christi*.[9]

Another possible source of assistance for young Barcelonan women was the royal almoner. A sample, drawn from the years 1378, and 1381–85, during the reign of Pere III, shows 106 grants to women, including 16 from Barcelona, 8 from Valencia and 4 from Saragossa. Like the parishes, the king preferred to subsidize the deserving poor, rather than dower the truly desperate. Thus, while there were a handful of large gifts, usually to poor relations of otherwise important families, the average subsidy was a mere fifty-five sous. For the most part, these were not for women of the lowest class, for example, ex-slaves, foundlings, or orphans, because in 75 percent of the cases a parent's name appears in the record. Several are children of workers in the royal household. Only about a fifth appear to have been real paupers — prostitutes or foundlings. Joan I was even less generous to the true poor than Pere III. His registers contain some thirty-two endowments that ranged in size from 275 sous to 3,000 sous. Most were given to the children of royal functionaries and domestics; of the total, only five recipients were genuinely needy.[10] The policies of Barcelona's municipal government mirror those of the royal almoner, poor shelters, and parish alms funds. Thus, the emphasis was on aiding the deserving poor by subsidizing dowries for girls of good family.

Municipal Assistance to Women

While councilors of Barcelona gave out no alms for dowries, except to the daughters of its own dependents, officials at Lleida were more generous and decided in 1303 to sponsor a municipal institution to dower orphaned girls, and this was given an initial endowment of twenty-five hundred sous by King Jaume II.[11] In Valencia, the major responsibility for dowering the poor was assumed by a confraternity composed of the heads of several of the city's leading mercantile families. Called the *almoina de los órfenes a maridar*, this was established in 1293 by ten merchants with an initial endowment of five hundred pounds. Bernat dez Clapers, the founder of the eponymous hospital, was its majordomo in 1309; other known members were prosperous merchants and professional men. The *almoina* invested its resources in various properties that yielded, by 1398, a yearly income of some four hundred pounds. From this, each of the ten members of the confraternity was permitted to disburse to young women gifts in the amount of sixty-six sous, with most of the rest used to purchase cloth, out of which trousseaux for brides-to-be could be fabricated. Given the size of the alms funds, it would seem that the confraters were able to help several dozen young women each year. But given the modest size of the confraternity's contributions, the preponderance of aid must have gone to the daughters of the working poor.[12]

Bordellos

In many respects, the special concern for women's welfare was a negative one, born out of a fear that in certain circumstances innocent girls would turn to prostitution and, as Francesc Eiximenis worried in his *Regiment de la cosa pública*, keep men from matrimony. Prostitutes (*meretrius, dones públiques*, or *putanes*) are castigated in Catalan documents as *viles mulieres, vilissimes mulieres, vils fembres*, or *inhonestes mulieres*, and in Valencia as *fembras públicas* or *fembres pecadrius*. In France they were called everything from *filles de joie* to *foles femmes* and *putains*. These terms, however, disguise the reality that there in fact existed many different kinds and degrees of prostitution. There was the practice of older professionals, who lived permanently in brothels or else in fixed areas of town. But many prostitutes were simply younger, unmarried girls — spinsters, cloth workers, serving maids — who supplemented their income by soliciting in taverns, at fairs, or on major feasts. In Valencia, these more discreet girls were called *fembres escuseres* and *fembres errades*.[13] Catalan social policy accepted most of these activities as a fact of life. Prince Joan, for example, wrote to his father King Pere III that "the Church permits bordellos as a way of diminishing sin and preventing more serious evils." Thus, even though prostitutes as individuals were held in low esteem, public policy tolerated certain forms of prostitution and treated harshly only those women who sought to evade civic regulation.[14] According to municipal ordinances in Barcelona and Valencia, for example, in public prostitutes always had to appear marked as dishonorable women and were forbidden to conceal their identity by wearing any type of cape, wrap, or overcoat, even in winter. Within these parameters, however, women were permitted to live in bordellos, some of which even existed under municipal ownership. But proscribed was prostitution of a more casual nature, the kind that might lure local girls into the profession or deter them from marriage, and its practitioners were subject to severe penalties.[15]

In the realms of Aragon, jurisdiction over prostitutes in the thirteenth century fell to the royal vicar, and afterward to municipal *consells*. The frequency of complaints in the thirteenth and fourteenth centuries from groups like the mendicant friars about prostitutes and brothels suggests that their activities were at first generally not regulated or else that restrictions were widely ignored.[16] In Barcelona, the first effort to segregate prostitutes dates from 1328, after a woman who lived near the leper hospice complained to the king that men and women of low estate loitered in the area.[17] In 1330, King Alfons III suggested to the municipal council that dishonest women have their own houses, and in 1332 the council established a curfew for prostitutes. In 1363, King Pere at the Cortes of Monzón decreed that the practice of prostitution anywhere in his realms should be limited to officially recognized bordellos. The first such municipal *bordellum* in Barcelona, located near the monastery of Santa Eulàlia, surfaced in 1361. Subsequently, a district for prostitution was established at the fringe of the old city, along the Ramblas. This grew into a network of licensed bordellos, each operated by a *hostaler*, or innkeeper, who was supposed to supply the women with food, drink, rooms, a bed, and bed linen at a reasonable price. Municipal officials, often men of high station, oversaw these establishments and collected rents for the city.[18] In Valencia, a district located outside the walls near the *morería*, or Muslim district, began to take shape early in the fourteenth century, perhaps at the instigation of King Jaume II, who in 1325 ordered that all prostitutes live in a designated location. In 1350, the municipal council decreed that all prostitutes should reside and ply their trade within this *Bordell* (or *Burdel* or *Pobla de les fembres pecadrius*), register themselves with the *maestre racional*, and observe a certain curfew. Subsequently, for the next four centuries, a distinctively organized community developed here within a walled compound, ruled by a regent appointed by the *justicia criminal* and a group of *hosteleros*, that is, men and women who operated the rooming houses in which the prostitutes resided.[19]

Reformed Prostitutes

Very often towns in the Mediterranean region operated some sort of shelter for women who wished, or who were compelled, to forsake their careers as prostitutes. In France, for example, such women were placed within a type of religious community as nuns. Such institutions served two functions. They rehabilitated women by substituting a regulated religious life for the former life of vice, but they also served as houses of charity, shelters, and places of retirement for women too old or sick to continue in the profession.[20] Barcelona and Valencia, and perhaps other towns within the Crown of Aragon, maintained such shelters as well, with little pretense, however, that they were houses of religion. In Barcelona, the municipal council established such a shelter for penitent women in 1365.[21] Twenty years earlier, in Valencia, the initiative came from Na Soriana, a Franciscan tertiary who is described as a *dona de penitència*. In 1345, she established a shelter for reformed prostitutes called the Casa de las Arrepentidas. It was given an initial grant of five hundred sous by the city council, and in 1362 the bishop ordered that all parishes take up a collection toward its support. The *casa* served two purposes. During Holy Week, and later on certain Marian feasts as well, it sheltered prostitutes who were rounded up, invited to meditate on their sinful lives, and fed at municipal expense. At other times of the year, the *casa* accommodated women who sought, for reasons of age or personal betterment, to give up prostitution. Those who ran the shelter, however, had little trust in these women's resolve because discipline in the house was extremely stringent. Upon entering, women would have to submit to total seclusion for at least a year; afterward they could leave the house with permission, but under the threat of expulsion and a public whipping should they ever return to their former habits. For those women who persevered, found a husband, and reentered society in an honorable estate, the municipal council agreed to provide a dowry.[22]

And at the beginning of the fifteenth century, the Consell de Cent of Barcelona, perhaps following the example of Valencia, also sought to prohibit the practice of prostitution during Holy Week.[23] From Wednesday of that week until mass on Easter Sunday, all the prostitutes of the city were to be confined in shelters on the street of *les Egipciaques,* where under the eyes of honest widows they were to be fed and invited to convert their lives through attendance at mass, sermons, and confession. To prevent escape, the women would be confined in rooms with bedding, firewood, and a serving girl who would fetch meals. At other times of the years, the shelters of *les Egipciaques* became a detention center for women and girls who plied their trade outside of the strict boundaries set by municipal regulation.[24]

Children

Perhaps the neediest segment of any society is its children, who depend upon adults for sustenance, shelter, and education. A study of medieval Girona and its environs, which is suggestive of all of Catalonia, concludes that the average family of the fourteenth century contained two children. The average is higher for patrician families (3), and for rural households (3.5). Urban artisans, on the other hand, seemed to have had fewer children, averaging between 1.3 and 1.8 per family. Perhaps as many as a fifth of all couples had no children at all.[25]

In order to understand the treatment of children in the Middle Ages, contemporary social scientists have discussed the attitudes of medieval people toward children and childhood, and particularly the amount of affection that parents exhibited toward their children and whether childhood was regarded as being a distinct stage of life. Out of this discourse has developed the "indifference and neglect" thesis, which argues that medieval society lacked affection for its children, and consequently parents did not bond with their offspring. Other writers, however, have rejected this view and argued that the primary differences between modern and medieval treatment of children has more to do with the much greater levels of poverty and mortality due to disease in the Middle Ages than to any difference in levels of affection. While this discussion, for the most part, has dealt with children who belonged to functional families and has not centered on the neediest children, it nonetheless bears upon the issue of why medieval people, individually and collectively, contributed to charities that assisted children. If the "indifference and neglect" thesis is correct, then such aid can be explained only in religious and ritualistic terms. If societal emotions, on the other hand, were more complex and closer to modern values, then a whole panoply of religious and social factors would have to be taken into account.[26]

Among medieval authors, it was customary to divide childhood into several stages: *infantia*, which lasted from birth to the age of seven; *pueritia*, which for boys encompassed the ages of seven to fourteen, and for girls seven to twelve; and *adolescentia*, which lasted until the onset of adulthood, which usually coincided with marriage and economic independence. The *Furs de València*, for example, established twenty as the age of majority.[27] Normally the rearing of children, particularly during the first two stages, was the exclusive responsibility of parents or other relations, and so medieval communities did not become concerned with their welfare unless or until they became orphaned. Then efforts were undertaken first to insure their survival, and afterward to provide them with the means to grow into functioning adult members of society.

Child Abandonment

Infantia, when children were at their most vulnerable, received the most attention from medieval authorities, primarily because of the problems of infanticide and child abandonment. There is not much direct evidence for the former, but it surely existed.[28] Legend has it, for example, that the sight of the bodies of children floating down the Tiber River motivated Pope Innocent III in 1202 to call Guy of Montpellier to Rome and to entrust the Hospital of Santa Maria in Sassia, which was located on the banks of the Tiber, to his Order of the Holy Spirit.[29] In 1294, a Florentine communal commission argued that the asylum of San Gallo played a vital role because, by providing shelter to foundlings, it helped the region "to avoid the many crimes committed against infants." Furthermore, several anecdotal studies of sex ratios among medieval children show an abnormal bias in favor of male children, suggesting the possibility that within some communities female children were murdered. In Spain, municipal legislation, aimed particularly at unwed mothers, suggests that deliberate neglect was a method employed for getting rid of unwanted children.[30] Furthermore, a synodal statute from Barcelona, dated 1354, reserved to the bishop's penitentiary the duty to absolve parents who found their children dead, next to them in bed, suggesting that smothering was yet another means.[31] Much better documented, however, and undoubtedly more prevalent is the phenomenon of abandonment.

Child abandonment is generally a product of illegitimacy and/or economic hardship, although Brian Pullan believes that medieval society itself was more conditioned than ours to accept the legitimacy of the abandonment of children into foundling homes because its social elite farmed its own children out to wet nurses.[32] Other historians cite factors of population growth and the loosening of sexual mores in the eleventh and twelfth centuries as contributing factors, but it seems that a worsening of economic conditions in the thirteenth precipitated the problem of abandonment.[33] The immediate reasons that led a parent to expose a child are varied. Poverty, ill health, deformity, or the death of a mother or both parents are well-known reasons. Some individuals abandoned children out of a sense of shame—to hide, for example, a sexual encounter that occurred during some forbidden period like Lent, or during menstruation, or else out of the fear that the progeny of illicit sex would have deformities. Among the more prosperous, in regions like Spain and Italy, where customs of partible inheritance prevailed, too many heirs could seriously dilute a family's wealth. Philip Gavitt, in his study of Florence's Hospital of the Innocenti during the fifteenth century, argues that a majority of the children who can be identified were connected in some fashion to prominent Florentine families, frequently the illegitimate offspring of a family member and a slave.[34]

Notes left alongside children abandoned at Barcelona's Hospital of Santa Creu in the first half of the fifteenth century, or earlier at Valencia's Hospital of En Clapers, add texture to these general observations. Genís Gil, abandoned in 1428 at eighteen months after she had been weaned, is the legitimate child of a married couple "who are poor like Job."[35] Ramon de Pla brought his eight-month-old son, Andreu Marc, because his wife, Na Johana, was sick and in a hospital. Baptized by hospitallers as Joan de

París, another infant was the son of a Barcelona slave, owned by the silversmith En Trullàs, and a French barber. Perhaps to prevent his son's enslavement, friends of the father stole Joan away from his mother and took him to the orphanage. Shortly thereafter, however, the administrators returned the child to his mother, but at the insistence of her master, who evidently saw Joan as more of a liability than an asset, he was brought back a second time to Santa Creu, where he survived until the age of two. Eulàlia, a girl of nine months, was abandoned by a mother who was sick with fever and whose husband was absent on a journey. A Valencian wet nurse ran off with a male servant, leaving a daughter at En Clapers. Aldonça de Sant Boi, the six-month-old daughter of a dead Aragonese beggar, was brought to the hospital, sent out to a wet nurse, who died in the epidemic of 1441, and then contracted to a squire as a serving girl until the age of eighteen. In 1384–85, Na Maria, widow of Martí d'Argent, left her daughter at En Clapers in Valencia; another widow, from the town of Cardona, abandoned her two-year-old daughter named Joneta.

As today, women who had lost their husbands were particularly vulnerable to poverty and so were put into the position of being forced to give up one or more of their children. This problem was exacerbated by a change in Catalan law at the Corts of Perpignan in 1351 that penalized women who remarried. In that eventuality, a widow would lose the lifetime usufruct of the first husband's property and retain only the initial sum of her dowry. Consequently, in Catalan towns like Girona, few widowed women, even those with children, felt able to remarry. With diminished resources, further eroded by inflation, such women might easily fall into poverty, and if she had a child, be forced by desperation to abandon it. Added misery was induced by the periodic famines that struck Catalonia in the years after 1333.[36]

Society seems to have accepted the legitimacy of abandonment, at least to some degree. Instances of legal prohibition are rare, and hospitals even encouraged the practice by affording those who left children the protection of anonymity.[37] Still it is interesting that the care of foundlings, like that of other social outcasts such as lepers, prostitutes, and vagrants, was the responsibility of hospitals and not of the parish alms funds that assisted the honest poor. While, in the main, such children were regarded as innocents and thus not personally responsible for their situation, nonetheless they were also in some fashion tainted by their supposed illegitimacy.[38] The law, both canon and civil, which was influenced by the tradition of Roman law, confined itself to the legal consequences of abandonment. For the child, it meant the severing of any legal tie to the parent; parents were condemned and suffered the ecclesiastical penalty of excommunication.[39] In some instances, however, the law provided parents with a justification for abandoning children. For example, Alfonso X of Castile's *Las Siete Partidas* argues that, while fathers and mothers in general have the responsibility to rear their offspring, they may be excused from doing so for reasons of poverty; in addition, a man has no obligation to support children who are born of a woman who is not his wife or an openly acknowledged mistress.[40] In a similar vein, Frederick II's Constitutions of Melfi (1231) severely penalized any Sicilian mother who sold her daughter into prostitution, but made an exception for poor women; and Castile's *Fuero real* imposed the death penalty only on those parents whose children died as a result of their abandonment. Other law codes, such as those from France, seem to have no interest in deterring the practice, and thus ignore the entire question of abandonment.[41] Because the Roman and Germanic traditions of adoption, which made adoptees full heirs to property, became rare after the eighth century, not to be revived until the nineteenth, the typical response to the phenomenon of abandonment was some form of institutional effort to provide shelter and care for the child, usually in a foster home. A series of early church councils like Vaison (442) required that priests announce to the community the discovery of children abandoned at churches; and ninth-century French bishops prescribed that unmarried women should bring their children to church for adoption by the faithful. When Gratian compiled his *Decretum* in the twelfth century, he merely reiterated this early legislation that suggested churches as appropriate points of abandonment. The earliest example of an asylum to house such children is said to have been founded by Bishop Dateo of Milan in 757.[42] It is difficult, however, to find further references to the care of exposed infants, either in law or practice, until the twelfth century, and concern does not appear to have become general until the thirteenth. Then, several thirteenth-century ecclesiastical councils in England, and also in France, began to address the issue, primarily out of a concern that such children be properly baptized. Indeed, Salimbene di Adam's *Cronica* consigns to hell hospital administrators in thirteenth-century Milan who permitted such orphans to die without baptism.[43]

Orphanages

The first solid evidence for the institutional care of abandoned children dates from the twelfth century. Among the religious orders, the statutes

promulgated by Roger Molins in 1181 for the Hospital of Saint John in
Jerusalem acknowledged as one of the order's responsibilities the reception
and care of orphans; and chapter 41 of its rule committed the Order of the
Holy Spirit to the care of both orphaned infants and pregnant women.[44]
The earliest civic facilities to care for orphans and foundlings appeared in
Italian towns. At Milan, for example, there was an eighth-century asylum,
which seems to have endured until the 1070s, the late-tenth-century orphanage at San Celso, and a foundling home established at Broglio in 1145.
During the next century, other shelters that accepted children were established in Florence, Siena, Pisa, and Mirandola. Information about these
becomes more abundant at the end of the thirteenth century. Florentine
records show Santa Maria de San Gallo functioning as a foundling home in
1294, and records from nearby Prato are extant from 1333. The port city of
Genoa had a hospital and a laic confraternity of free aliens and freed slaves
that took charge of abandoned children and orphans from their own community. In the fifteenth century, substantial foundations devoted entirely to
the care of abandoned children were established in Florence (1445) and
Bologna (1450).[45]

   In France, as in Italy, municipal shelters also seem to have taken in
orphans and abandoned children, but here there seems to have been less
willingness to do so. For example, some municipal shelters, such as those at
Troyes and Angers, refused to admit any children on the grounds that they
were too numerous for institutional resources and that orphans were a
parochial responsibility. In a similar vein, the Hôtel-Dieu of Saint-Pol, near
Châtillons, would support only children actually born within its precincts.
Paris, given its large size, accommodated parentless children in a number of
ways. The Hôpital du Saint-Esprit-en-Grève was founded in 1363 to house
orphans, but not abandoned or illegitimate children; in the next century,
however, its administrators came under royal and municipal pressure to
admit foundlings as well. Because Saint-Esprit had a capacity of only fifty
children, other abandoned children had to be taken to the municipal shelter,
the Hôtel-Dieu at Notre Dame, while others were assigned to the care of the
parish in whose territory the child was first discovered. Capitular records of
the fifteenth century show that some children were placed in foster homes
and their guardians paid some sort of subsidy. In northern France, bishops
and chapters also aided children, called here *bons-enfants,* through the distribution of alms in the form of coin, food, and clothing, presumably also to
foster parents; the clergy also reared some children as choirboys. Approximately twenty-four hospices for children, dating from the 1240s and patron-

ized both by prelates and laypeople, have been discovered in northern France and in the Low Countries. Outside of Paris, they seem to have served male children between the ages of nine and sixteen, who studied Latin and religious chant. In Paris, these shelters seem to have served an older clientele of young undergraduate students at the University of Paris, including those of foreign origin. In Montpellier, on the other hand, municipal authorities accepted responsibility for children, but otherwise adhered to the general pattern of seeking out paid foster parents from among the women of the town rather than institutionalizing the children.[46]

In Castile, shelters for abandoned children began to appear in the fourteenth and fifteenth centuries. Among the earliest known is the Hospital de Santo Tomé in Astorga, which was functioning in 1344 and which, according to later sources, took in children abandoned at the door of the cathedral. The Church of San Pedro and San Ildefonso in Zamora in the mid-fifteenth century maintained the *capellanía de los enechados* for abandoned children, and in the sixteenth century the cathedral canons assumed responsibility for their care. Palencia in the sixteenth century had the Hospital San Antolín, and in the towns of Salamanca and Valladolid caring for abandoned children was the work of various confraternities.[47]

The pattern of care in the Aragonese Crown followed the Italian and French models. At first, abandoned children were the responsibilities of the community shelters that housed the broad spectrum of the needy. At Barcelona, these children, *infants de comú* as they were called, were parceled out in the fourteenth centuries among the hospitals of En Marcús, Sant Macià, Santa Eulàlia, and En Colom; and in Vic they were housed in the hospitals of Sant Bartolomeu and Ramon de Terrades. At Valencia, the hospitals of La Reyna, En Clapers, and Sant Vicent counted children among their inmates; in Lleida, abandoned children were housed alongside the insane and penitent women in the hospital of the Order of the Holy Spirit. Another hospital of the Holy Spirit, one operated by the Trinitarians, was established at Palma, in Majorca, circa 1270, and this served abandoned children. After the foundation of Barcelona's general hospital of Santa Creu in 1401, children became one of its responsibilities. Shelters specifically for children came late — in Valencia not until the establishment of the Hospital de Ignoscents in 1409, and in Barcelona with the hospital established circa 1370 by a resident named Guillem de Pou. It is doubtful, however, that these new foundling homes were ever adequate to the need. In Valencia, for example, between a third and a half of all children under care continued to be housed in the hospitals of En Clapers and La Reyna throughout the fifteenth century.[48]

Public Wardship

In addition to hospitals and shelters, municipal governments and the king, through the establishment of an official entitled the *pare dels òrfens*, acknowledged a responsibility toward needy children. The earliest example of this is the directive addressed by King Pere III on March 6, 1338, to the magistrates of Valencia. In this, the king accepted an obligation to protect the children of poor beggars and to ensure that they be reared in such a fashion that they become useful citizens. To this end, he ordered the council to name suitable *curadores* to ensure that minors, with or without parents, be profitably employed according to their wish and aptitude. Clearly the king's intent was to reduce begging, since the penalty demanded for those who refused work was expulsion from the city. In May of 1338, the council, which had requested Pere's intervention, appointed two citizens and charged them to deter youths from becoming thieves, drunkards, and gamblers; in 1351, or just after the plague, these officers were empowered to compel parentless children to take a master. By the end of the century, the official charged with the oversight of children was called the *pare dels òrfens*; virtually all of its incumbents were merchants of the city. The idea, based on an Italian model, spread to other towns in the Crown of Aragon, such as Castelló de la Plana (1376), Saragossa (1475), and Lleida, as well as to various Navarrese towns.[49]

Foundlings and Orphans

Recent studies have given us some idea of the social origins, and even identities, of the children who were abandoned. Gavitt's study of Florence's Hospital of the Innocenti, for example, reveals that 90 percent of the children admitted were received between a few hours and three weeks old, 56 percent were female and 44 percent male, and 60 percent born of a mother who was a domestic servant or slave. Because most of these seem to have been connected to some prominent family, the possibility existed that the birth father would eventually acknowledge his offspring and reclaim the child from the orphanage. This happened to 10 percent of the boys, but only 3 percent of the girls. The children of nonresidents also seem to have been born to those of high rank, so despite a rough correlation between grain prices and admissions, poverty here does not seem to have been the principal reason for abandonment at Florence.[50]

The records of Santa Creu in Barcelona, which are roughly contemporaneous to those of the Innocenti, indicate a somewhat more diverse population. Indeed, Santa Creu did not discriminate on the basis of residence,
condition, race, health, or social status, although the vast majority of admissions were the children of Barcelonans.[51] As at Florence, most children
were no more than a few days old, and some were still covered in blood and
attached to the umbilical cord. Only 23 percent of the children were older
than a month; 18 percent were between one and twelve months; and only 4
percent were older than a year. For the most part, abandonments were
spaced fairly evenly throughout the year, indicating that cyclic factors like
the weather and the availability of food were not prime factors in the decision to give up a child. At Valencia, a study of children assisted at the
Hospital of En Clapers shows little difference of gender: 52 percent girls
and 48 percent boys.[52]

Among the approximately forty children received by Santa Creu each
year, there were seven categories of children, according to the study of
Teresa-María Vinyoles and Margarida González. As at both Florence and
Valencia, the largest group was composed of illegitimate children. Rubio
Vela notes, for example, that *bort* or bastard is the usual synonym in Valencian records for parentless children; typically, medieval and premodern society throughout Europe assumed that foundlings were illegitimate. These
infants for the most part were poorly dressed and abandoned at a very young
age, often hours after birth. Their birth mothers favored names like Bona-
ventura or Ventura; a few were the offspring of clergy. Among legitimate
children, there were genuine orphans, the sick and retarded, children of the
desperately poor, those with mothers who for various reasons could not care
for them, and those with honest fathers (*pobres vergonyants*) who temporarily left their children until economic conditions improved. Records at
Valencia in 1396–97, for example, speak of the children of poor women who
were physically unable to breast-feed. There were also children such as
Catalina who became En Claper's responsibility when her mother, a patient
at the hospital, died without known family, or those temporarily entrusted
to the hospital for nursing by widowed fathers. Barcelona also accepted the
offsprings of slaves, who were sent to the hospital to spare the birth father
embarrassment and responsibility, or on the initiative of the slave mother to
save her offspring from servitude. Among a group of fifteen for whom the
reason for abandonment is known, five had foreign fathers, two were children of women recently widowed, another was the son of a female slave, two
were children of battered wives (one of whom was beheaded by her spouse),

two more were orphans, and another was an illegitimate child brought to the hospital by friends of the birth father. This small sample suggests a multiplicity of motives, but there is a sense that at Barcelona economic deprivation was a more significant factor than at Florence. Poverty, whether that of the beggar or widow, is a stated issue in several cases. There is also the sense that many abandonments were the result of some temporary emergency because the rate of reclamation at Barcelona is also higher, 10 percent as opposed to 6.3 percent in Florence, or even more impressively 30 percent of all children who survived the hazards on infancy.[53]

Despite the fact that municipal hospitals did not appear to discriminate against the children of noncitizens, foreign communities, especially those of a servile character, organized protective benevolent associations that collected, fed, and attempted to find foster homes for children within their group. At Valencia and Barcelona, for example, there were confraternities of freed black slaves called respectively the Cofradia de San Jaime Apostol de Negros Libertos and the Confratia Nigrorum Libertate Datorum Civitatis Barchinione.[54] At Barcelona, it is impossible to estimate the number of orphans who were the offspring of slaves or of ex-slaves because the municipal orphanage kept no record of the mother's social status, out of a concern that any servile condition would pass onto the child. Nevertheless, the proliferation of female slaves in Barcelona after 1270 and their utilization as domestic laborers in the city's wealthiest households certainly created an environment conducive to the production of unwanted and socially embarrassing offspring.[55]

While in most instances, it was the decision of parents whether to rear or to abandon their children, in the case of slaves the authority resided in the hands of the master. The child could remain within the household, be abandoned at the gate of the municipal hospital, or be placed somewhere else. In some instances, a master might apprentice the offspring of a servant to someone else, as Elisenda, widow of the Barcelonan merchant Jaume Texander, did in 1412. She handed over the young infant daughter of her slave Magdalena to one Francesca, on the understanding that the young girl serve until the age of twenty when she was to be freed, married, and given a dowry. In another instance, also at Barcelona in 1401, the widow Juana sold the two young daughters of her slave Caterina to the butcher Francesch Ferrari, who had fathered them.[56]

Whenever possible hospitals sought to avoid undertaking full responsibility for the care and rearing of a child. In order to empower parents who might otherwise be unable to raise their own children, hospitals such as En

Clapers in Valencia and Sant Macià in Barcelona were willing to pay a small subsidy in money directly to the parents. Thus, evidently when some parents were discovered leaving their children at the hospital's gate, hospitaller officials attempted to persuade them to keep the child and return home with the promise of a certain amount of ongoing assistance. While such care was certainly less expensive for the hospital, it could only be applied to children within functional families. In the case of children abandoned anonymously, the hospital at times attempted to discover the mother's identity, or that of a parent's family. But evidently, fewer than 16 percent of those assisted had relations willing to rear their kin. Nonetheless, hospital administrators would go to some lengths to avoid taking on a child by attempting to convince others to undertake its care. For example, a newborn son of a Majorcan woman, who was on the verge of death, was brought in 1374 to En Clapers by her neighbors. But the administrator refused to take the child and instead suggested that the neighbors, in return for a small subsidy, rear the child themselves.[57]

In the majority of instances, however, hospitals could not turn away the children, who then had to be given into a type of formal care. In doing this, hospitals pursued three principal objectives: the salvation of their souls through the sacrament of baptism,[58] their survival through the provision of care and nourishment, and, if they lived through the perils of infancy, enough training to transform them into productive members of the community. The Hospital of Santa Creu at Barcelona was typical in its procedures for receiving abandoned children. The prior, the principal religious official, maintained *llibres d'infants*, in which registrars recorded all the information that could be discerned about the foundling: a name if any, age, date and time of discovery, clothing, the presence of any other objects or food, a verbatim copy of any accompanying note, and signs of whether the child was baptized. At Valencia's En Clapers, scribbled notes accompanying the child could reveal not only the baby's name but the fact of baptism; in one instance in which the child was not baptized, the note requested that the child be given the name of Tristan. The purpose of this examination was twofold. If there was no evidence of baptism, the infant was immediately given the sacrament conditionally and named frequently after the staff person who stood as godparent or else for the saint of the day. Subsequently the record of admission could be used as a means of identification should a birth parent or relative seek to claim the child, and as a justification for the hospital to charge a child's family for expenses should it ever be identified.[59]

Wet-Nursing

In most instances, the hospital's first priority, after baptism, was to see that the infant was fed. Because the use of animal milk was rare, this meant that a woman would have to be employed to nurse the child. Although a majority of women who belonged to the rural and urban laboring classes nursed their own child, wet-nursing in the Middle Ages was common at both ends of the social scale.[60] Alfonso X of Castile, in his *Siete Partidas*, troubled himself to describe at length the qualities of the nurses who would tend the male and female offspring of the royal family.[61] The well-to-do in Italy, Germany, and Catalonia would purchase slaves or employ live-in women recruited from town or the countryside.[62] Montpellier, which in the fifteenth century had no orphanage, regularly employed local women to nurse orphans and abandoned children for a year or so.[63] In Florence, children were retained at the orphanage and nursed by rented slaves or by country women for six to twelve days, and then sent out to rural villages until they had attained the age of eighteen to twenty-four months.[64] In Iberia, the principal restriction imposed on wet nurses was a religious one. Castilian law, for example, forbade Muslim and Jewish women from nurturing Christian children, and Christians from suckling the children of non-Christians.[65]

For urban hospitals that took in children, wet-nursing was obviously a major preoccupation. At Florence, the Hospital of the Innocenti had a few resident wet nurses (some were slaves and others local women under contract), who fed the children temporarily until they could be placed in foster care with a wet nurse; in large measure, this seems to have been the practice in Catalonia as well. Mortality rates for these children were extraordinarily high. At Florence's Innocenti, between 27 and 55 percent of infants died within their first year; and at Santa Creu in Barcelona, between 52.2 percent and 67 percent had perished before the age of two. Valencia's En Clapers had a mortality rate of 42 percent. Gavitt contrasts these elevated mortality rates with an average of 20 percent for Florentine children sent out to wet nurse by their own parents. Compared with an overall estimate of 50 percent mortality for all children in preindustrial Europe up to the age of five, and specific sixteenth-century estimates of 20 to 30 percent for England and 57 percent for France, however, these medieval institutional statistics seem slightly less horrific. Nonetheless, the discrepancy between institutional and general rates of medieval child mortality has led scholars to pay particular attention to the institution of the wet nurse.[66]

At Barcelona, the Hospital of Santa Creu always maintained at least one wet nurse on hand to feed children until they could be placed with someone else, usually a farm woman. The picture that emerges here is one of great instability. While some children stayed with their nurse for as long thirty or forty months, many stayed less than a month; consequently, many who survived infancy must have been passed from woman to woman. The *llibres d'infants*, in fact, record an average of three or four wet nurses per child. In 1426, for example, a farmer's wife named Francesca nursed an infant named Antoni for eight days, then Lancelot for four days, Eulàlia for a day and a night, and then Joan Robí for six months. The death of the child was most often the cause of this turnover, but lack of milk, illness, and pregnancy on the part of the wet nurses also contributed to the instability.[67]

In Valencia, the hospital of Sant Vicent itself housed nursing children; En Clapers, with the help of a broker, farmed them out to wet nurses in the community, but continued to provide clothing, medicine, and even medical care to the child. The women employed as wet nurses were a mixture of rural and urban; some were slaves rented out by their masters. Some seem to have been full-time wet nurses; Na Salvadora, the daughter of a manuscript illuminator, for example, received a new child on May 15, 1375, the day after the one previously in her care had died. As at Barcelona, babies were often shunted back and forth due to the condition of either the nurse or the child. In one instance, for racial reasons, Benenguda, a black child abandoned in June 1396, had ten nurses over the next ten months. The administrator noted that "the child was as black as a cooking pot and no wet nurse wanted to have her." After the children had been weaned, at around the age of three, and introduced to solid food, they were returned to the hospital.[68]

There is no way to know why so many children died, but contemporaries were ready to suspect negligence on the part of the nursing women. Castilian town law, for instance, imposed fines and banishment on nurses who fed contaminated milk to infants.[69] By all accounts, most nurses undertook their work for pay, but the amount was low and the supervision of their care minimal. In Florence, for example, these women earned only between two-thirds and three-quarters of what the lowest paid hospital worker was given and would be visited by the hospital's chaplain at most once or twice a year. Barcelona women seem to have fared somewhat better. Town nurses were paid one and a half sous per day for short-term care; resident nurses as well as rural women received about twenty sous per month for full-time care. Here there was no system of on-site inspection, but children were supposed to be returned to the hospital for this purpose annually on All Saints' Day (November 1). Thus, there was a fear that a nurse, unsupervised, underpaid, and poor, would accept more children than she could feed or else give priority to her own children over those receiving foster care. Consequently, the commune of Florence in 1415 forbade wet nurses to stop breast-feeding a child before the age of thirty months, subject to a fine or public whipping. In fact, because the principal documented fraud seems to have been the nurse's failure to report the death of a child in order to keep collecting the monthly stipend, neglect alone is not an adequate explanation for the high rates of mortality.[70]

Another aspect of this issue that has received considerable attention is the higher mortality of female, over male, infants. At Florence's Innocenti, for example, between 1445 and 1466, girls represented 60.4 percent of the recorded deaths, somewhat in excess of the 56.4 percent that was the female proportion of admissions for the same period. Richard Trexler has argued that the differential might be explained in two ways: infanticide through the suffocation of girls, and better care for boys. He believes that a higher percentage of girls were sent out into the countryside to be nursed, where presumably they might be neglected by unsupervised wet nurses. On the other hand, because there was a greater expectation that male infants might be reclaimed by a parent and the hospital thus reimbursed for their upkeep, boys were more likely to receive residential care at the hospital itself. Gavitt dismisses both arguments but does see a difference in the quality of care that resulted from the larger number of female infants entrusted to the hospital. At Barcelona, however, the situation may well have been different. Because the Hospital of Santa Creu did not attempt to collect accrued expenses from parents who reclaimed their children, there was not only a higher rate of reunion but less incentive to discriminate by gender.[71]

Disease, particularly the plague, was an important cause of childhood death in the Middle Ages. Some studies in Italy, for example, have shown that half to two-thirds of the victims of the plague were children.[72] This situation is confirmed in the records of Barcelona. For example, in the first half of 1430, some twenty-three children died of a disease variously described as granuloma or the plague in and around Barcelona. Between April and September of the following year another eighteen children perished from the plague. The plague was an important factor in infant deaths in Valencia as well; here the records of the Hospital of En Clapers show elevated mortality rates during May and June 1383, a period of plague. Another recurrent malady, although less fatal, was ringworm, a fungal inflection of the skin or hair, but the most serious of all childhood diseases were dysentery and diarrhea. Such illnesses, however, were difficult to diagnose, and most children were not treated at all because they were in foster care. Most often the only concrete evidence that we have of a child's fate is the certificate of burial wet nurses were required to produce for charges who had perished.[73]

On average, wet nurses cared for children during the first two years of life. Social status does not seem to have been a factor in setting this term, since it appears to have been the same for the *infants* of the Catalan royal court and the charges of Barcelona's municipal hospitals.[74] Once weaned, children might remain in foster care, in which instances the subsidy paid for their care was reduced by half or more. Records at Barcelona, and also at Montpellier, indicate that this stage of care might last until the age of eight; French and English hospitals acknowledged a responsibility for children up to the age of seven, at which time they were sent out into homes. At Florence all the children were returned to the hospital after weaning to await adoption. Thus, the Hospital of the Innocenti had a large resident population of 20 nursing children, and some 150 older boys and girls, as contrasted to Barcelona's resident population of some 25 children between the ages of two and six. These institutionalized children would be clothed and fed under the supervision of female attendants (Barcelona) or married couples (Florence).[75] At Valencia, however, children rarely stayed for more than a few days at hospitals like En Clapers. Immediately after nursing, the hospitaller sought out a family to take the child on, and only the sick and handicapped would actually be housed at the hospital for any length of time.[76]

Apprenticeship and Child Labor

Guillem de Pou, the founder of an orphanage at Barcelona in 1370, expressed what must have been an important sentiment that explains why his society provided continuing care for orphaned and abandoned children: "Many children and other adults, who might die of hunger and become wicked and men of a depraved life, are with time honorable men, choice and good workers."[77] Thus, once a child had been baptized and supported through the vulnerable years of infancy, steps had to be taken to make sure that the individual would become a useful member of society. For boys, this usually meant an apprenticeship of some sort; girls, on the other hand, were pressed into domestic service, often with the promise of marriage and a dowry at the end of its term.

The age at which children entered service varied according to opportunity and circumstances. In Florence, the "adoption" of boys typically occurred between the ages of five and ten, but in Barcelona (perhaps because Santa Creu was less equipped for a resident population of children) and Valencia the age could be considerably younger. Fifteenth-century examples show Catalan children as young as six months being contracted as apprentices, with 31.5 percent of all children apprenticed being under the age of five. At one extreme are Mateu Esteve, a poor orphan of six months who was admitted on April 29, 1427, and apprenticed to an apothecary on July 29, and Caterina Llorença who was apprenticed to a seamstress at the age of six months. At Valencia's En Clapers, all children who survived nursing and attained the age of three were returned either to their families or to other members of the community. At Barcelona, the oldest children awaiting families were ten and eleven, but these might well be juveniles whose initial contracts had not worked out well. In theory, at least, the boys would enter an apprenticeship that would last between nine and sixteen years, during which they were to learn a trade, receive food, clothing, and shelter at the master's home, and earn a modest stipend that would be paid at the termination of the apprenticeship. Boys, at times, were also taught to read, but girls never were. Unlike Florence, where many girls wound up in the cloth industry, Barcelonan girls rarely learned a trade; most became domestic servants. At the age of eighteen, young men and women would be given their freedom, the former with enough money to buy a suit of clothing and perhaps some tools, and the latter with a sufficient dowry.[78]

In general, foundlings and orphans appear to have been apprenticed or contracted at a younger age than the children of artisans, who normally seem to have started nearer the ages of eleven or twelve. The term of an apprenticeship itself was the product of a number of variables. It would vary, for example, by craft, by locale, and by social status. The *Livre des métiers* of thirteenth-century Paris established a term of only two years for cooks, but ten years for silversmiths. Here and in England, crafts like glove making, butchering, and tanning required between seven and eight years. In Tuscan towns, however, terms were nearer three or four years, and in fourteenth-century Girona they varied by craft — only one year for leather workers, but three for a glove maker, six for those who fabricated bags or parchment, and as many as twelve for shoemakers. Because apprentices were a source of cheap labor, the length of the contract, furthermore, could be shortened if the parent was willing to make a cash payment to the master. Because foundling homes were eager to reduce their own expense and certainly were unwilling to make extra payments, the terms for these children, as with the offspring of laborers, tended to begin earlier and last longer. Similarly, the terms of domestic service for girls seem to have extended to the age of eighteen, a year or two beyond the usual age of marriage.[79]

Apprenticeships, whether arranged by a family or a caritative institution, were the subject of detailed contracts that outlined the mutual responsibilities of the master and the child.[80] For Valencia, Rubio Vela has studied a series of 161 charters of apprenticeship that were negotiated by the municipal *pare dels òrfens* between 1379 and 1389 on behalf of orphans and abandoned children. Most of these (72.7 percent) dealt with boys because, Rubio Vela speculates, they were harder to place than girls and so were more likely to need the intervention and assistance of the municipality. Almost 86 percent of the children are identified by family, which suggests that in Valencia orphaned children outnumbered abandoned ones. Furthermore, in many cases the mother or some relative is alive; it was the death of the father that led families to seek assistance. While most children were not abandoned, many, in this city of immigrants, were the children of outsiders. Of those who can be identified, only 29 percent were offspring of natives. Thirty percent had parents from Castile, 20 percent from elsewhere within the Kingdom of Valencia, 8 percent each from Catalonia and Aragon, and others from France, Portugal, and Andalusia. Those who were not identified by family (14 percent) were abandoned children, the children of slaves, and the children of Muslims and Jews who, once abandoned, had been baptized.

Only five of the contracts speak of the children's age, and most of these were very young, between one and three years. Undoubtedly most children were far older, to judge by the terms of service that were specified. Over three-quarters of the boys were obligated for between one and six years, and of all contracts only 9 percent were for terms longer than ten years. Thus, boys in the main do not seem to have served apprenticeships appreciably longer than the offspring of artisans. Girls, on the other hand, tended to be apprenticed earlier and to serve for longer periods as domestics. Francesca, for example, who was of Jewish background, was sent to the household of the notary Berenguer de Peramola for a full ten years.

Of those individuals who took in these children, 85.6 percent were Valencian males of diverse professions, with textiles (cloth-cutters and weavers) being the most prevalent. Another 6.8 percent of the contracts were negotiated with widows, who usually requested orphaned girls. In two instances, wet nurses gained custody of children that they had nursed for the Hospital of En Clapers. While there was no formal adoption in the legal sense, a girl Alienor was taken as if she had become a daughter. Most girls, however, became mere domestic servants; boys were taught a trade. Only three contracts required instruction in reading and writing. Children were obligated by the city to complete their terms of service and would be apprehended if they ran away. Some children were evidently mistreated, but, despite legislation in 1350 that permitted the *curadores* to remove abused children from the custody of their masters, Ramon de Palou, the *pare dels òrfens* in 1374, claimed that he lacked the economic resources to care for boys and girls who had suffered from harsh treatment. Apart from the obligation that the child be supported, there are few details concerning the period of service itself; presumably this passed much as would any apprenticeship. But, at the end of the contract, the master had certain obligations toward the youths. Girls received dowries, a substantial sum that averaged about fifteen pounds. Boys were rarely promised much, if any, money but were to be provided with a complete wardrobe (tunic, long gown, hat, and shoes) and in a few instances the tools of a trade.[81]

*   *   *

In terms of modern values, the character of medieval social policy toward women and children was very conservative and traditional. At its heart was the promotion of marriage and the family, the ideal state for Christians who had not entered some form of the religious life and for the citizen who would thereby be a productive and contributing member of the community. Just as disease, physical handicaps, or indolence might prevent a man from assuming his proper role as a husband, an inability to offer the expected dowry kept some women from becoming wives. Without marriage, the individual would lose status, become a burden on society, and be marginalized as an outcast or criminal. While various punishments — whipping, banishment, and so on — were devised to keep men from crime, women were assisted in a more positive fashion. Young girls, particularly those from established families, could receive assistance toward a dowry; orphans and foundlings could earn the same reward, but at the price of long years of domestic service. Women who were forced or fell into prostitution as an alternative to marriage had at least some prospect for rehabilitation, if it was desired. Those who continued as prostitutes certainly did not have a pleasant life in brothels, where they were often financially exploited by their housemasters, but legally they were tolerated, if segregated and regulated. Little of this, however, was for the benefit of women, who by accepting this status had lost their honor. Like Hawthorne's Hester, their shame was marked on their clothing. For men, however, many of whom were presumably married and honorable members of the community, legalized prostitution offered an opportunity to enjoy sex without obligation.[82]

The attitude toward children is ambivalent, although it does not seem to have been one of "indifference and neglect." On the one hand, children had an unconditional right to life and survival. Infanticide was condemned, and there is little indication that Catalan society absolutely refused help to any orphans or foundlings, whatever their origins or circumstances. This assistance, furthermore, was owed to the child until he or she reached the age of marriage and entry into the world of work. On the other hand, however, this obligation had limitations. There was the prejudice, often true, that the child under care was illegitimate; the term *bastard*, in the Middle Ages or in our society, is not one of endearment. Then there was the question of finance. Hospitals, even those with municipal affiliation, were supported in the main by private alms and could not afford full-time institutional care for their charges. Consequently, a makeshift system of wet nurses, foster parents, apprenticeships, and contract labor had to be stitched together. It is difficult to gauge exactly how children fared under this system. There is little doubt that their prospects for survival were somewhat worse, particularly in the early years, than for children from the general population. It would be interesting, but undoubtedly impossible, to know how well foster care prepared them for entry as adults into the world.

Late Medieval Assistance

A Religious or Secular Model?

MEDIEVAL CATALAN INSTITUTIONS OF CHARITY underwent a significant evolution between the emergence of small cathedral shelters and *almoinas* in the eleventh century and the establishment of general hospitals in the fifteenth century. Foundations grew in number, size, and complexity. They became more specialized in function, broader in purpose, and more discriminating in terms of the clientele they intended to serve. A desire to serve "Christ's poor," or to gain pardon for sin, did not disappear after 1300, but religious motivation became bound up with a myriad of other intentions that sprang from more temporal concerns. Loosely organized structures that grew out of the often pious intentions of twelfth-century founders gradually coalesced into institutions that had defined hierarchies and were governed by written ordinances and statutes, subject to the scrutiny of episcopal visitation and municipal auditors. In short, what began as an effort to provide the needy with the barest of essentials had evolved into something with the semblance of a welfare policy.

Historians who have surveyed this development in Iberia, as well as elsewhere in Europe, agree on the broad outlines of the evolution of medieval charity. Michel Mollat, in his influential study of medieval poverty, established the basic model wherein there were, he argued, four ages. The first, from the fifth to the eleventh century, was characterized by monastic hospitality; a second, extending to the early thirteenth century, brought the involvement of bishops, canons, religious orders, and confraternities, who attended to the poor as a spiritual and ritualistic obligation; the third, stretching to the onset of the great plague, saw a profusion of new institutions, attempts at their reform, and a growth in the numbers of the poor and of efforts to understand them as individuals; and a fourth period that ends circa 1500 develops a more cynical and discriminatory attitude toward

the poor, as the institutions of charity become overwhelmed by the needy.[1]
For Iberia, Carmen López Alonso argues that these four periods can be
conflated into only two, with the year 1200 being the general divide. Prior
to the thirteenth century, the works of charity were organized by bishops,
secular lords, and, in the twelfth century, by Cluniac and Cistercian monasteries. Afterward, there is a proliferation of urban hospitals, supported
however inadequately by the bourgeoisie, which practiced increasing discrimination in the character and type of assistance rendered to the poor.[2]

This latter model, however, is more appropriate to Castile than to
Catalonia, a region whose urban character places it closer to developments
in France and Italy than to the interior of Iberia. In Catalonia, the first
stirring of organized charity dates from the eleventh century, with the establishment of cathedral shelters in Barcelona and Urgell, and probably also in
Girona and Vic. The movement accelerates in the twelfth century, but principally in towns such as Lleida, Tarragona, and Tortosa, which were newly
conquered and occupied by the count of Barcelona. Of the principal urban
centers, only Barcelona sees additional foundations in the twelfth century.
The largest number of new hospitals date from the mid-twelfth to the mid-
thirteenth century. A portion of these reflects Catalan territorial expansion
into Majorca and Valencia, where royal and lay largesse and the advent of
several religious orders played the crucial role in the establishment of a
caritative infrastructure. But there was also significant development within
Catalonia itself, which was experiencing a rapid increase in its population
and fundamental changes in the structure of its rural society.[3] Lleida's
capitular-controlled hospitals, for example, were joined by several under
the aegis of various religious orders. The mendicant orders, whose growth
in Catalonia was explosive, however, held few hospitals, and then only in
smaller towns such as Olesa de Bonesvalls and Montblanc. Elsewhere, cathedral chapters continued to occupy a prominent position, with their
establishment of *almoinas* in Barcelona and Girona and their assumption of
control over each of the three new hospitals established in Barcelona. Gradually, municipal councils, still in their infancy, began to assume some responsibility as well, as seen by the establishment of new hospitals under
their direction in Urgell, Girona, Reus, Cervera, and Tortosa. During the
fourteenth century, the majority of new foundations was established after
the onset of hard times in the mid-1330s and these were undoubtedly a
response to wars, famine, and disease characteristic of this era. Most of
these new hospitals operated under some sort of municipal governance.
Conciliar control, furthermore, was extended over *almoinas* on Majorca

and in Vic, and over hospitals in Barcelona, Manresa, Cervera, Tarragona, and Valencia. Town councils also became involved in the regulation of prostitution and in the care of orphaned and abandoned children. After 1300, moreover, there were few new ecclesiastical initiatives in Catalonia and only a handful in Valencia. It is particularly significant that cathedral chapters, perhaps precisely because they already bore a heavy burden of administration, sought no new responsibilities and in fact began to shed them. One hospital, En Marcús in Barcelona, was surrendered to municipal control in 1339, and in 1401 the diocese agreed to merge several capitular and municipal hospitals into the new general hospital of Santa Creu. During the decades that followed, similar consolidations occurred in Lleida, Urgell, Tarragona, Montblanc, Majorca, and Valencia.

While the physical and institutional dimensions of the medieval hospital movement have gradually come into focus, the human and moral aspects are still subject to debate. The fundamental questions are these. To what degree did medieval assistance to the poor, as it evolved, remain religious in motivation, and to what degree was it a response to social conditions? Or, in slightly different terms, is there a major paradigmatic shift from religious to secular relief, or from charity to welfare? Ultimately, we must ask ourselves whether there is a fundamental difference between medieval and modern notions of charity and public assistance, whether a decisive change of direction occurred at some point during the fifteenth and sixteenth centuries, or whether there is a remarkable continuity in Western society's attitude toward the poor.

These are difficult questions because the forces that originated, sustained, and changed the institutions of charity are themselves so multifaceted. At issue are factors of population, urbanization, legal and institutional structures, the economic cycle, spiritual values, and *mentalité* that affected and influenced each other in ways perhaps too subtle and complex for us to understand fully. Attempts to verbalize change, and to see therein consistent patterns of development, are hampered by ambiguities of language. Just as medieval definitions of poverty and the poor differ from the income-based standards of contemporary statistics, thirteenth or fourteenth-century understandings of *religious* and *secular* differ in important ways from late-twentieth-century usage. With all of these complications in mind, we can now apply the experience of the medieval Crown of Aragon, and in particular of Catalonia, to the discussion concerning the motivation and purposes of medieval poor relief.

In Catalonia, as elsewhere, most initiatives of an eleemosynary nature had an ecclesiastical character, and even those that were laic in their origin were soon placed under some sort of ecclesiastical tutelage. Why was this so? For the most part, in the twelfth century the new institutions of charity were urban, and they were frequently founded by the bishop, the chapter, or individual canons. Catalonia was undergoing an economic and social transformation that laid the foundations for the principality's future success as a commerical power in the western Mediterranean, and that awakened older urban centers such as Barcelona and Girona. In addition, as a consequence of the wars against the Muslim south, new urban centers were added: Balaguer (1105), Tarragona (1118–30), Tortosa (1148), and Lleida (1149).[4] The expansion of old towns and the creation of new ones reflected a demographic upsurge, one of whose consequences was the emergence of a class of urban poor. Why were these taken as the particular responsibility of the cathedral chapter? While the antecedents of such episcopal and capitular alms can be traced to the earliest beginnings of Christianity, in the twelfth century this obligation to help the poor was given special urgency by the reforming ideas unleashed by the Gregorian reform movement.

The new spirituality of the late eleventh century resonated throughout the Church and produced a torrent of new religious movements. While they all partook to some degree of the model of the *vita apostolica*, there was a fundamental difference in the response of monks and secular clerics, or canons. The latter became more conscious of their responsibility toward others, and exhibited a concern for neighbors.[5] Efforts to reform the secular, or diocesan, clergy date from the pontificate of Innocent II (1030–43) and the Lateran synod of 1059, and they gained momentum during the pontificate of Urban II (1088–99), who encouraged clergy to adopt a common life under the Rule of Saint Augustine. While the attempt met with only indifferent success, apart from the establishment of independent communities of canons (e.g., the Premonstratensians, Saint Victor of Paris), the effort had a lasting impact on how members of the clergy viewed themselves and their role in society. Increasingly important to them were preaching, teaching, and service.[6]

The attempt in Spain to impose a common life on cathedral chapters, likewise, was generally short-lived; the Catalan church particularly showed itself hostile to the Gregorian reforms.[7] Nonetheless, as we have seen in Chapters 2 and 3, both cathedral chapters and individual canons were especially active in establishing and maintaining houses of charity. In Urgell, Girona, and Barcelona, during the twelfth and most of the thirteenth centuries, the cathedral bore the principal responsibility for poor relief, in terms of providing both food and shelter. Only in towns of recent conquest, like Lleida in the twelfth century and Valencia in the thirteenth, was the obligation more diffuse. On the frontier, the absence of a preexisting diocesan structure meant that more hospitals were operated by religious orders or else remained in the hands of their founding families. But even in the older centers the weak, corporate nature of the chapter meant that often the actual initiative for endowing hospitals and meals came from individual canons, such as Joan Colom in Barcelona or Gerald Zacosola in Lleida. In the dioceses of Urgell and Barcelona, the capitular obligation toward the poor assumed a ritualistic form, as seen in the custom of donating the bedding of deceased clergy to shelters for the poor.

While chapters did not begin to relinquish control over hospitals for which they were responsible until the early fifteenth century, a different dynamic is discernible by the middle of the thirteenth century, after which no new hospitaller foundation can be traced to a bishop or his chapter. One suspects that chapters, now immersed in their own institutional development and less influenced by reform impulses, were content to leave new foundations to others. While some of this would continue to have a private character, for example, the hospital established in 1338 at Vic by Ramon de Terrades or that of 1311 at Valencia by Bernat dez Clapers, much of the initiative now passed to corporate bodies of laypeople — confraternities and municipal councils.

In Catalonia, municipal institutions predominated over confraternities, or craft associations, because of the power and attitude of the count-kings, who were suspicious of all unauthorized lay associations and formally prohibited the formation of confraternities. The thirteenth century, on the other hand, was the era during which municipal institutions began to emerge in Catalonia.[8] At the beginning of the century, towns were still under the authority of a royal magistrate, the *veguer,* but during the latter half of Jaume I's reign more complex municipal institutions were developed. Valencia (1245), Tarragona (1255), Tàrrega (1242), Montpellier (1246), Palma de Mallorca (1249), Barcelona (1249), Lleida (1264), Cervera (1267), Perpignan (1273), and Girona (1284) acquired the right to elect *jurats* who came to share authority within their towns with royal officials. In a series of privileges, for example, the wealthy burghers of Barcelona were permitted to select a council, first of two hundred, but fixed in 1274 at one hundred, and to place executive power in the hands of five councilors. King Pere II at a meeting of the Corts in 1283 extended similar privileges to all municipalities and accepted new limits upon the powers of royal *veguers* and *batlles*. What followed upon these privileges was the development of municipal governments and bureaucracies that began to take responsibility for several aspects of municipal life, among which was the care of the poor.[9]

Beginning in the thirteenth century, Catalan municipalities began to establish town hospitals and assume responsibility for other caritative institutions that had been founded by individual citizens. But the pattern is inconsistent. For example, a few towns such as Urgell (1247), Reus (circa 1250), and Tarragona (1362) appear to have directly established municipal hospitals. Much more typical, however, was the assumption of control over a preexisting institution. In some cases, this was due to the decision of the founding family to relinquish its authority to a permanent institution. So, as we have seen, Pere Desvilar in 1308 conferred control of his foundation upon Barcelona's Consell de Cent, and in the nearby towns of Granollers and Manresa the council assumed responsibility for the hospitals of Bertran de Seva and Pere Salvatge. By 1300, Girona's *jurats* were also responsible for the New Hospital that had been initially founded by a local confraternity. Insolvency could be an issue, as it was in the transfer of the Hospital of En Marcús from the bishop to the city of Barcelona in 1339. In Valencia, where most thirteenth-century hospitals were operated by religious orders, the municipal *jurats* were given charge of the hospitals of En Clapers and the Beguins in the early fourteenth century, the Hospital de la Reyna in 1379, and in 1409 established an asylum for the mentally disturbed. Yet towns like Montblanc and Vic had no municipally governed hospitals, and the council of Lleida only began to assume responsibility after the general consolidation of 1453.

Municipal councils were not the only corporate bodies to become active dispensers of charity in the period after 1250. In addition, numerous laic groups organized into confraternities and parish relief agencies. Confraternities, while noticeably weaker in Catalonia than in Castile, nevertheless, established hospitals in Girona, Lleida, and Montblanc, and in Valencia provided dowries to the poor.[10] Like the confraternity of poor cripples and the blind in Barcelona, they provided a myriad of services to their members and families, which included burial and various forms of assistance.[11] Of a similar nature are the parochial *bacís* and *arcas de misericordia* that were established between the late thirteenth and fifteenth centuries to assist the poor of the neighborhood with food, clothing, subsidies, and loans, and which gradually supplanted the clergy as the chief providers of local relief. Unlike municipal councils, which were forced to deal with the problem of vagrants and immigrants, these agencies focused their efforts upon the *pauperes verecundi*, the deserving poor. Like municipal charity, however, this was conducted entirely by laypeople, by *baciners* who were selected by their fellow parishioners to collect and distribute communal alms.

The prevalence of these lay institutions — municipal, confraternal, and parochial — has led some to argue that an important shift of paradigm took place at the end of the thirteenth century. Before this, charity had been the responsibility of the Church; now it passed into the hands of merchants and tradesmen, and in the process had thereby become secular. For England, the studies of Patricia Cullum in York and Miri Rubin in Cambridge agree that after 1300 new foundations were the work of guilds, individual merchants or artisans, and municipalities; Rubin believes that all hospitals had now moved into the secular sphere.[12] Philip Gavitt cites the will of 1407 in which Francesco Datini, the benefactor of Florence's Hospital of the Innocenti, gives this description for the charitable trust from which this and other benefactions were to be paid:

The Casa del Ceppo [or trust] and its aforementioned goods [are] to be private and not sacred, and in no way said to be ecclesiastical, but thought of secularly, for the love of God, to the aforementioned perpetual use of the poor, and to be subject neither to the church nor to clerics in any way.[13]

Carmen López Alonso sees this trend toward secularization applying to Iberia as a whole, arguing that the urbanization of hospitals in the fourteenth century made them secular institutions. Consequently, for society as a whole, the poor were cast less as a means to salvation than as objects, and this in turn created new and negative images of hospitals as "dung heaps," uncaring in their attitudes toward the poor.[14] Agustín Rubio Vela, on the other hand, in his study of Valencian hospitals, sees this secularization in a more positive light. For him the bourgeoisie's assumption of responsibility for charity is a witness to its empowerment, to the dominant role that merchants and artisans had attained in commercial cities like Valencia. While he recognizes that hospitals continued to have the trappings of religion, for example, chapels, for him the essential element is that they had assumed a civil character in terms of their foundation and governance.[15]

Within Catalonia, late medieval authors such as Ramon Llull (d. 1315) and Francesc Eiximenis (d. 1409) depict charity as an enterprise of the urban wealthy. The former in his *Llibre d'Evast e Blanquerna* describes the couple Evast and Aloma as washing the hands and feet of thirty paupers, providing them with new clothing, operating a hospital to serve the sick, and conferring alms in secret to the deserving poor. Evast, a man of fortune, feels the obligation to share a portion of his wealth with the poor.[16] Carme Batlle, whose study of charity in Barcelona and Urgell began with an examination of wills, emphasizes the broad support for the works of charity among Catalan laypeople, which spanned divisions of gender, profession, wealth, and social class. She, however, does not argue in favor of the secularization thesis. Instead, Batlle holds that the works of charity throughout the entire era remained the primary responsibility of the bishop, although gradually the burden would be shared in a cooperative spirit with the municipality, as exemplified by their dual responsibility for the Hospital of Santa Creu. The lay population, she argues, saw no fundamental distinction between hospitals operated by the Church and those by municipal officials; both types of institutions benefited equally from bequests in the wills.[17]

Evidence from Urgell and Girona, however, contradicts Batlle's conclusions about charity at Barcelona. While Batlle's own study of Urgell provides no exact statistics, the suggestion is that townspeople there favored the New Hospital of the town over the Old Hospital of the cathedral. Guilleré, furthermore, offers precise data that show that in the decade of the 1330s Girona's town hospital was remembered in 40 percent of wills, while the cathedral institution was favored in only 10 percent.[18] At Urgell, this discrimination might well be explained by the fact that shortly after the establishment of the New Hospital, the older institution itself changed and became a shelter for needy clergy. This, however, was not the case in Girona, where the capitular hospital was an ample structure that contained among its eleven rooms a dormitory for poor women and so was not exclusively a clerical hospice.[19] Thus, Girona might provide some evidence of a preference for municipally sponsored charity, but this must be set aside data from the town's Almoina del Pa, which though governed by the chapter remained an exceedingly popular charity in the wills of fourteenth-century Gironans.[20]

The argument that has engaged historians about the relative religious or secular character of charity is very much one of definition and grows out of a confusion of the words *secular* and *laic*. The evidence from Catalonia and elsewhere clearly shows increased participation by laymen, both as individuals and as organized groups (confraternities, *consells*), in the works of charity, particularly after the mid-thirteenth century. Steven Epstein, in his study of medieval Genoa, finds nothing remarkable in this. He argues that the initiative for establishing a network of charity naturally belonged to the Church because, in the twelfth and thirteenth centuries when material conditions favored such a development, it had the personnel and ideology to accomplish the goal. Municipal institutions, on the other hand, were in their infancy, and town officials had other tasks to perform. The key question is whether the gradual shifting of responsibility from religious to laic leadership is merely a reflection of institutional developments and rivalries or a sign of a deeper shift away from a religious toward a social justification for poor relief. Views on the issue have been diverse. Miri Rubin, for example, while observing the same institutional shift in medieval Cambridge that Epstein has noted in Genoa, is skeptical that religion was ever the primary motive behind charity, even in the twelfth century. Bronislaw Geremek, on the other hand, in his study of the poor in late medieval Paris, believes that religion continued to justify charitable giving, although he allows that there was an evolution from the practice of an indiscriminate charity to one increasingly focused on the distinction between worthy and unworthy beggars.[21]

Various recent studies of Italian confraternities and their role as agents in the dispensing of charity agree that assistance to the poor retained a religious character well into the sixteenth century, even if individual authors disagree on the importance of the Church's participation. Brian Pullan's study of *Scuole Grandi* in Venice, for example, shows that laic confraternities assumed a principal responsibility for serving the deserving poor. Even when the task began to exceed their resources, the confraternities were not replaced by public agencies but instead were co-opted and subsidized by the Venetian state. James Banker studied the commune of San Sepolcro, and through the confraternity of San Bartolomeo demonstrates that charity was a cooperative effort between pious lay associations, the town, and the bishop, and that assistance for the poor was closely linked to ideas of merit, propitiation, and remembrance. While Italian confraternities in the fourteenth century established new hospitals and assumed responsibility for those once operated by the clergy, they did so within a religious context, as associations that were both laic and religious and that derived their institutional legitimacy not from episcopal approval but from their service to the poor of Christ. Likewise, Christopher Black in his analysis of sixteenth-century confraternities concludes that the alleviation of misery required the cooperative efforts of state officials, parish priests, monasteries, and confraternities. In reviewing the recent scholarship concerning Italian confraternities, Andrew Barnes argues that, if anything, these studies have undervalued the participation of the clergy, particularly as spiritual advisers, in these various laic associations, and he concludes with a warning about the dangers of excluding the clergy from any assessment of lay Catholic behavior.[22]

These examinations of confraternities are paralleled by other analyses of early modern Italian and French hospitals. They also stress the complexity of motivation that operated within late medieval society. In her discussion of the "language of relief," Miri Rubin, who tends to dismiss the importance of religious impulses, argues that charity was not so much a direct response to the needs of the poor but a reaction to an elite's perception of its social obligations. Katherine Park, however, in demonstrating the medieval origins of the medical hospital, believes that fourteenth-century Florentines were moved by multiple impulses: a genuine concern for the needy, a fear of God's retribution, and a desire to protect the supply of industrial workers. Sandra Cavallo, whose work centers on early modern Turin, argues that conflicts within the social and political elite were an important motivating force behind poor relief but acknowledges that this aspect is just a piece in a larger jigsaw puzzle. Furthermore, she believes that the case for excluding religion as a motivating factor for charity has been adequately demonstrated only for post-Reformation England. Cissie Fairchilds, on the basis of her study of Aix-en-Provence, concludes that the desire "to buy salvation" was the principal motivating force behind charity in this region until the last decades of the eighteenth century. An emerging consensus seems to be that the older models that sought to differentiate between medieval and modern notions of relief by opposing the ideas of charity and welfare, care and cure, and religious and secular motivations no longer seem to accord with reality.[23]

Turning to Catalonia and the realms of Aragon, the image that emerges is of just such a mosaic of lay and clerical participation, religious and secular purposes. Because, as Carme Batlle has pointed out, religious orders, and other organized communities of hospitallers played only a minor role in the administration of assistance in Catalonia, there never was a clear-cut boundary between clerical and lay spheres of activity.[24] On the one hand, the rectors of ecclesiastically governed hospitals in Barcelona and Girona for the most part were priests, often because duties of a sacerdotal nature were associated with these posts. But Clement V's bull of 1311, *Quia contingit*, by declaring that the office of hospital administrator was not to be considered as an ecclesiastical benefice, fully sanctioned the appointment of lay men and women as rectors of ecclesiastically governed hospitals. As we have seen, this permitted Bishop Ponç de Gualba of Barcelona in 1326 to separate the office of administrator from that of chaplain for the city's leper hospital and appoint a layperson to the former position.[25] Similarly, municipal hospitals most often had lay administrators, but there were exceptional cases like the appointment of a priest as rector of the newly established municipal hospital at Tarragona in 1370. Furthermore, examples (from Barcelona, Lleida, Urgell, and elsewhere) of the merger and then joint operation of capitular and municipal hospitals indicate a degree of cooperation between diocesan and town officials.[26]

Traditionally medicine, an increasingly important part of the late medieval hospital, has been thought to be one area that clearly separated laymen from the clergy, because various decretals of the thirteenth century forbade the study and/or practice of medicine to various categories of the clergy. Reexamination of the sources, however, indicates that in fact nothing prevented the diocesan clergy from either the study or practice of medicine at the start of the fourteenth century, and even the restrictions on monks and canons were not absolute. Within the Crown of Aragon, Michael McVaugh has identified nine clerics who practiced medicine within the half century prior to 1335. While none of these can be tied directly to any of the hospitals under study, it indicates that medical practice was not regarded as incompatible with clerical status and thus evidence for the secularization of hospitals.[27]

The analysis of the internal operation of all Catalan hospitals, including those under private or secular governance, reveals an overlay of religious observance and intent. As Agustín Rubio Vela admits, despite his insistence on the secularist thesis, fourteenth and fifteenth-century establishments maintained chaplains and chapels and exhibited "a curious worldly-spiritual duality."[28] For example, our examination of both hospices and foundling homes has revealed that such institutions provided not only nurture and care but also the sacraments of the Church — baptism for the newborn, confession, and anointing for the terminally sick or old. Indeed, the sacred received a certain priority over the temporal. Those finding children were always first supposed to detect evidence of baptism, and at Barcelona's Hospital of Santa Creu inmates were visited by a priest before they saw a physician. Hospitals were also responsible for the burial of dead inmates, a duty that involved not only the provision of a shroud and place of interment but also in some instances commemorative masses. Yet another example would be municipal shelters for prostitutes, like *les Egipciaques* in Barcelona, where women were not only taken off the streets but subjected to a regimen of sermons and religious devotions.[29]

Despite the continued interplay of the sacred and profane, it is indisputable that the influence and importance of municipal institutions and lay elites in the distribution of charity from the thirteenth to the fifteenth century expanded. While the maturation of urban institutions and the increased demands placed on charity by the plagues, disorder, and economic hardships of the late Middle Ages help us to understand the forces that impelled greater municipal participation, do these same forces also signal a change in how society viewed the ends of charity? George Rosen, for example, has argued that hospitals were initially religious in purpose and throughout the medieval era retained the legal status of religious places, even when administered by municipalities. Yet, by the end of the Middle Ages, they had also become social instruments, with a secular agenda to ameliorate suffering, diminish poverty, eradicate begging, and maintain public order.[30]

One of the arguments made by those who distinguish between religious and secular assistance is that the former, because it is concerned principally with the effects on the benefactor, is indiscriminate in character and does not consider the merit or need of the recipient. Secular relief, on the other hand, is highly selective in nature since its primary purpose is to encourage industry, repress idleness, and provide help only to the genuinely deserving.[31] Such a distinction is fundamental to any understanding of Catalan charity. The deserving poor, the *pauperes verecundi*, appear in the sources as a category from the early thirteenth century and were the particular focus of parochial charity. Fourteenth-century legislation, furthermore, in cities such as Barcelona and Valencia discouraged begging, especially by outsiders, and hospitals made attempts to distinguish between those in genuine need and mere vagrants.[32] The question at issue here is whether the distinction between the deserving and undeserving poor is evidence of a fundamental shift in motivation and intent from religious to secular. For several reasons, this does not seem to be so. The distinction, first of all, was fundamental in the writings of medieval canonists and was the largest topic of discussion under the heading of charitable giving. Among these canonists is the Catalan Dominican, Ramon de Penyafort, who compiled the decretals of Pope Gregory IX. Citing texts from Saint Ambrose, the fourth-century bishop of Milan, Ramon argues that charity should be indiscriminate only when "you have enough for all." When resources are insufficient, on the other hand, he argued that preference should first be given to family and friends. The *Glossa ordinaria* explained that "if we do not have enough for all, then we should give rather to the good than to the evil, to a relative rather than a stranger."[33] Fourteenth-century Catalan sources also allowed for some discrimination in assisting poor people. Saint Vicent Ferrer, for example, in his sermon for the feast of Saint Lawrence argued that, among the observances that must be kept by all Christians, was the obligation to "bank treasure with the poor," and elsewhere he lists charity as one of the ten ways of obtaining grace. Yet the Franciscan Francesc Eiximenis argued that it was not desirable for cities to support beggars; even the handicapped, he says, can find honorable work. Charity, he believed, should be systematic but discriminating.[34] Thus, the restrictions on begging and vagabondage that we have noted in municipal legislation reflect attitudes common among both the clergy and the laity and thus indicate no fundamental rift between these two groups in their attitude toward the poor.

There is, however, a significant change in how assistance to the poor was to be financed. Charity in the twelfth century was entirely voluntary, supported in large measure through endowments conveyed by an affluent elite. By the thirteenth and fourteenth centuries, there is greater participation by the lower orders, both in the form of small pious bequests as well as in the offerings collected in poor boxes put out by representatives of parochial *bacís*, religious orders and other charitable organizations. The statutes of Barcelona's Hospital of Santa Creu testify to continued importance of legacies, endowments, alms, and other gifts into the fifteenth century.[35] Yet, in the later Middle Ages, evidence begins to mount that voluntary offerings had become insufficient to sustain the work of existing charities.

During the fourteenth century, with the onset of hard times, municipal councils in both Barcelona and Valencia began to pay direct subsidies to individual hospitals. The first instance, just six years after the first of the bad years, was that of En Marcús in Barcelona, which was ceded in 1339 by its insolvent administrators to the Consell de Cent. Valencia's Hospital of Sant Guillem, operated by the Trinitarian Order, suffered as a consequence of the War of the Two Pedros (1356–69). Beginning in 1361, it received a series of cash gifts from the municipality to repair its damaged structure and to compensate for patrimonial income lost as a consequence of damage to its rural, agricultural lands. Another Valencian institution, the Hospital de la Reyna suffered economic shortfalls beginning with the famine of 1333. During the plague of 1375, the *consell* paid out thirty pounds so that the hospital could afford to bury its dead. Ultimately, in 1383, the hospital became the property of the city, which then had to make payments on its debt and provide funds for its day-to-day operation. In 1380, a third institution, the leprosarium of Sant Llàtzer, petitioned the Valencian council for fifty pounds to relieve a deficit brought on by high prices.[36] In Barcelona, hard times forced the merger of several institutions in 1401 to form the

Hospital of Santa Creu, which became the joint responsibility of the chapter and municipal council. While neither bishop nor town accepted any direct obligation to finance the new hospital, which in theory would be supported by its consolidated endowments, the Consell de Cent, following the bank failures and currency devaluations of 1406, was forced in 1407 to extend a line of credit to Santa Creu. For the rest of the century, until 1482, the municipality guaranteed to make available sufficient monies, up to two or three thousand florins, to compensate for unexpected shortfalls in revenue.[37] The story is much the same in small cities like Urgell where the unrest of the mid-fifteenth century not only forced the consolidation of hospitals but also compelled the surviving institution to turn to the municipal consuls for operating subsidies.[38]

Municipal contributions were a sign that income from endowments had been adversely affected by Catalonia's deteriorating economy. In 1362, for example, during the War of the Two Pedros, tenants of the Hospital of En Clapers in Valencia petitioned the city council for a reduction in their rents, under threat of abandoning their holdings altogether. In 1409, furthermore, the trustee, or *procurator menor*, charged with collecting income from the *censales* owed to the *almoina* of Lleida received only 68 percent of what was due.[39] This phenomenon is a reflection of the long and profound decline that set in, particularly within Catalonia, between 1333 and 1500. First there were years of famine in the 1330s, followed by the Unionist revolt in the 1340s. The Black Death struck in 1348, 1362, 1374–75, 1380, 1383–84, and 1395. The War of the Two Pedros lasted from 1356 to 1369. In 1381, 1383, and 1406, Barcelona suffered a series of bank failures, which caused a rise in unemployment and a serious devaluation of the currency. All of these calamities, which led to a decline in Catalonia's population of as much as 38.5 percent between 1330 and 1381, had a depressing effect on rents. The currency devaluations caused *censales*, or bonds, to lose between 22.8 and 28 percent in value.[40]

Charitable institutions were particularly vulnerable to declines such as these in land rents (*censos*) and bonds (*censales*) because the preponderance of their revenues came from these sources. In 1306, Barcelona's Hospital of En Colom received only 10 percent of its income from alms and sales of its produce; the remainder came from investments. Between 1374 and 1397, En Clapers in Valencia derived 95 percent of its revenue from *censos*, rights of lordship, and bonds; alms amounted to a mere 3.5 percent. Studies of two parochial alms funds in Barcelona reveal a similar pattern. The *bací* of Santa Maria del Pi, between 1434 and 1454, gained 83.8 percent of its income from investments, 7.2 percent from legacies and donations, and only 9 percent from direct collections. The statistics from the richer and more aristocratic parish of Santa Maria del Mar in 1421 suggest that the entire income came from investments, 72.6 percent from *censales* and 27.3 percent from *censos*. The situation for Sant Llàtzer's in Barcelona was somewhat different; here 55 percent of revenue came from offerings of different sorts, but still 45 percent of income was derived either from rents or the sale of agricultural produce.[41]

The relative insignificance of monies collected from the general community broaches the broader question of the depth of society's commitment to works of relief. Was this an endeavor supported by a broad spectrum of the population, or was it, as Sandra Cavallo has argued in the case of early modern Turin, an affair of the elite that had as much to do with power and status as assistance to the poor? Carme Batlle, on the basis of her extensive analysis of Barcelonan wills, believes that the charitable impulse was shared by all social classes and that giving was practiced by all but the destitute themselves. Yet the amount dedicated to charity in the thirteenth-century wills that Batlle studies was relatively small, typically a few sous and only in exceptional cases amounting to more than a hundred sous.[42] The scattered statements that survive of hospitaller income, furthermore, demonstrate that only a minor portion of annual budgets was derived either from legacies such as these or from alms. The preponderance of revenue came from *censos* and *censales*. While no one has studied these in any detail, the initial impression is that patrimonies derived in large measure from the endowments conferred by an institution's founder, the founding family, and then by subsequent benefactors, both large and small. While administrators typically capitalized even small gifts and alms into *censos* and *censales*, no one has yet determined what proportion of the subsequent endowment derived from the gifts of the rich or from the smaller offerings of those with modest means.[43]

Another issue that touches on the question of societal attitudes toward the poor is the varying degrees of support allotted to the working poor and the so-called "deserving" poor vis-à-vis migrants and outsiders. John Henderson, in his study of Florentine charity, argues that the deserving poor were principally the concern of charitable confraternities, which in the fourteenth and fifteenth centuries had broad support within the community and close connections to the governing elite. More peripheral to the communal consciousness were the hospitals, which in large measure seem to have served rural workers and foreigners, who had migrated into the city looking for work, or else servants and freed slaves who were generally excluded from confraternal charity. These institutions survived on their endowments and received municipal subventions only when they were strapped for cash. In the main, he believes that Florentines preferred to assist, above all, working families with children.[44]

In Barcelona, unlike Florence where various confraternities devoted themselves to this work, the deserving poor were the particular concern of parish charity, which, as we have seen, became an organized vehicle for charitable assistance at the beginning of the fourteenth century. It is noteworthy that even during the difficult decades of the fifteenth century, when the city was suffering through a period of profound economic crisis and decline, the *bacís* of Santa Maria del Pi and Santa Maria del Mar were able to maintain their income and consequently their support for the needy of the parish.[45] A similar bias toward relatives and friends has been detected in the policies of *almoinas* in towns such as Barcelona, Lleida, and Urgell, and in hospitals like Barcelona's Pere Desvilar, where many places were subject to rights of presentment and nomination. Only the town of Girona seems to have made a genuine effort to distribute bread to all or most of the needy, but even here surely the preponderance of those fed were permanent residents of the town.

Discrimination in favor of the deserving poor by episcopal and municipal hospitals, on the other hand, is more difficult to detect because these institutions had a greater obligation toward outsiders—abandoned or orphaned children, pilgrims and other travelers, the old and terminally ill. Yet, when care would imply a long-term commitment, as at the leprosarium of Sant Llàtzer in Barcelona, clear preference was given to local lepers, and at the end of the fifteenth century the Consell de Cent decided not to construct a new and larger leprosarium precisely because it would only encourage the immigration of outsiders into the city. Evidence from Girona, furthermore, shows at least some effort to exclude from shelter and care vagrants who made a habit of public charity.[46] Yet, on the other hand, Barcelona was willing to erect, during the difficult decades of the fifteenth century, a monumental gothic structure for the Hospital of Santa Creu that was financed at least in part by public subscription. This is of some significance because the patient population at Santa Creu, unlike Valencia's En Clapers, for example, contained a substantial proportion of foreigners.[47] Furthermore, both establishments accepted foundlings and orphans irrespective of their origins. Thus, the line delineating charity to neighbors and to foreigners is not always easy to draw.

Whatever kindness was extended to outsiders, however, seems to have been limited to Christians. While Jews and Muslims might have mingled with Catalan or Valencian Christians in the course of their daily business, they formed self-contained communities separated from Christian society by real, if invisible, boundaries of religion, culture, and history. David Nirenberg, in his discussion of the Holy Week violence perpetrated by Christians against Jews, has underscored how important it was for the dominant group to remember and reinforce these social boundaries. Jews, like the Christian prostitutes of Barcelona and Valencia, were segregated and kept physically confined during the culminating days of Holy Week. Their exclusion from the community, however, ran year round when it came to matters of solidarity and assistance. Thus Jews and Muslims alike articulated their own institutions of charity that paralleled those of their Christian neighbors. The only known application of Christian assistance to Jews or Muslims involved their orphaned and abandoned children, but these young ones were always baptized and raised as Christians.[48]

Among Christians, Catalan communities in the fourteenth century began to discourage begging and the immigration of those likely to become beggars and thieves. Barcelona's Consell de Cent in 1322, for example, permitted nonresidents to beg within the city for only a day and attempted to restrict the time and locale of such activities.[49] In Valencia, in 1338 and 1339, a public wardship for orphans was created, lest these children, most of whom were the offspring of migrants, would become beggars, drunkards, or thieves; youths who evaded such supervision were to be expelled from the city.[50] Teresa-María Vinyoles argues that the undeserving poor (*pobres captaires*), by reason of their dress or social status (slaves, serfs, Jews, Muslims, prostitutes, pimps, bastards, the blind, the deaf, foreigners) were simply more visible than the deserving poor, who lived intermingled among their more fortunate neighbors, and were thus more likely to generate suspicion and ill-feeling in the minds of urban residents. At best, such poor became public spectacles, as gray-robed pallbearers who conveyed the bodies of wealthy citizens to the cemetery, at times performing macabre dances in the streets. But most often they were associated with crime and violence simply because those areas of the city where they congregated were more likely locales for these phenomena than residential neighborhoods.[51] Furthermore, the term customarily applied to foundlings in Valencia, *bort* or bastard, was scarcely more endearing in the fourteenth century than it is today.[52] The sense is that whatever public assistance was provided to such marginalized groups sprang more from an enlightened selfishness — whether the desire for spiritual reward or more pragmatically the maintenance of public order — than from any sense of affection or concern for their welfare.

As a consequence, some distinction can be made between the types of

relief rendered to the *vergonyants* and *captaires*. The former were eligible for
a broad array of assistance: distributions of food, clothing and money subsidies, assistance with dowries, admission to leprosaria, shelters, and hospitals, and care for dependent children. With the exception of lepers, most of
the aid was of a temporary, emergency nature that assisted families and
individuals to survive an economic downturn, the death of a parent or
spouse, an injury or illness, or to face an extraordinary expense like a dowry.
The intent went beyond mere benevolence; it sought to preserve individuals in their status as functioning members of the community. Those without roots in the neighborhood, however, received far less. They were not
eligible for parochial largesse, and the limited places available at cathedral
almoinas seem to have been reserved for more deserving souls. At most, the
rootless were eligible for funereal and other "extraordinary" handouts of
food and clothing. The restrictions noted against begging, in fact, suggest
that mendicancy was their principal means of support. It was not until
1584, for example, that Barcelona established a shelter specifically for beggars and even this does not seem to have functioned very successfully.[53] The
municipality, however, would care for the abandoned children of the marginalized, perhaps out of a sense of moral and religious decency, possibly
because uncertainty over their origin would make discrimination difficult,
and certainly to give those children who survived the chance to become
productive members of the community. Hospitals, given the numbers of
transients within their population, also provided a measure of care, an
honorable place to die, and the promise of a decent burial for those lacking
the support of a family. But, given the growing emphasis on medical care in
the fourteenth and fifteenth centuries, the modest populations of patients,
and a seeming decline in mortality rates among inmates, the very desperate
must not have had ready access even to this level of assistance.

To return to the question that began this discussion, these observations suggest that the fourteenth and fifteenth centuries saw no major paradigmatic shift in intent from religious to secular purposes. The evidence
from Catalonia provides yet additional confirmation that the old distinction between Catholic and Protestant charity is not a useful or accurate tool
for the analysis of late medieval and early modern relief. While Catalan
charity did not absolutely exclude anyone from assistance, it did show a
marked preference for friends, neighbors, and those perceived as deserving.
These attitudes of the fifteenth century, as expressed by Francesc Eiximenis,
appear little different from the sentiments of twelfth and thirteenth-century
canonists, including those of the distinguished Catalan Dominican Ramon
de Penyafort. Thus, it is difficult to argue that late medieval society hard-

ened in its attitude toward the poor. The evolution was less one of attitude than of actual service. Assistance in the fifteenth century was more specialized and directed than it was in the twelfth century. The later period saw in Valencia a hospital specifically for the mentally ill; Santa Creu in Barcelona provided a complete regimen of medical care, in addition to the bed, board, and religious solace of its thirteenth-century predecessors. Foundling homes in Barcelona and Valencia not only cared for infants but articulated a program for their nurture that led children through apprenticeships toward their reinsertion as full members of the community. *Almoinas* in Barcelona and Lleida in the fifteenth century began to substitute cash payments for actual meals, marking their evolution from soup kitchen to relief agency. Throughout Catalonia, older foundations were consolidated into larger municipal or general hospitals, often with expanded and specialized facilities. In short, as Jonathan Barry and Colin Jones have argued, the line between traditional and modern ideas of assistance, between charity and welfare, care and cure, private and public assistance, is not only difficult to draw but also lacks any clear chronological demarcation.[54]

Support for these programs of assistance rested on the traditional resources and endowments, which derived from collections, gifts, and wills that were given for conventional, religious motives. As Cissie Fairchilds has shown in her studies of Aix-en-Provence, or Linda Martz for Toledo and Maureen Flynn for Zamora, religious motivation remained an important underpinning of charitable activity beyond the medieval into the early modern period.[55] Beginning in the fourteenth century, in addition to private, religiously inspired benefaction, municipal governments also began to direct certain centers of relief and to subsidize others. But, as we have seen, this led not to the establishment of rival and competing institutions, but instead to a high degree of cooperation and coordination between religious and secular agencies. Religious foundations such as Valencia's Hospital de la Reyna or Barcelona's En Marcús could look to the city for financial aid. Municipal authorities, for their part, recognized the legitimatizing value of religion in the control of undesirable elements of the population, such as beggars and prostitutes. What the dual nature of assistance seems to show is that, however limited was the concept and practice of charity in late medieval Catalonia, voluntary contributions were not sufficient to sustain any but purely neighborhood and parochial institutions. Hospitals and other types of charity required for their survival an infusion of public funds.

Appendix

Selected Hospitals, Shelters, and Relief Agencies in Catalonia, Majorca, and Valencia

FIRST CITATION	LOCALITY	TYPE/CLIENTELE	NAME/FOUNDER
Eleventh Century			
995–1011	Barcelona	Cathedral shelter	Hospital de la Seu/En Guitard
1048	Urgell	Cathedral alms	Pia Almoina
1054–63	Vic	Cathedral shelter	Sant Jaume dels Malalts
1059	Urgell	Cathedral shelter	Old Hospital/ Poor Clerics
1095	Girona	Cathedral shelter	Sant Pere/Old Hospital
Twelfth Century			
1141	Vilafranca del Penedès	Poor shelter	Hospital de Sant Valentí
1149–68	Lleida	Cathedral alms	Pia Almoina
1156	Lleida	Shelter for poor	En Nicolau
1161	Barcelona	Cathedral alms	Pia Almoina
1166	Barcelona	Shelter	En Marcús
1170	Lleida	Shelter for poor	Pere Moliner
1171	Tarragona	Cathedral shelter	Hospital of the Poor
1172	Tortosa	Cathedral shelter	Santa Maria
1174	Lleida	Capitular shelter for clergy	Unknown
1180	Lleida	Clerical shelter	Casa de la Caritat
1185	Lleida	Leper Shelter	Sant Llàtzer
1185	Lleida	Shelter	Hospitallers of Saint John
late 12th c.	Barcelona	Leper shelter	Sant Llàtzer
late 12th c.	Cervera	Leper shelter	Santa Magdalena

FIRST CITATION	LOCALITY	TYPE/CLIENTELE	NAME/FOUNDER
Thirteenth Century			
1200s	Barcelona	Jewish hospice	Samuel ben rabí Isaac Ha-Sardí
Ca. 1200	Cervera	Victims of ergotism	Antonines
1211	Girona	Confraternal/town shelter	New Hospital
1212	Barcelona	Confraternal/capitular shelter	Santa Eulàlia
1214	Lleida	Women and children	Order of the Holy Spirit
1216	Lleida	Shelter for poor and captives	Trinitarians
1217	Vic	Poor shelter	En Cloquer
1228	Girona	Capitular relief	Almoina del Pa
1229	Barcelona	Capitular hospital	En Colom
1230	Majorca	Sick poor	Sant Andreu
1235	Cervera	Poor shelter	Joan de l'Hospital
1238	Valencia	Royal hospital	Sant Vicent (Sant Victorian/Merced)
1240	Valencia	Poor shelter	Roncesvalles
1242	Valencia	Sick poor	Sant Guillem (Trinitarians)
1247	Urgell	Municipal hospital	New Hospital
1248	Majorca	Canonical shelter	Sant Antoni Abad
1248	Majorca	unknown	Santa Magdalena
1248	Xàtiva	Poor shelter	Friars of the Sack
Ca. 1250	Reus	Town hospital	Sant Joan
1251	Valencia	Leper shelter	Sant Llàtzer
1256	Barcelona	Capitular hospital	Sant Macià (Pere Desvilar)
1262	Olesa de Bonesvalls	Mendicant shelter	Unknown
1265	Xàtiva	Poor shelter	Pere Soler
1266	Montblanc	Poor shelter	Santa Magdalena
1266	Montblanc	Mendicant shelter	Franciscans
1270	Tortosa	Town hospital	La Grassa
1271	Lleida	Victims of ergotism	Antonines
1275	Vic	Poor, sick, lepers	Santa Trinitat (Ramon de Malla)

FIRST CITATION	LOCALITY	TYPE/CLIENTELE	NAME/FOUNDER
1284	Urgell	Leper shelter	Santa Maria Magdalena
1290	Castelló de la Plana	Shelter for the sick	Town Hospital
1277	Barcelona	Jewish *almoina*	Abraham of Alexandria

Fourteenth Century

1300s	Vilafranca del Penedès	Poor shelter	Trinitarians
1300s	Barcelona	Parochial alms funds	Bacís, Plats
1300s	Vic	Municipal alms	Almoina
Ca. 1300	Xàtiva	Poor shelter	Bernat de Bellvís
1300	Manresa	Municipal shelter	Pere Salvatge
1301	Valencia	Franciscan hospital	La Reyna
1308	Barcelona	Municipal shelter	Pere Desvilar
1310	Tarragona (Cambrils)	Royal hospital	L'Enfant
1311	Valencia	Municipal hospital	En Clapers
1328	Cervera	Poor travelers	Onze Mil Verges
1333–40	Valencia	Victims of ergotism	Antonines
1334	Valencia	Municipal shelter	Beguins
1338	Valencia	Orphans and foundlings	Pare dels òrfens
1338	Vic	Pilgrims, sick, foundlings	Santa Creu (Ramon de Terrades)
1339	Montblanc	Shelter for the poor	
1345	Majorca	Poor shelter	Santa Catarina dels Pobres
1345	Valencia	Prostitute shelter	Casa de las Arrepentidas
1356	Valencia	Diocesan shelter	Poor Priests
1362	Tarragona	Municipal hospital	New Hospital
1365	Barcelona	Municipal prostitute shelter	Les Egipciaques
1370	Barcelona	Orphans and foundlings	Guillem de Pou
1377	Majorca	Poor Jews	Moisés Cabrit
1377	Valencia	Castilian refugees	Confraternity of Sant Jaume
1390s	Valencia	Hospital for the sick	Francesc Conill
1390s	Valencia	Fishermen shelter	Pere Bou

FIRST CITATION	LOCALITY	TYPE/CLIENTELE	NAME/FOUNDER
Fifteenth Century			
1401	Barcelona	General hospital	Santa Creu
1409	Valencia	Municipal insane asylum/children's shelter	Ignoscents, Folls e Orats
1411	Solsona	Private shelter	Llobera
1440	Majorca	Leper shelter	Massells
Pre-1445	Urgell	General hospital	Hospital of the City
1453	Lleida	General hospital	Santa Maria
1456–58	Majorca	General hospital	Hospital general
1464	Tarragona	General hospital	Santa Tecla
1475	Majorca	Clerical shelter	Poor Priests (Antoni Lana)
1495	Valencia	General hospital	Hospital general

Notes

Preface

1. These early works include: for England, Rotha Mary Clay, *The Mediaeval Hospitals of England* (1909; reprint ed., New York, 1966); for Spain, Fermin Hernández Iglesias, *La beneficencia en España*, 2 vols. (Madrid, 1876), and Manuel de Bofarull y Sartario, *Gremios y cofradías de la antigua Corona de Aragón*, Colección de documentos inéditos del Archivo General de la Corona de Aragón, vols. 40–41 (Barcelona, 1876–1910); for France, *Statuts d'Hôtels-Dieu et de Léproseries. Recueil de textes du XIIe au XIVe siècle*, ed. Léon LeGrand (Paris, 1901).

2. See, for example, Jean Imbert, *Les hôpitaux en droit canonique* (Paris, 1947); and Brian Tierney, *Medieval Poor Law: A Sketch of Canonical Theory and Its Application in England* (Berkeley and Los Angeles, 1959).

3. See Paul Bonenfant, "Hôpitaux et bienfaisance publique dans les anciens Pays-Bas des origines à la fin du XVIIIe siècle," in *Annales de la Société Belge d'Histoire des Hôpitaux*, 3 (1965): 1–195.

4. Mollat's work was first published in France as *Les pauvres au moyen âge* (Paris, 1978), and in English translation as: *The Poor in the Middle Ages: An Essay in Social History*, trans. Arthur Goldhammer (New Haven, Conn., 1986). See also *Études sur l'histoire de la pauvreté*, ed. Michel Mollat, 2 vols. (Paris, 1974). For Geremek, see *Les marginaux parisiens aux XIVe et XVe siècles* (Paris, 1976), published in English as *The Margins of Society in Late Medieval Paris*, trans. Jean Birrell (Cambridge, 1987); and *Poverty: A History*, trans. Agnieszka Kolakowska (Oxford, 1994).

5. Philippe Ariès, *Centuries of Childhood: A Social History of Family Life*, trans. Robert Baldick (New York, 1962); Shulamith Shahar, *Childhood in the Middle Ages* (London, 1990); and John Boswell, *The Kindness of Strangers: The Abandonment of Children in Western Europe from Late Antiquity to the Renaissance* (New York, 1988).

6. For example, see Leah Otis, *Prostitution in Medieval Society: The History of an Urban Institution in Languedoc* (Chicago, 1985); Françoise Bériac, *Histoire des lépreux au Moyen Âge, une société d'exclus* (Paris, 1988); *Aging and the Aged in Medieval Europe: Selected Papers from the Annual Conference for Medieval Studies, University of Toronto, Held 25–26 February and 11–12 November 1983*, ed. Michael M. Sheehan, C.S.B. (Toronto, n.d.); and Charles Verlinden, *L'esclavage dans l'Europe médiévale*, 2 vols. (Bruges, 1955–77).

7. See, for example, *Violència i marginació en la societat medieval*, Vol. 1 of *Revista d'història medieval* (Valencia, 1990); Danielle Jacquart and Claude Thomasset, *Sexuality and Medicine in the Middle Ages*, trans. Matthew Adamson (Princeton, N.J., 1988); *Women and Work in Preindustrial Europe*, ed. Barbara A. Hanawalt (Bloomington, Ind., 1986); and R. I. Moore, *The Formation of a Persecuting Society: Power and Deviance in Western Europe, 950–1250* (Oxford, 1987).

8. Luis Batlle Prats, "Inventari dels Bens de l'Hospital de la Seu de Girona," *Estudis Universaris Catalans* 19 (1934): 58–80; César Martinell, "Els hospitals medievals catalans," *Pratica medicina* (1935): 109–32; Joseph Maria Roca, *L'hospital migeval de Sant Macià* (Barcelona, 1926).

9. Pedro Sanahuja, O.F.M., *Historia de la beneficencia en Lérida* (Lérida, 1944); Antonio Rumeu de Armas, *Historia de la previsión social en España: Cofradías, gremios, hermandades, montepíos* (Madrid, 1944).

10. J. Tolivar Faes, *Hospitales de leprosos en Asturias durante las edades media y moderna* (Oviedo, 1966); Robert I. Burns, S.J., "Los hospitales del reino de Valencia en el siglo XIII," *Anuario de estudios medievales* 2 (1965): 135–54.

11. The proceedings are published as *A pobreza e a assistência aos pobres na península ibérica durante a idade média. Actas das 1.ᵃˢ jornadas luso-espanholas de história medieval. Lisboa, 25–30 de Setembro de 1972.* 2 vols. (Lisbon, 1973) (hereafter cited as *A pobreza*).

12. See Luis Martínez García, *La asistencia a los pobres en Burgos en la baja edad media* (Burgos, 1981) and *El Hospital del Rey de Burgos: un señorío medieval en la expansión y en la crisis (siglos XIII y XIV)* (Burgos, 1986). See also Adeline Rucquoi, "Hospitalisation et charité à Valladolid," in *Les sociétés urbaines en France méridionale et en Péninsule Ibérique au Moyen Âge. Actes du Colloque de Pau, 21–23 Septembre 1988* (Paris, 1991), 393–408; Rafael Martínez San Pedro, *Historia de los hospitales en Alicante* (Alicante, 1974); Antonio García del Moral, *El Hospital Mayor de San Sebastian de Córdoba: Cinco Siglos de Asistencia Médico-sanitaria Institucional (1363–1816)* (Córdoba, 1984); Carmen López Alonso, *La pobreza en la España medieval* (Madrid, 1986).

13. *La pobreza y la asistencia a los pobres en la Cataluña medieval*, ed. Manuel Riu, 2 vols. (Barcelona, 1980–82) (hereafter cited as *La pobreza*). For a discussion of the project, see 1: 7–16.

14. See, for example, Carme Batlle i Gallart, *La Seu d'Urgell medieval: La ciutat i els seus habitants* (Barcelona, 1985) and Christian Guilleré, *Girona al segle XIV*, trans. Núria Mañé, 2 vols. (Barcelona, 1993–94).

Chapter 1. Hospitals and the Poor

1. For a discussion of the idea of poverty in the Middle Ages, see Mollat, *Poor in the Middle Ages*, 1–9; see also Geremek, *Poverty*, 3–4.

2. Geremek, *Poverty*, 20. Francesc Eiximenis at the start of the fifteenth century says much the same. See José Luis Martín, "La pobreza y los pobres en los textos literarios del siglo XIV," in *A pobreza*, 2:595.

3. For a history of the *matricularii*, see Michel Rouche, "La matricule des pauvres. Evolution d'une institution de charité du Bas Empire jusqu'à la fin du Haut Moyen Âge," in Mollat, *Études sur l'histoire de la pauvreté*, 1:83–110.

4. Among the practitioners of ritualistic charity would be Cluny, which maintained eighteen paupers in residence; in addition, the monks fed a fixed number of the poor, typically twelve, at ceremonies honoring benefactors and those of high rank but even more for exalted patrons like the kings of León. Lester K. Little,

Religious Poverty and the Profit Economy in Medieval Europe (Ithaca, N.Y., 1978), 67–68. For a review of monastic customs regarding the poor, see Willibrord Witters, "Pauvres et pauvreté dans les coutumes monastiques du Moyen Âge," in Mollat, *Études sur l'histoire de la pauvreté,* 1:117–216. See also Mollat, *Poor in the Middle Ages,* 20–23, 40–42, 46–48, 53; Marvin Becker, *Medieval Italy: Constraints and Creativity* (Bloomington, Ind., 1981), 101.

5. For Bernard of Clairvaux, see Little, *Religious Poverty,* 95. See also ibid., 41, 99–112; Geremek, *Poverty,* 62–66; Pierre Toubert, "La vie commune des clercs aux XIᵉ–XIIᵉ siècles: Un questionnaire," *Revue historique* 231 (1964): 11–26; Caroline Walker Bynum, *Jesus as Mother: Studies in the Spirituality of the High Middle Ages* (Berkeley, Calif., 1982), 22–56; Giles Constable, "Renewal and Reform in the Religious Life: Concepts and Realities," in *Renaissance and Renewal in the Twelfth Century,* ed. Robert L. Benson and Giles Constable (Cambridge, Mass., 1982), 56, 62; M.-D. Chenu, *La théologie au douzième siècle* (Paris, 1966), 225–40.

6. The right to free legal counsel is a feature of the Castilian *fuero* of Soria, Alfonso X's *Las Siete Partidas,* and the *acta* of various Cortes. In the Cortes of Zamora, for example, Alfonso X established in his court two advocates of the poor, and in 1312 Fernando IV paid an advocate six thousand maravedis to defend orphans, widows, and other poor people who made pleas in the royal court. In Valencia and Murcia, the public defender was a municipal officer. The institution became widespread in both Spain and Italy during the fifteenth century. See Agustín Bermúdez Aznar, "La abogacía de pobres en la España medieval," in *A pobreza,* 1:142; Tierney, *Medieval Poor Law,* 12–14; and López Alonso, *Pobreza en la España medieval,* 395–403.

7. Mollat, *Poor in the Middle Ages,* 57–58. See also Tierney, *Medieval Poor Law,* 15–18, 33–44. The concept of right can also be seen in Thomas Aquinas's *Summa theologiae:* "He who suffers from extreme need can take what he needs from another's goods if no one else will give them to him" (Little, *Religious Poverty,* 179).

8. In 1167, Pere Queralt left the castle of Roderico "pauperibus Hospitalis Iherusalem," that is, to the paupers of the Hospital of Jerusalem. Clearly, Pere here meant the members of the Order of Saint John, not the inmates of their Jerusalem hospital. See *Cartulari de Poblet: Edicio del manuscrit de Tarragona* (Barcelona, 1938), 140–42, no. 234. A century later, however, the notion of who constituted "Christ's poor" had changed dramatically, as seen in the will of Master Llorenç, a canon of Barcelona, who directed in 1267 that the residue of his estate be divided among "the poor of Jesus Christ, orphans, widows, girls to be married, and captives to be redeemed who come to the notice of my manumissors, having made those poor of Jesus Christ . . . my heirs." See Arxiu de Sant Pere de les Puelles [hereafter, ASPP], carp. 33, no. 518; carp. 38, no. 585.

9. Geremek, *Poverty,* 25.

10. Eiximenis argues in his *Regiment de la cosa pública* that integration into the community requires that an individual contribute to the public good in a positive fashion: "Each one in the community ought to be employed—rich or poor . . . male or female." Quoted in Martín, "La pobreza y los pobres," 2:590–95. See also John Henderson, *Piety and Charity in Late Medieval Florence* (Oxford, 1994), 346.

11. "For under the pretext of hospitality and the guise of piety, they [i.e.,

religious charlatans] become alms-collectors, improperly extorting monies by lies and deceptions and by every means of which they are able, feasting themselves from the poor, not caring for them except when they, by giving a little bit to the poor and infirm, are able to demand alms from the faithful, so that these crafty businessmen and sly hucksters may profit much through fraud from a certain type of prey" (Jacques de Vitry, *The* Historia occidentalis *of Jacques de Vitry: A Critical Edition*, ed. J. F. Hinnebusch [Freibourg, 1972], cap. 29, pp. 148–49). For *Glossa ordinaria* and the canonists, see Tierney, *Medieval Poor Law*, 54–61. Alfonso X of Castile, in his *Las Siete Partidas*, makes a distinction between the truly poor and those who "by means of their labor are able to earn what they and others can live upon, but do not do so, but rather prefer to resort to the houses of others, and support themselves in this way." The king advises the clergy that it would be better, short of actually permitting those individuals to starve to death, "to deprive them of food than to give it to them, since they avoid earning it, though able to do so, but, not being willing, choose to obtain it by knavery" *(Las Siete Partidas*, trans. Samuel Parsons Scott [Chicago, 1931], 1.5.40, p. 67). See also Geremek, *Poverty*, 47.

12. Geremek, along with Brian Pullan, believes that social concern over the dimensions of poverty that becomes evident in new public policies of the sixteenth century has its roots in the crises of the fourteenth and fifteenth centuries. The *matricularii*, or registered poor, in late Roman and Merovingian times were those aided by the cathedral; indeed, in Carolingian times the position developed into a kind of office as church warden (Mollat, *Poor in the Middle Ages*, 40–41). For early use of the term *pauperes verecundi*, see Immaculada Ollich i Castanyer, "Les entitats eclesiastiques de Vic al segle XIII," *Ausa* 8 (1976): 93; Carme Batlle and Montserrat Casas, "La caritat privada i les institucions benèfiques de Barcelona (segle XIII)," in *La pobreza*, following 1:182; *Cartulario de «Sant Cugat» dels Vallés*, ed. José Rius Serra (Barcelona, 1945–47), 3:401, no. 1284 (August 27, 1214). With regard to restrictions upon the poor, the *Établissements* of Louis IX of France, for example, state that folk without steady income who loitered about in taverns could be seized and, if they led an evil life, expelled from town. In France, the first laws against vagabondage, per se, date from the mid-fourteenth century when John II ordered hospitals not to shelter vagrants. In Castile, Fernando IV ordered that beggars who were unwilling to work be expelled from Burgos; in 1351 Pedro I promulgated a more general law against vagabondage. See Geremek, *Poverty*, 73–76, 100–102; idem, *The Margins of Society*, 30–31; and Brian Pullan, *Rich and Poor in Renaissance Venice: The Social Institutions of a Catholic State to 1620* (Cambridge, Mass., 1971), 198, 200, 636–37. In 1300, the Grand Council of Venice decreed that paupers were not to wander the street begging, but instead were to be put into shelters. Street people like prostitutes, swindlers, and ruffians were liable to a public whipping; Florence in 1294 expelled poor, blind beggars from the city (Henderson, *Piety and Charity in Florence*, 244). Geremek's argument that restrictions on the nonresident poor and on begging originated in southern German cities in the fourteenth century would seem to be an overstatement, given the parallel practices in France and Barcelona; see his *Poverty*, 46–47.

13. Teresa-Maria Vinyoles i Vidal, *La vida quotidiana a Barcelona vers 1400* (Barcelona, 1985), 119.

14. Josefina Mutgé Vives, *La ciudad de Barcelona durante el reinado de Alfonso el*

Benigno (1327–1336) (Barcelona, 1987), 317; Martín, "La pobreza y los pobres," 618–19.

15. Guillermo Aramayona Alonso, "El cuaderno de 1421 de «El Bací dels Pobres Vergonyants» de la parroquia de Santa María del Mar, de Barcelona," in *La pobreza*, 2:175; Richard C. Trexler, "Charity and the Defense of Urban Elites in the Italian Communes," in *The Rich, the Well-Born and the Powerful: Elites and Upper Classes in History*, ed. Frederic Cople Jaher (Urbana, Ill., 1973), 75; Giovanni Ricci, "Naissance du pauvre honteux: Entre l'histoire des idées et l'histoire sociale," *Annales: économies, sociétés, civilisations* 38 (1983):168–69; Geremek, *Poverty*, 40. This distinction survives into the twentieth century, as witnessed by Provident Loan Society, a pawnshop founded for the *worthy poor* that still operates in New York City. See *New York Times*, March 14, 1993, 19.

16. Berenguer Borell, for example, was the brother and executor of a Barcelonan who in traditional fashion left the residue of his estate to Christ's poor. Berenguer successfully sought permission from the bishop's court to use this money to pay his own educational expenses. In another case, the court allowed one hundred sous to Guillem ça Tria of Vilafranca from the estate of his sister-in-law who had left money to dower unmarried girls so that he could dower his own two daughters. See Kristine Utterback, *Pastoral Care and Administration in Mid-fourteenth Century Barcelona: Exercising the "Art of Arts"* (Lewiston, N.Y., 1993), 180–81; and Robert I. Burns, S.J., *The Crusader Kingdom of Valencia: Reconstruction on a Thirteenth-Century Frontier* (Cambridge, Mass., 1967), 1:246–47.

17. The *Doctrina Compendiosa*, an anonymous treatise of the early fifteenth century, argues that God will not only glorify individuals who give alms, but increase their earthly goods while diminishing those of individuals who do not practice charity. See Martín, "La pobreza y los pobres," 596; and Geremek, *Poverty*, 48. Speaking of King Alfonso VIII's foundation of the Hospital del Rey in Burgos, Ximénez de Rada states: "To such an extent that the works of piety in that same hospital could be contemplated by anyone as if in a mirror, and [he] who in life merited universal praise for his excellent works, because of the multiplication of [his] intercessors, would deserve to be crowned by God after his death." See his *Historia de rebus Hispanie sive Historia Gothica*, ed. Juan Fernández Valverde (Turnhout, 1987), 7.34.10–13, 256.

18. Brian Pullan argues that it was not until the sixteenth century that charity's focus began to shift away from the devotional demands placed upon the poor, to be replaced with the goal of improving their discipline and moral behavior. See his *Renaissance Venice*, 635.

19. Mollat and Miri Rubin, among others, make this argument. Patricia Cullum, on the basis of her study of charity in York, disagrees; but all of these authors seem to make the unwarranted assumption that society ever looked with great kindness upon the poor. Pullan and Geremek, on the other hand, assert that poverty itself was never regarded as a virtue (only a taste for it!); to the contrary the poor were typically stigmatized as idle or dissolute. Patricia Cullum, "Hospitals and Charitable Provision in Medieval Yorkshire, 936–1547" (D. Phil. thesis, University of York, 1989), 439. Geremek, *Poverty*, viii, 28–29, 68. On Eiximenis, see Martín, "La pobreza y los pobres," 604.

20. Henderson argues that into the late thirteenth century Florentines con-

tinued to identify the practitioners of voluntary poverty, like monks and friars, as the *pauperes Christi*; it is not until after the subsistence crises of the early fourteenth century that Florentine society became interested in helping the lay poor, and especially the poor family. He notes that in 1324 the Orsanmichele confraternity conferred 94 percent of its alms on the urban poor, 4 percent on beggars and only 2 percent on pious institutions; see his *Piety and Charity*, 252–54. For a discussion of the fourteenth-century economic crisis, the persistence of unemployment, and the efforts to restrict wage demands, see Geremek, *Poverty*, 78–90, 100–114.

21. See Pullan's "'Support and Redeem': Charity and Poor Relief in Italian Cities from the Fourteenth to the Seventeenth Century," in Brian Pullan, *Poverty and Charity: Europe, Italy, Venice, 1400–1700* (Aldershot, England, 1994), 5: 181.

22. Geremek, *Poverty*, 26; Tierney, *Medieval Poor Law*, 55–56, 68.

23. Theorists of the nineteenth century attempted to distinguish between Catholic and Protestant approaches to charity. The former was said to focus upon religious merit for the giver, and thus to be indiscriminate and lack any incentive to end poverty. The latter is said to have produced a rational and secular system of poor relief designed to reduce poverty and to improve society. Still others have argued that charity, with a focus on care, is a medieval phenomenon, while welfare, which aims at cure, is a modern idea. For a discussion, see Pullan, *Renaissance Venice*, 11–12; Jonathan Barry and Colin Jones, Introduction to *Medicine and Charity before the Welfare State*, ed. Jonathan Barry and Colin Jones (London, 1991), 1–3.

Chapter 2. Feeding the Poor in Medieval Catalonia

1. For a general discussion of the rise of the poor as a permanent social class, see Mollat, *Poor in the Middle Ages*, 57–69. On the obligation to assist the poor, as related in patristic texts and then adapted by the twelfth and thirteenth-century canonists, see Tierney, *Medieval Poor Law*, 44–54, 68–75.

2. The almonry at Jaca was founded by Bishop García in 1076, that at Roda by Bishop Dalmau in 1092, and that at Huesca by Bishop Esteban in 1108. See J. Boix Pociello, "Les persones pobres e miserables a la Ribagorça medieval," *Acta historica et archaeologica mediaevalia* 5–6 (1984–85): 194–95; and Antonio Ubieta Arteta, "Pobres y marginados en el primitivo Aragón," *Aragón en la Edad Media* 5 (1983): 20–21.

3. Stephen P. Bensch sees the period 1140–1220 as crucial in the development of Barcelona's economy and urban patriciate. See his *Barcelona and its Rulers, 1096–1291* (Cambridge, 1995), 232–33.

4. Josep Baucells i Reig, "La Pia Almoina de la seo de Barcelona," in *A pobreza*, 1:81–82.

5. The ritual of monastic hospitality included the *mandatum*, or washing of the feet. See: Mollat, *Poor in the Middle Ages*, 47; and Josep Baucells i Reig, "Gènesi de la Pia almoina de la Seu de Barcelona: Els fundadors," in *La pobreza*, 1:19.

6. Baucels, "Gènesi," 26–33; Baucells, "Pia Almoina," 87–90.

7. Evidence suggests that Bernat de Santa Eulàlia was able to use Bishop

Berenguer's endowment to feed fourteen poor, two more than originally intended. Baucels, "Pia Almoina," 93–94, 98.

8. The Plegamans was the most prominent family in thirteenth-century Barcelona; Ramon was vicar of the city, and then royal vicar and bailiff of Catalonia. In 1240, he asked that as many poor be fed on his anniversary as funds permitted; in 1241, the canon Ramon de Riera endowed daily meals for two poor persons and special meals for fifty others on his anniversary and also on the first Friday of Lent; Bishop Berenguer's estate initially fed fourteen daily and another hundred on his anniversary (ibid., 96, 98). The smaller amount of a single morabetin was left by the canon Larrentius in his will of 1267 to feed the poor in the cathedral refectory (ASPP, carp. 25, perg. 333). On Plegamans, see Bensch, *Barcelona*, 321–22.

9. The bishop's will directed: "We assign the alms for the alms of the aforesaid poor, so that those poor may henceforth be fed in the refectory of the Church of Barcelona, all in such manner that they be able to be suitably refreshed, under the direction of one cleric, or canon or benefice holder of this Church, who is to be called the 'Almoner,' appointed by the bishop or chapter of Barcelona, and who is held to answer once a year to the authority of the chapter and bishop." Sebastián Puig y Puig, *Episcopologio de la sede barcinonense* (Barcelona, 1929), 442, no. 96. The layman Pere Grony in 1264 placed his endowment in the hands of the curate of the parish of Sant Miquel. Baucells, "Pia Almoina," 99.

10. Baucells, "Pia Almoina," 104.

11. Ibid., 99, 106–7.

12. Ibid., 110–12.

13. Antonio Pons, *Los judios del reino de Mallorca durante los siglos XIII y XIV* (Palma de Mallorca, 1984), 2:126.

14. Sanahuja, *Beneficencia en Lérida*, 42–45; Josep Lladonosa i Pujol, *Història de la ciutat de Lleida* (Barcelona, 1980), 138.

15. See Agustín Prim Tarragó, *Cosas viejas de Lérida* (Lleida, 1893), 6. Sanahuja counters by arguing that the reason for this is that those tithes were diverted from the *almoina* in 1237 by Bishop Pere de Albalat to the cathedral construction fund (*Beneficencia en Lérida*, 48–50).

16. The dining room contained rude tables, probably arranged in a rectangle, with stools and chairs. Food was served on ceramic platters; wine was in pottery jars, from which it was poured into individual bowls. Prim Bertrán i Roigé, "El menjador de l'almoina de la catédral de Lleida. Notes sobre l'alimentació dels pobres lleidatans al 1338," *Ilerda* 40 (1979): 110–11.

17. An example of an endowment is the will of Ramon de Montanyana, an archdeacon and canon of the cathedral, which in 1309 provided funds for the alimentation of seven poor persons in the *almoina* of Lleida, and three others in that of Valencia. In addition four large loaves of white bread (two more in Valencia) were to be distributed to the poor at the onset of winter, and in June one hundred measures of rough linen cloth were to be given out. See Sanahuja, *Beneficencia en Lérida*, 62–64, 68–76. See also Prim Bertrán i Roigé, "L'Almoina de la Seu de Lleida a principis del segle XV," in *La pobreza*, 2:349–52, 355; and his "El menjador," 110. The custom of distributing food to external constituencies was not unusual. In the English town of York, for example, the Hospital of Saint Leonard, in addition to

feeding its own inmates, distributed food at its gate to regular dependents and itinerant beggars and to the inmates of the local leper hospices and the prisoners of York Castle. See Patricia Helen Cullum, *Cremetts and Corrodies: Care of the Poor and Sick at St. Leonard's Hospital, York, in the Middle Ages* (York, 1991), 29.

18. Batlle, *Urgell medieval*, 112–13, 119–21.

19. Ibid., 123–25.

20. For the grain trade between Urgell and Barcelona, see Mutgé, *La ciudad de Barcelona*, 49.

21. Bread in the amount of a hundred sous was to be given out on All Souls' Day, and two hundred sous worth on Good Friday. Christian Guilleré, *Diner, poder i societat a la Girona del segle XIV* (Girona, 1984), 158.

22. Christian Guilleré, "Assistance et charité à Gérone au début du XIVᵉᵐᵉ siècle," in *La pobreza*, 1:194; Christian Guilleré, *Girona medieval: L'etapa d'apogeu, 1285–1360* (Gerona, 1991):10, 89.

23. Christian Guilleré, "Une institution charitable face aux malheurs du temps: La Pia Almoina de Gerone (1347–1380)," in *La pobreza*, 2:318–21; 324.

24. Christian Guilleré, "La peste noire à Gérone," *Annals de Institut d'Estudis Gironins* 27 (1984): 132.

25. Guilleré, "Institution charitable," 314–15.

26. Ibid., 326.

27. Enrique Bayerri y Bertomeu, *Historia de Tortosa y su comarca* (Tortosa, 1956), 7:580; Guilleré, "Institution charitable," 313n.

28. In time of need, for example, Tortosa would keep the grain for itself and embargo sales to Barcelona (Mutgé, *La ciudad de Barcelona*, 70).

29. Lawrence J. McCrank, "Restoration and Reconquest in Medieval Catalonia: The Church and the Principality of Tarragona, 971–1177" (Ph.D. dissertation; University of Virginia, 1974), 586.

30. Eduard Junyent, *La ciutat de Vic i la seva història* (Barcelona, 1976), 124.

31. Alvaro Santamaría, "La asistencia a los pobres en Mallorca en el bajomedievo," *Anuario de estudios medievales* 13 (1983): 388–93; 398.

32. Michel Mollat, "Pauvres et assistés au Moyen Âge," in *A pobreza*, 1:17; Carme Batlle, *L'expansió baixmedieval (segles XIII–XV)*, vol. 3 of *Història de Catalunya*, ed. Pierre Vilar (Barcelona, 1988), 90. Estimates of poverty in Italy range from 10 to 30 percent in the late thirteenth century, and upwards of 50 percent by the mid-fourteenth century (Henderson, *Piety and Charity*, 246–47).

33. In general, Catalonia in the fourteenth century suffered from the problem of underproduction, so food was never plentiful. But the degree of crisis varied. A contemporary source, for example, states that in 1333, a year of great hunger, more than ten thousand people died in Barcelona, but in 1328–29, when shortages were not so severe, the king permitted some wheat to be sent to Valencia where shortages were greater. Mutgé, *La ciudad de Barcelona*, 42–44.

34. The *Llibre Vert*, an account book of the *almoina*, dating from 1317 lists 176 poor people being fed daily, and another 975 individual, endowed rations; Baucells's accounting for that year is 178 daily meals and 1,920 individual meals. Fourteenth-century sources speak of a more or less constant 288 poor people; in 1536 the number was 279. In terms of endowments, Baucells counts 88 places established between

1200 and 1299, 186 for 1300–1399 and 40 in the fifteenth century; the peak period for the establishment of new endowments was the decade 1290–99. Baucells, "Pia Almoina," 102–3. At the end of the fifteenth century, the number of places grew to 288 per day. Josep Baucells, "L'església de Catalunya," *Acta historica et archaeologica mediaevalia* 13 (1992): 433.

35. Batlle, *Urgell medieval*, 123.

36. Sanahuja, *Beneficencia en Lérida*, 84–85; Bertrán, "El menjador," 93–94.

37. Bertrán, "Almoina de la Seu de Lleida," 355; Sanahuja, *Beneficencia en Lérida*, 68–69, 102.

38. Guilleré, "Institution charitable," 329–31; Batlle, *L'expansió baixmedieval*, 255.

39. Sanahuja, *Beneficencia en Lérida*, 71, 114.

40. Josep Baucells i Reig, *El maresme i la Pia Almoina de la Seu de Barcelona: Catàleg del fons en pergamí de l'Arxiu Capitular de la Catedral de Barcelona* (Barcelona, 1987), 27–30.

41. Baucells, "Pia Almoina," 108.

42. Sanahuja, *Beneficencia en Lérida*, 61; Batlle, *Urgell medieval*, 123.

43. Mutgé, *La ciudad de Barcelona*, 34.

44. Baucells, "Pia Almoina," 97, 107–8.

45. See her "La alimentación de los pobres asistados por la Pia Almoina de la catedral de Barcelona según el libro de cuentas de 1283–84," in *Alimentació i societat a la Catalunya medieval* (Barcelona, 1988), 186.

46. Bertrán, "Almoina de la Seu de Lleida," 361–63. Students, particularly in educational centers, were not uncommon recipients of this sort of largesse. In fifteenth-century Valladolid, for example, the monastery of San Benito handed out some ninety meals a day — sixty to beggars and thirty to students: Rucquoi, "Hospitalisation et charité à Valladolid," 396.

47. Sanahuja, *Beneficencia en Lérida*, 80.

48. Bertrán, "Almoina de la Seu de Lleida," 355.

49. Equip Broida, "El àpats funerais segons els testaments vers al 1400," in *Alimentació i societat a la Catalunya medieval* (Barcelona, 1988), 264.

50. Bertrán, "El menjador," 91.

51. Baucells, "Pia Almoina," 102–3.

52. Ibid., 96–98.

53. Bertrán, "El menjador," 93.

54. Guilleré, "Institution charitable," 329–31.

55. Guillem Tor in 1347 left twenty pounds for the repair of the bridge of Sant Esteve, with the stipulation that if the work were not completed within four years that the money be instead given to the Pia Almoina for the distribution of bread to the "poor of Christ." See Batlle, *Urgell medieval*, 124.

56. Agustí Altisent, *L'Almoina reial a la cort de Pere el Cerimoniós. Estudi i edició dels manuscrits de l'almoiner Fra Guillem Deudé, monjo de Poblet (1378–85)* (Abbey of Poblet, 1969), xix–xx, xli–xlii. The kings of Castile did not have a similar royal almoner, although there are instances of such alms, as when Juan I in 1387 ordered that forty poor people be clothed and three hundred be fed (López Alonso, *Pobreza en la España medieval*, 477).

57. Within the Low Countries, "tables of the poor" that were established by parishes also played a prominent role in aiding the poor; see M.-J. Tits-Dievaide, "Les tables des pauvres dans les anciennes principautés belges au Moyen Âge," *Tijdschrift voor geschiedenis* 88 (1975): 562–75. On the general obligation of parishes to provide hospitality to the poor, according to canon law, see Tierney, *Medieval Poor Law*, 75–78.

58. Mollat, *Poor in the Middle Ages*, 141.

59. See wills of 1348 and 1366 in Salvador Vilaseca Anguera, *Hospitales medievals de Reus* (Reus, 1958), 28–29.

60. Santamaría, "Asistencia a los pobres en Mallorca," 391, 400.

61. Junyent, *Vic*, 124; Guilleré, "Charité à Gérone," 195.

62. López Alonso, *Pobreza en la España medieval*, 392–93.

63. Others were located at the parishes of Santa Maria del Pi, Sant Pere de las Puelles, Sant Jaume Apostol, Sant Miquel, Sant Just.

64. Carme Batlle i Gallart, "La ayuda a los pobres en la parroquia de San Justo de Barcelona," in *A pobreza*, 1:65–67. We have this 1344 description of the institution: "Likewise, there is another praiseworthy custom, whereby in each of the seven parish churches of this city certain upright men are chosen each year who have the responsibility of collecting on behalf of the deserving poor, and who distribute in secret what they collect to the deserving poor of the said parochial churches." Quoted in Miguel Pardo Fernández, "'El bací des pobres vergonyants' de la parroquia de Santa María del Mar," *Estudios històrics i documents dels Arxius de Protocols* 8 (1980): 149–53.

65. Joan-F. Cabestany and Salvador Claramunt, "El «Plat des pobres» de la parroquia de Santa María del Pí de Barcelona (1408–1428)," in *A pobreza*, 1:160–71.

66. Ibid., 167, 171. Similar categories of the "shamed" poor have been identified as the principal objects of charity in late medieval Florence: Henderson, *Piety and Charity*, 257, 266, 272, 340, 393.

67. Mutgé, *La ciudad de Barcelona*, 42–44; Batlle, *L'expansió baixmedieval*, 288, 424.

68. The poorer neighborhoods are identified by their lack of prominent residents, or of artisan families, churches, and religious or municipal structures. See Salvador Claramunt, "Una primera aproximación para establecer un plano de la pobreza vergonzante en el arrabal de la Rambla, de Barcelona, a lo largo del siglo XV," in *La pobreza*, 2:380–82.

69. For example, there are accounts from Santa Maria del Pi from 1401, 1402, 1423, and 1428; and from Santa Maria del Mar for 1404, 1416, 1421 and 1425. See Salvador Claramunt, "Los ingresos del «Bací o Plat dels Pobres» de la parroquia de Santa María del Pí de Barcelona, de 1434 a 1456," in *La Pobreza*, 1:373; and Aramayona, "Santa María del Mar," 173.

70. While the giving of pious legacies dates back many centuries, the legal procedures for the disposition of such bequests do not appear in Barcelona until the fourteenth century. Synodal legislation of 1354, which may in fact reflect the reforms of Bishop Ponç de Gualba (1303–34), placed the administration of legacies destined for spiritual uses in the hands of the clergy. Executors were given one year to fulfill the terms of the will, at which time they would have to make an accounting to the

bishop, on penalty of being placed under interdict; for a variety of reasons this goal seems rarely to have been attained. See Utterback, *Pastoral Care*, 70–71, 164–90.

71. The principal risk, it seems, came from currency devaluation that lessened the real value of the return. See ibid., 164–65; Claramunt, "Los ingresos," 374–75, 378–79, 383; Batlle, "San Justo," 69. In Valencia, beginning in 1368, hospitals like En Clapers and La Reyna began to invest endowments in municipal bonds, the *censal de la ciutat*, earning a return between 7.7 and 8.3 percent. See Agustín Rubio Vela, *Pobreza, enfermedad y asistencia hospitalaria en la Valencia del siglo XIV* (Valencia, 1984), 62–63. In fourteenth-century Venice, charitable trusts were strongly encouraged by the municipality to invest in bonds rather than directly in real estate. The government evidently feared that the latter strategy would remove tax-paying property from the rolls and would obligate charities to excessive maintenance expense. In Venice, however, given the interest defaults of the next century, real estate proved to be the better investment. See Brian Pullan, "Houses in Service of the Poor in the Venetian Republic," *Poverty and Charity: Europe, Italy, Venice, 1400–1700* (Aldershot, England), 4.

72. These statistics are all from the first half of the fifteenth century. See Batlle, "San Justo," 71; Claramunt, "Los ingresos," 376; Aramoyona, "Santa María del Mar," 188.

73. Cabestany and Claramunt, "Santa María del Pí," 165.

74. Ibid., 166, 170. This is essentially verified by the more comprehensive studies of charitable confraternities in Florence. Normally, institutions of the Orsanmichele provided the bulk of their assistance to women; in the second quarter of the fourteenth century, two-thirds to three-quarters of all of its clients were women — widows, married women burdened with children, and, after the plague, young women needing dowries. But during the hard times of the mid-fifteenth century organizations like the Buonomini di S. Martino gave the bulk of their alms to men, many poor migrants who had entered the city looking for work. See Henderson, *Piety and Charity*, 260–61, 288, 340, 384, 388–89, 399.

75. For example, it is reported that King Joan II in 1478, when he was in his eighties, awoke at 5 A.M., ate between 8 and 9 A.M., supped at 6 P.M. and went to bed around 10 P.M. Salvador Claramunt, "Dos aspectos de l'alimentació medieval: Dels canonges a les «miserabiles personae»," in *Alimentació*, 171. A study of Castilian peasants reflects a similar pattern, two meals a day — in the morning and the evening — although in places this increased to three in the summer, particularly during the harvest. See: P. Martínez Sopena and María J. Carbajo Serrano, "L'alimentation des paysans castillans du XIᵉ au XIIIᵉ siècle d'après les «fueros»," in *Manger et boire au Moyen Âge: Actes du colloque de Nice* (Nice, 1984), 1:340.

76. The Rule of the Hospitaller Order of the Holy Spirit, interestingly, permitted members to eat twice a day (but no more); in speaking of the *hora prandii pauperum*, however, it suggests that the poor were fed but once. "Regula ordinis S. Spiritus de Saxia," *Patrologiae cursus completus, series latina* (hereafter, *PL*), ed. Jacques-Paul Migne (Paris, 1844–85) 217:1141, caps. 10, 13.

77. The fifteen holidays were Christmas, New Year, Epiphany, Candlemas, the Annunciation, Easter, Ascension Thursday, Pentecost, Corpus Christi, Saint John the Baptist in June, Santa Margarita, Marian feasts in August and September, All

Saints, and Sant Llàtzer. See Aurora Pérez Santamaría, "El hospital de San Lázaro o Casa dels Malalts o Masells," in *La pobreza*, 1:111–12. Sant Macià served wine, salsa, honey, dove, fowl, pork, and other foods that were donated by the hospital's rural tenants. See Roca, *Sant Macià*, 10.

78. Rubio Vela, *Pobreza, enfermedad y asistencia*, 142–43.

79. Bertrán, "El menjador," 95. French calendar iconography of the twelfth and thirteenth centuries shows peasants eating bread shaped into large and small round loaves. See P. Mane, "L'alimentation des paysans en France et en Italie aux XIIᵉ and XIIIᵉ siècles à travers l'iconographie des calendriers (sculpture, fresques, mosaïques et vitrail)," in *Manger et boire au Moyen Âge: Actes du colloque de Nice* (Nice, 1984), 1: 321; Mutgé, *La ciudad de Barcelona*, 30.

80. Bertrán, "El menjador," 96; Batlle, *Urgell medieval*, 125.

81. Fifteenth-century sources rarely mention rye; this study concludes that wheat bread predominated. See María del Carmen Carlé, "Alimentación y abastecimiento," *Cuadernos de historia de España*, 61–62 (1977): 255–56.

82. The disease is caused by ergot, a fungus that infests grain such as rye and produces a toxin that attacks the circulatory and nervous system. It is not destroyed by baking or cooking, although it does produce a bad taste. The disease is manifested by the swelling and blackening of the feet, leading to gangrene, and accompanied by prolonged and excruciating pain.

83. Echániz, "Alimentación de los pobres," 179; Guilleré, *Girona medieval*, 89.

84. Guilleré, "Institution charitable," 331; Bertrán, "El menjador," 106; Baucells, "Pia Almoina," 110. By comparison, the Hospital del Rey in fifteenth-century Burgos served pilgrims and its sick inmates a loaf of bread made of unsifted flour that weighed about six hundred grams, called a *panchón*. See Luis García Martínez, "La asistencia material en los hospitales de Burgos a fines de la Edad Media," in *Manger et boire au Moyen Âge: Actes du colloque de Nice* (Nice, 1984), 1: 335. At Toledo, the confraternity of San Pedro fed poor folk at sites throughout the city on February 2 with a meal that included two loaves of bread weighing 690 grams. See J. P. Molénat, "Menus des pauvres, menus des confrères à Tolède dans la deuxième moitié du XVᵉ siècle," in *Manger et boire au Moyen Âge: Actes du colloque de Nice* (Nice, 1984), 1:316. Carme Batlle i Gallart, *L'assistència als pobres a la Barcelona medieval (s. XIII)* (Barcelona, 1987), 51. For example, a study from Provence suggests a daily diet of closer to one thousand grams; privileged consumers like the residents of the Spanish college at the University of Bologna ate approximately double that amount. Rubio Vela, *Pobreza, enfermedad y asistencia*, 145–47.

85. Bertrán's estimate is that the 715 grams of bread at Lleida provided 1,861 of the 2,372.9 calories provided per day in his sample week: see his "El menjador," 106; Echániz, "Alimentación de Barcelona de 1283–1284," 185. Loaves at Girona were to weigh 800 grams, but these presumably were to be shared four ways: Guilleré, *Girona medieval*, 89.

86. Leo Moulin, more broadly, has estimated that inmates of medieval religious houses of average wealth ate between 1.5 and 2 kilograms of bread per day, much more than either the Catalan poor or the canons from Lleida seem to have enjoyed (Claramunt, "Dos aspectos," 167–69).

87. In more northern latitudes, the wine would be substituted with beer or ale;

at Saint Leonard's of York in 1287, the ration amounted to a half gallon of beer, with a like amount as an extra portion on feast days (Cullum, *Cremetts and Corrodies*, 16).

88. Echániz, "Alimentación de los pobres," 179–80; Baucells, "Pia Almoina," 110; Bertrán, "El menjador," 97–98, 107; Batlle, *L'assistència*, 51.

89. Molénat, "Menus des pauvres," 314. Bertrán estimates that the fourteenth and fifteenth centuries average daily consumption of wine was one to two liters ("El menjador," 98). Martínez García contrasts the .75 liter given to the poor with the 4 liters allotted to the brothers of the Hospital del Rey ("Asistencia material," 353). Lleida's canons in 1168 were allocated 1.3 liters per day, close to Leo Moulin's estimate of 1.5 liters for the average religious in medieval Europe. See Claramunt, "Dos aspectos," 168–69. and Rubio Vela, *Pobreza, enfermedad y asistencia Valencia*, 147.

90. The consumption of meat was also a statement of religious orthodoxy, particularly since groups like the Albigensians, who were present in Catalonia, forbade meat and all dairy products to their adherents. See Josep Hernando, "Els moralistes i l'alimentació a la Baixa Edat Mitjana," in *Alimentació*, 276. The records of the leper hospital of Sant Llàtzer in Barcelona show that the typical quantity of meat purchased was a half pound, for an inmate population and staff that numbered perhaps two dozen. Surely, here at least, the meat was little more than a flavoring agent in some sort of stew of beans and/or vegetables (Pérez Santamaría, "San Lázaro," 100).

91. Guilleré, *Girona medieval*, 22.

92. Bertrán, "El menjador," 99; Echániz, "Alimentación de los pobres," 180.

93. Claramunt, "Dos aspectos," 168.

94. Bertrán, "El menjador," 99–101; Echániz, "Alimentación de los pobres," 180–81; Martínez and Carbajo, "L'alimentation des paysans castillans," 1:339. The confraternity of San Pedro at Toledo in the late fifteenth century served the poor exclusively beef, reserving mutton for the sick. But the beef was undoubtedly from old cows, since it served its own members veal stew and roasted chicken (Molénat, "Menus des pauvres," 315, 317). Only in the early fourteenth century did municipal legislation address the problem of diseased meat; Barcelona enacted an ordinance against its sale in 1301, Valencia in 1295, and Lleida in 1340. See Michael McVaugh, *Medicine before the Plague: Practitioners and Their Patients in the Crown of Aragon, 1285–1345* (Cambridge, 1993), 226.

95. While the *almoina* at Lleida served no poultry, the records of the visitation made by the commander of Gardeny in 1409 show 13.9 percent of his meals to have contained poultry (chicken, partridge, capon, or turkey): Bertrán, "El menjador," 101. In Castile, chicken was considered a luxury food everywhere except Galicia and Asturias. Sumptuary laws forbade its consumption at feasts except for those of confraternities, ecclesiastical chapters and important people; the giving of chickens as charity, on the other hand, was encouraged (Carlé, "Alimentación y abastecimiento," 270). As to price, in Barcelona in 1331, lamb, veal, and fresh pork sold for eight diners per pound, ham for seven diners; ox, cow, or mutton for six diners. Meat with off smells could command no more than five diners. By contrast, chickens cost one sou each and capons 2.6 sous. Butchers who specialized in the meat of diseased or damaged animals were grouped together at the meat market located near the Boquería gate (Mutgé, *La ciudad de Barcelona*, 21–24).

96. Like the Catalan establishments, the hospital at Burgos served mostly mutton, although chicken was given to the sick (Martínez García, "Asistencia material," 355). In 1494–98, the confraternity of San Pedro at Toledo gave out a much more generous portion: 759 grams of beef and another 50 grams of different meat; but this meal was intended as a feast, not a normal meal (Molénat, "Menus des pauvres," 315). By contrast, wealthy consumers like the canons of Lleida were served three meats at special meals, with one sheep for each ten canons, a large ham for each dozen canons, a cow for each twenty-four, a large duck for each four or a young duck for each two, a year-old hen to be shared by two canons, and a younger hen allotted each participant (Claramunt, "Dos aspectos," 169).

97. This estimate is based on the price of bad meat at five diners to the pound, and the *òbol* or half penny that was at times given to the poor in lieu of a meat or fish course. For Desvilar, see Batlle, *L'assistència*, 51.

98. In 1329, a half diner (or *òbol*) would purchase a quarter pound of the cheapest fish, dolphin, or tuna. Sea bass and sardines cost four diners per pound. Mullet at six diners and sturgeon at eight diners were certainly out of reach for the poor (Mutgé, *La ciudad de Barcelona*, 20).

99. Bertrán, "El menjador," 102, 109; Echániz, "Alimentación de los pobres," 181; Baucells, "Pia Almoina," 110.

100. Bertrán, "El menjador," 102; Martínez García, "Asistencia material," 355.

101. There is no mention of eggs as a menu item at Lleida (Bertrán, "El menjador," 106). At Barcelona, cheese was the main course for 12 percent of the meals, eggs for 2 percent (Echániz, "Alimentación de los pobres," 182). Portions for the canons of Lleida in 1168 were specified at five eggs and three large pieces of cheese on Mondays, Wednesdays, Fridays, and Saturdays; Leo Moulin, on the other hand, estimates that medieval religious typically ate between 70 and 111 grams of cheese at a meal, a portion close to that served to the poor (Claramunt, "Dos aspectos," 168–69). On fast days at the Hospital of Pere Desvilar in Barcelona, the poor were to be given fish, cheese, or eggs at the cost of one diner (Batlle, *L'assistència*, 51). Synodal regulations at Barcelona (1354) recommended that all the faithful should eat cheese and eggs on days of abstinence (Utterback, *Pastoral Care*, 66).

102. Juan Ruiz, *The Book of True Love,* trans. Saralyn R. Daly, ed. Anthony Z. Zahareas (University Park, Pa., 1978), 299, verses 1162–69.

103. See McVaugh, *Medicine before the Plague,* 147.

104. Echániz, "Alimentación de los pobres," 182–83; Bertrán, "El menjador," 103–5. It seems that vegetables were only slowly introduced in the diet. Sources before 1200 rarely mention anything beyond garlic, onions, and colewort, but at Avila in the thirteenth century, for example, the chapter is recorded to have received leeks, garlic, onions, vetches (as fodder for animals), and garbanzos, and later asparagus, spinach, lentils, and beans (Carlé, "Alimentación y abastecimiento," 254, 273–74). See also Rubio Vela, *Pobreza, enfermedad y asistencia*, 83.

105. Echániz, "Alimentación de los pobres," 184–85; Bertrán, "El menjador," 107–9; Claramunt, "Dos aspectos," 169. Girona's bread allotment has been estimated to have provided only a quarter of the calories needed by the poor (Guilleré, "Institution charitable," 331).

106. Cullum, *Cremetts and Corrodies*, 17.

Chapter 3. The Origins of Hospices and Hospitals

1. The Rule of Benedict states: "All guests who present themselves are to be welcomed as Christ. . . . The kitchen for the abbot and guests ought to be separate, so that guests — monasteries are never without them — need not disturb the brothers when they present themselves at unpredictable hours. . . . The guest quarters are to be entrusted to a God-fearing brother. Adequate bedding should be available there." *RB 1980: The Rule of St. Benedict*, ed. Timothy Fry (Collegeville, Minn., 1981), 53.1,16, 21, 255–59. The Spanish Rules of San Fructuoso and Isidore of Seville mandated that a third of monastic goods be reserved for the poor. The Benedictine Rule called upon the monastic porter to welcome all regardless of class, but by the ninth century this function was frequently divided between a *limosnero* who welcomed the poor, and a *custos hospitum* who had charge of those of higher estate (López Alonso, *Pobreza en la España medieval*, 421–23).

2. For a general discussion of the functions of early hospitals, see Timothy S. Miller, "The Knights of Saint John and the Hospitals of the Latin West," *Speculum* 53 (1978): 709–17.

3. Gregorio del Ser Quijano, "Algunos aspectos de la caridad asistencial altomedieval. Los primeros hospitales de la ciudad de León," *Studia historica* 3 (1985): 160. The earliest reference to pilgrims in Aragonese documentation was an exemption from customs duty given them by Sancho Ramírez (1076–94) (Ubieto Arteta, "Pobres y marginados," 17).

4. López Alonso, *Pobreza en la España medieval*, 410–13; Gérard Jugnot, "Deux fondations augustiniennes en faveur des pèlerins: Aubrac et Roncevaux," in *Assistance et charité* (Toulouse, 1978), 323; Narciso Hergueta, "Noticias históricas del maestre Diego de Villar . . . , de los hospitales y hospederías en la Rioja en los siglos XII y XIII, y de la villa de Villar de Torre," *Revista de Archivos, Bibliotecas y Museos* 11 (1904): 433; Ubieto Arteta, "Pobres y marginados," 18; Antonio Durán Gudiol, *El hospital de Somport entre Aragón y Béarn* (Saragossa, 1986).

5. Martínez Garcia, "Asistencia material," 1:349–50; Ser Quijano, "Primeros hospitales," 161ff.

6. López Alonso, *Pobreza en la España medieval*, 449.

7. Juan Ignacio Carmona García, *El sistema de hospitalidad publica en la Sevilla del antiguo Regimen* (Seville, 1979), 26, 49–51. Rucquoi, "Hospitalisation et charité," 399–400.

8. García del Moral, *Hospital Mayor*, 39.

9. Rubio Vela, *Pobreza, enfermedad y asistencia*, 29–30, 41; Mercedes Gallent Marco, "Aproximación a un modelo medieval de institución sanitaria: el Hospital de la Reyna," *Saitabi* 31 (1981): 76; José Sanchez Herrero, "Cofradías, hospitales y beneficencia en algunes diócesis del valle del Duero, siglos XIV y XV," *Hispania* 34, no. 126 (1974): 34.

10. C. A. Ferreira de Almeida, "Os caminhos e a assistência no norte de Portugal," *A pobreza*, 51–52.

11. Geremek, *Margins of Society*, 169–75; Jacqueline Caille, "Assistance et hospitalité au Moyen Âge," *Bulletin de la Société des Études Littéraires, Scientifiques et Artistiques du Lot* 102 (1981): 297.

12. Villani is cited in George Rosen, "The Hospital: Historical Sociology of a Community Institution," in *The Hospital in Modern Society*, ed. Eliot Freidson (New York, 1963), 9. Henderson's recent study counts thirty-three Florentine hospitals in the fifteenth century; see his *Piety and Charity*, 375. Pullan, "Support and Redeem," 5:188.

13. Bonenfant, "Hôpitaux et bienfaisance," 13–15.

14. Edward J. Kealey, *Medieval Medicus: A Social History of Anglo-Norman Medicine* (Baltimore, 1981), 83.

15. Joan-Albert Adell i Gisbert, "L'hospital de pobres de Santa Magdalena de Montblanc i l'arquitectura hospitalària medieval a Catalunya," *Acta historica et archaelogica mediaevalia* 4 (1983): 240.

16. Manuel Riu, "Presentación," in *La pobreza*, 1:10–11; Junyent, *Vic*, 404; Martinell, "Hospitals medievals catalans," 110–12; Sanahuja, *Beneficencia en Lérida*, 28.

17. One estimate counts 113 hospitals in England in 1154, and 700 in the fourteenth century, excluding monastic *infirmaria* and the many small institutions for which no documentary evidence survives. Of these twenty-one were established prior to the twelfth century; ninety-two others date from 1100–1154 (Kealey, *Medieval Medicus*, 83).

18. Documents from the territory of Roda in Aragon use names like *limosnas*, *pías almoines*, *limosnerías*, *hostalet*, and *hospitalet* to describe such shelters; similar terms were commonly found elsewhere as well. See Francisco Castillón Cortada, "El limosnero de la catedral de Roda de Isábena (Huesca)," *Cuadernos de Aragón* 21 (1990): 66.

19. Catalonia, lying within the Carolingian sphere of influence, may have responded to the decree of the Council of Aachen (816), which decreed that shelters for the poor be established by cathedral chapters and other religious communities. Elsewhere in the Carolingian world such hospices began to appear between the ninth and eleventh centuries (Rosen, "Historical Sociology," 7).

20. Baucells, "Pia Almoina," 84–86; Batlle and Casas, "Caritat privada," 1:121–22; Tómas Sivilla, "Apuntos históricos sobre el hospital de Barcelona," *Memorias de la Academia de Buenas Letras de Barcelona* 3 (1880): 48–50. Legacies for this hospice are extant for 995, 1011, 1038, 1077, 1082, 1087, and 1092. See Pierre Bonnassie, *La Catalogne du milieu du Xe à la fin du XIe siècle, croissance et mutations d'une société* (Toulouse, 1975–77), 172, 304, 955–56. See also Batlle, *L'assistència*, 28. On the wealth of the Barcelona church, see Bensch, *Barcelona*, 50–53. The clerical obligation to donate bedding persisted until at least the mid-fourteenth century to judge by a suit brought by the cathedral hospital against the estate of a deceased canon in 1349. See Richard Gyug, *The Diocese of Barcelona during the Black Death: The Register Notule Communium 15 (1348–1349)* (Toronto, 1994), 341, no. 905.

21. There is evidence that a couple, Pere Prim and his wife, had already been using one of the small houses on the property as a shelter for the indigent sick. See Dolors Pifarré Torres, "Dos visitas de comienzos del siglo XIV a los hospitales barceloneses d'en Colom y d'en Marcús," in *La pobreza*, 2: 83; Batlle, *L'assistència*, 29–34; Bensch, *Barcelona*, 36.

22. For example, in 1286 Guillem Ribau, a nonresident of Barcelona, died here, and with enough possessions to make a will (Batlle, *L'assistència*, 23, 41).

23. Batlle and Casas, "Caritat privada," 1:123–32, 168–71, no. 3; Pifarré, "Dos visitas," 2: 84–89; Batlle, *L'assistència*, 42, 44. There are many examples elsewhere in Europe of assistance, in the form of room and board, being given to students. See Rosalina Manno Tolu, "La «Domus pauperum scolarium Italorum» a Parigi nel 1334," *Archivo Storico Italiano* 146 (1988): 49–56.

24. This was established in 1396 by Pere Bou, a member of a Valencian burgher family: Rubio Vela, *Pobreza en la Valencia*, 38–39, 46. The Crown of Aragon, however, generally did not have the sort of specialized shelters that appeared in Italian municipalities like Florence, which had institutions that served specific trade groups like porters (San Giovanni Decollato), dyers (Sant'Onofrio), and shoemakers (Santissima Trinità). See Katherine Park, "Healing the Poor: Hospitals and Medical Assistance in Rensaissance Florence," in *Medicine and Charity before the Welfare State*, ed. Jonathan Barry and Colin Jones (London, 1991), 31.

25. Batlle and Casas, "Caritat privada," 1:132–35; for Pere Desvilar's will, see 171–73, no. 4.

26. Ibid., 1:176–78, no. 6.

27. The family, as owner of extensive lands in the city's suburbs, farms and gardens in the surrounding region, and a share of the royal mint, was Barcelona's wealthiest. Bernat's son, also named Bernat, received in 1178 the office of *mostolaf* from King Alfons I, which gave him exclusive right to exchange Muslim and Christian captives, a license for which he was willing to pay the king five hundred sous of Barcelona: Stephen P. Bensch, "From Prizes of War to Domestic Merchandise: The Changing Face of Slavery in Catalonia and Aragon, 1000–1300," *Viator* 25 (1994): 73, 87; Bensch, *Barcelona*, 162–63.

28. Batlle and Casas, "Caritat privada," 1:137–41; Pifarré, "Dos visitas," 2:83–90; Batlle, *L'assistència*, 52–59.

29. For the Hospital of En Clapers, see Rubio Vela, *Pobreza, enfermedad y asistencia*, 25–26, 41.

30. Batlle and Casas, "Caritat privada," 1:135–37, 178–80, no.7; Batlle, *L'assistència*, 51. In 1348, the hospital had two administrators; a priest in that year was given the benefice in the chapel of Santa Marta upon nomination of Romeus Lulli, a *conseller* of the city (Gyug, *Diocese of Barcelona*, 87, no. 27, 164, no. 298).

31. For the documents of 1210, 1213, 1221, and 1237, see Lluís G. Feliu, "L'hospital de Santa Eulàlia del Camp," *Analecta sacra Terraconensia* 11 (1935): 299–305.

32. Batlle and Casas, "Caritat privada," 1:141–44; Feliu, "Santa Eulàlia del Camp," 291–306; Batlle, *L'assistència*, 60–64.

33. Martinell, "Hospitals medievals catalans," 120.

34. Ibid., 112–13; Gyug, *Diocese of Barcelona*, 363, no. 966.

35. Baucells, "Pia Almoina," 1:79–80.

36. Josep Danon, *Visió històrica de l'Hospital General de Santa Creu de Barcelona* (Barcelona, 1978), 17.

37. Ignasi Aragó, *Els hospitals a Catalunya* (Barcelona, 1967), 174.

38. A. Cardoner Planes, "El 'hospital para judios pobres' de Barcelona," *Sefarad* 22 (1962): 373–75; Batlle and Casas, "Caritat privada," 1:147–49; Abraham A.

Neuman, *The Jews in Spain: Their Social, Political and Cultural Life during the Middle Ages* (New York, 1969), 2:163.

39. Nùria Coll Julià, "Documentación notarial relativa a los pobres en la Cataluña del siglo XV," in *La pobreza*, 2:294–96. Barcelona had no equivalent of Paris's Quinze-Vingts, a hospice established by Saint Louis that housed three hundred blind persons born in Paris (Geremek, *Margins of Society*, 172–73). Kings Pere the Ceremonious, in 1353, and Martí, 1408, did attempt to restrict the blind and other physically handicapped individuals to certain sections of Barcelona (Vinyoles, *Vida quotidiana*, 119). For examples of material assistance rendered by confraternities at Valladolid to members and their families, see Rucquoi, "Hospitalisation et charité," 397–98.

40. Fermín Hernández Iglesias ties the establishment of hospitals in the eleventh century to the construction of bridges and the development of pilgrim traffic to sites like Santiago de Compostela. Bishop Ermengol of Urgell, for example, constructed a bridge over the Segre. See his *Beneficencia en España*, 1:16. The earliest legacy for the poor that is extant here dates from 1048, with others from 1068, 1084, and 1092/3 (Bonnaissie, *Catalogne*, 955–56).

41. Batlle, *Urgell medieval*, 108–18; B. Marquès, "Fundació d'un hospital a Organyà en 1156," *Església d'Urgell* 108 (1982): 7–8.

42. Batlle, *Urgell medieval*, 126–32.

43. In England, at least three such hospices were in operation in the thirteenth century, and in 1312 what turned out to be the largest, to house a dozen clerics, was established by the bishop of Exeter. See Nicholas Orme, "Medieval Almshouse for the Clergy: Clyst Gabriel Hospital near Exeter," *Journal of Ecclesiastical History* 39 (1988): 1–3. Fourteenth-century Valencia had its Hospital of Poor Priests, established before 1356 by the cathedral's confraternity of Santa Maria, and, in addition, the hospital of En Bou served the clergy; on Majorca, a will of 1475 endowed the Hospital of Sant Pere and Sant Bernat for indigent priests. See Rubio Vela, *Pobreza, enfermedad y asistencia*, 35, 46; and Santamaría, "Asistencia a los pobres en Mallorca," 387.

44. Batlle, *Urgell medieval*, 137–38.

45. The election took place on Christmas Eve before 1440, when it was moved to New Year's Day (Batlle, *Urgell medieval*, 149–50).

46. Coll Julià, "Documentación notarial," 2:287–94.

47. Sanahuja dates the old hospital, which he calls the Hospital de Sacerdotes, from the twelfth century; see his *Beneficencia en Lérida*, 28. See also Bonnassie, *Catalogne*, 955–56.

48. The hospitaller had to remember the anniversaries of some sixty priests and distribute alms to the poor in remembrance of several others. Additional support almost certainly came from alms, since in 1321 the hospitaller was obliged to distribute coins in remembrance of one Guillem de Lafone and to observe other anniversaries. Batlle Prats, "Inventari dels Bens," 55–60.

49. Guilleré, *Girona medieval*, 89. Of the seventy-three testaments studied for the decade 1320–30, 40 percent contained legacies for the new hospital, but only 10 percent for the episcopal establishment (Guilleré, "Charité à Gérone," 1:197–99). The reforms of the previous decade or the worsened conditions after 1330 resulted in

even greater support for the new hospital. It was remembered in 60 percent of the wills that survive from the years 1330–47, in 67 percent of those from 1348, the year of the plague. At the same time, approximately a fifth of wills redacted in the countryside also contributed to the hospital (Guilleré, "La peste noire à Gerone," 52).

50. Maria-Mercè Costa i Paretas, "Els antics ponts de Girona," *Anales del instituto de Estudios Gerundenses* 22 (1974–75): 139–40.

51. Bonnassie, *Catalogne*, 955–56; Danon, *Visió històrica*, 17.

52. Junyent, *Vic*, 87–88, 124; Martinell, "Hospitals medievals catalans," 115, 122–23; Ollich, "Les entitats eclesiastiques de Vic," 92–93; Sanahuja, *Beneficencia en Lérida*, 28–29.

53. Castillón, "Limosnero de la catedral de Roda," 63.

54. José Fernando Tarragó Valentines, *Hospitales en Lérida durante los siglos XII al XVI* (Lérida, 1975), 19–21, 72–74; José Trenchs Odena and Federico Lara Peinado, "La casa de caridad y la cofradia de los clerigos pobres, dos instituciones medievales leridanas," *Ilerda* 36 (1975): 8–17. Similarly, in the early thirteenth century the monks of the Cistercian monastery of Grandselve transformed a hospital that had been given them within the city of Toulouse into a residence for traveling monks. See John H. Mundy, "Charity and Social Work in Toulouse, 1100–1250," *Traditio* 22 (1966): 213–15.

55. Tarragó, *Lérida*, 22–24. The provisions of this agreement seem to exclude from any right of burial a secular oblate, that is, a benefactor who in return for monetary donation would be granted status as a religious of the house. See Josep Ferran Tarragó i Valentines, *Noves aportacions a l'historia dels antics hospitals de Lleida* (Lleida, 1977), 7–9.

56. Tarragó, *Lérida*, 24–29; Federico Lara Peinado and José Trenchs Odena, "Documento inedito sobre la venta del Hospital de Pedro Moliner de la ciudad de Lerida (1459)," *Ilerda*, 37 (1976): 59–68.

57. Tarragó, *Lérida*, 45, 48.

58. Ibid., 39, 44, 47. The first documents referring to the latter two are of the early thirteenth century (Tarragó, *Noves aportacions*, 12, 14, 18, 21).

59. Tarragó, *Lérida*, 69.

60. The Trinitarians were required to maintain a chantry in the see of Lleida, with the obligation to be enforced by the chapter. Gerald, on the other hand, consented to the requirements of the Trinitarian Rule that divided all income into three parts — for maintenance, for the poor, and for the ransoming of captives. Tarragó, *Noves aportacions*, 16–18; Arxiu de la Corona d'Aragó (hereafter, ACA), Gran Priorat, pergs., arm. 28, no. 264.

61. Tarragó, *Noves aportacions*, 18.

62. Tarragó, *Lérida*, 30, 58–60, 65–66; Josep Lladonosa i Pujol, *La pediatria als antics hospicis de Lleida* (Lleida, 1978), 8.

63. Augustí Duran i Sanpere, *Llibre de Cervera* (Barcelona, 1977), 213–14, 223–24; Danon, *Visió històrica*, 16.

64. César Martinell, "L'antic hospital de Santa Tecla, de Tarragona," *Butlleti arqueologic* 3, no. 49 (1934): 390–96. See also José María Miquel Parellada and José Sánchez Real, *Los hospitales de Tarragona* (Tarragona, 1959), 24–43, 149–51; and Martinell, "Hospitals medievals catalans," 116–18.

65. Martinell, "Hospitals medievals catalans," 121.
66. Danon, *Visió històrica*, 16.
67. E. Fort i Cogul, "Sant Bernat Calvó i l'Hospital de Pobres de Santes Creus," *Miscel.lània Història Catalana: Homenatge al Pare Jaume Finestres, Historiador de Poblet* (Abbey of Poblet, 1970), 181–213.
68. Adell i Gisbert, "Montblanc," 240, 244–54.
69. Martinell, "Hospitals medievals catalans," 127.
70. The hospitallers in 1329 and 1339 were Guillem Cayró and Ferrera, his wife. In 1368 Pere de Bellvy and his wife Geralda directed the hospital; the same pattern holds true for the fifteenth century. See Vilaseca, *Hospitales medievals de Reus*, 26–29, 33, 38, 60–61.
71. Ibid., 52, 55, 65.
72. Bayerri, *Historia de Tortosa*, 7:579–82; Marc-Aureli Vila i Comaposada, *Tortosa al segle XIII: vida i costums dels tortosins* (Barcelona, 1986), 115. A will of 1183 bequeaths 2 morabetins each to the infirm of Tortosa, and to the Hospital of the Poor. See L. Pagarolas, *La comanda del Temple de Tortosa* (Tortosa, 1984), 255–56, no. 80.
73. Pablo Cateura Bennasser, *Sobre la fundación y dotación del Hospital de San Andrés, en la Ciudad de Mallorca, por Nuño Sans* (Palma, 1980), 16–22.
74. Santamaría, "Asistencia a los pobres en Mallorca," 385, 399.
75. Pons, *Judios del reino*, 2:126, 134–35. Santamaría gives 1387 as the date for the endowment of Sayt Mill's foundation: "Asistencia a los pobres en la Mallorca," 387.
76. For an overview of Valencian hospitals in the thirteenth century, see Burns, *Crusader Kingdom*, 1:188, 237–43, 282–94.
77. Rubio Vela, *Pobreza, enfermedad y asistencia*, 25–47; Jill R.Webster, *Els Menorets: The Franciscans in the Realms of Aragon from Saint Francis to the Black Death* (Toronto, 1993), 94–96.
78. Vicente Pons Alós, *El archivo histórico del Hospital "Major de Pobres" de Xàtiva: Catálogo y estudio* (Valencia, 1987), 10–16; *Llibre del Repartiment de València*, ed. Antoni Ferrando i Francés (Valencia, 1979), 290, no. 3048.
79. Luis Revest Corzo, *Hospitales y pobres en el Castellón de otros tiempos* (Castellón de la Plana, 1947), 16–37.
80. Rubio Vela, *Pobreza, enfermedad y asistencia*, 136.
81. A recent study of the expense accounts of the small fleet that protected the waters off the island of Majorca during the first half of the fourteenth century, for example, shows that sailors were regularly housed in private homes, hostels and taverns, some large enough to accommodate as many as one or two dozen boarders. See Gabriel Llompart, "La hostelería mallorquina en el siglo XIV," in *XIII Congrés d'història de la Corona d'Aragó, Comunicacions* (Palma de Mallorca, 1990), 2:83–93.

Chapter 4. Hospitals and Hospitallers

1. Batlle, *L'assistència*, 36–37.
2. Ibid., 50–51. A similar situation prevailed at Valencia where Bernat dez

Clapers entrusted the task of nominating the administrator and chaplains of his eponymous hospital, after the death of his executors, to the *jurats* of Valencia (Rubio Vela, *Pobreza, enfermedad y asistencia*, 107–8).

3. Coll Julià, "Documentación notarial," 2:287–89.

4. In the instance of Bertran's heirs, control of his hospital, which had been established circa 1325, was transferred to the town council (Danon, *Visió històrica*, 17).

5. For a discussion of this at Toulouse, see Mundy, "Charity and Social Work in Toulouse," 240–46; see also Rosen, "Historical Sociology," 12. Of the more than twenty hospitals and hospices identified in the Kingdom of Valencia circa 1300, all but Valencia City's leprosarium fell under some sort of ecclesiastical control; the fourteenth century was characterized by municipal and laic initiatives. See Luis García Ballester, *La medicina a la València medieval: Medicina i societat en un país medieval mediterrani* (Valencia, 1988), 111–12. An example of a mixed regime would be that of Valencia's Hospital of Sant Vicent, operated by Cistercian monks under royal patronage, but subject after 1370 to visitations by delegates of the municipal council. The city council itself directed only the leprosarium in 1300, but by 1400 had added three other institutions. One of these was the Hospital of En Clapers, whose administrator was appointed by the *jurats* and who had to render account to the council twice a year. Furthermore, the founder requested, but did not require, the *jurats* to check once a week that the sick were being properly cared for. See Rubio Vela, *Pobreza, enfermedad y asistencia*, 51–52, 54, 108–10.

6. In Barcelona, by the fourteenth century, the power of appointment was in fact exercised by the bishop's vicar general, as a document of January 8, 1349, naming Bernat Domenge as administrator of the Hospital of Santa Maria de Bonesvalls (Cervelló) makes clear (Gyug, *Diocese of Barcelona*, 241, n. 576).

7. Rubio Vela, *Pobreza, enfermedad y asistencia*, 39–43. Philip Gavitt, in his study of Florentine hospitals, essentially comes to a similar conclusion, but places the shift from a religious to a secular emphasis in the late fourteenth century. He notes, for example, that testators now turned to guilds or the commune to realize their charitable objectives, not to churchmen. See his *Charity and Children in Renaissance Florence: The Ospedale degli Innocenti, 1410–1536* (Ann Arbor, Mich., 1990), 18.

8. The administrators, as they were called, were chosen for two-year terms on the feast of the Holy Cross in May, with one cleric and one citizen chosen each year. See Danon, *Visió històrica*, 21–22. *Ordinacions del Hospital General de la Santa Creu de Barcelona (any MCCCCXVII), Copiades textualment del manuscrit original y prologodes* (hereafter *Ordinacions*), ed. Joseph María Roca (Barcelona, 1920), viii; for Girona, see Guilleré, *Girona al segle XIV*, 1:165. Such sharing of authority was not unique to Catalonia. At Amiens, in the fifteenth century, the master of the Hôtel-Dieu was elected by the town council and then installed by the bishop (Rosen, "Historical Sociology," 14). On the broader issue of lay versus clerical influence over charity, see Andrew Barnes's critique of the secularist thesis: "Poor Relief and Brotherhood," *Journal of Social History* 24 (1991): 603–11.

9. Rosen, "Historical Sociology," 13; Tierney, *Medieval Poor Law*, 86.

10. Pérez Santamaría, "San Lázaro," 1:83–90.

11. Rubio Vela, *Pobreza, enfermedad y asistencia*, 51; 169–70, n. 7.

12. The *racional* or auditor was to review all accounts every six months. Those

found guilty of any impropriety would be liable for any damage done, through the garnishment of their salary, and subject to any other penalty, corporal punishment, or fine levied by the administrators. *Ordinacions*, vi–vii, xxxvii, xlv.

13. "Nos, itaque, Arnaldus, Dei gratia episcopus Barchinone, et capitulum eiusdem, attendentes laudabilem propositum et pie devotionis affectum tui dicti Bernardi Ferrarii comendamus tibi predictum hospitale." Batlle and Casas, "Caritat privada," 1:176–78, no. 6.

14. Amada López de Meneses, "Documentos acerca de la peste negra en los dominios de la Corona de Aragón," *Estudios de la edad media de la Corona de Aragón* 6 (1956): 354–55, no. 75 (June 15, 1349).

15. At Toulouse, *minister* was the preferred term, but *gubernator* and *infirmus* were also used (Mundy, "Charity at Toulouse," 239). At Aix-en-Provence, *commander* was the title of choice in the thirteenth century (Jean Pourrière, *Les Hôpitaux d'Aix-en-Provence au Moyen Âge: XIIIᵉ, XIVᵉ et XVᵉ siècles* [Aix-en-Provence, 1969], 89). A municipal ordinance at Valencia in 1319 mandated that the rector of the municipal leper house serve for two years, while King Alfons III in 1333 gave Miquel Sánchez del Coro a lifetime appointment to the nearby Hospital de la Reyna (Rubio Vela, *Pobreza, enfermedad y asistencia*, 163–65, nos. 1–2). At Girona's Hospital Nou, commanders served indeterminate but lengthy terms. Bonanat Nadal and his wife served, for example, from 1319 to 1331 (Guilleré, *Girona al segle XIV*, 1:166).

16. Batlle, *L'assistència*, 47.

17. J. N. Hillgarth and Guilio Silano, *The Register* NOTULE COMMUNIUM 14 *of the Diocese of Barcelona (1345–1348)* (Toronto, 1983), 184, no. 498; see a similar document in Gyug, *Diocese of Barcelona*, 241 n. 576 (January 8, 1349).

18. Pérez Santamaría, "San Lázaro," 1:84; Guilleré, *Girona al segle XIV*, 1:292.

19. Guilleré, *Girona al segle XIV*, 1:166; *Ordinacions*, viii–xviii.

20. Rubio Vela, *Pobreza, enfermedad y asistencia*, 165.

21. Complaints the rector's regime was ineffective date from 1384 (Tarragó, *Noves Aportacions*, 25–26).

22. *Ordinacions*, xli–xlv.

23. Batlle, *L'assistènica*, 28–29.

24. Batlle Prats, "Inventari dels Bens," 79–80.

25. The new chaplain was obligated to say mass daily for the lepers, hear their confessions, administer to them the other sacraments, bury them in the hospital cemetery, and serve as deputy to the lay administrator (Pérez Santamaría, "San Lázaro," 1:86–87, 90).

26. Rubio Vela, *Pobreza, enfermedad y asistencia*, 192–93, n. 24.

27. The Hospital's confraternity was confirmed by King Martí in 1405. *See Ordinacions*, x–xii; Danon, *Visió històrica*, 158.

28. Rubio Vela, *Pobreza, enfermedad y asistencia*, 112–5. A similar division of responsibility is noted at Valencia's Hospital de la Reyna by the fifteenth century. Batlle, *L'assistència*, 67–69.

29. Batlle, *Urgell medieval*, 126–33.

30. For example, Na Camp, a female attendant, in 1300 and 1301 was paid a salary of sixty-five and seventy sous, plus articles of clothing. In 1379, Na Alamanda,

the porter, received eighty sous, while two of the bread collectors were paid one hundred ten sous, and a third, who had additional duties, was given a hundred twenty sous. See Pérez Santamaría, "San Lázaro," 1:85, 104–5. Hillgarth and Silano, *Register*, 184, no. 498; Sanahuja, *Beneficencia en Lérida*, 75.

31. Batlle, *L'assistència*, 38; Rubio Vela, *Pobreza, enfermedad y asistencia*, 111; Gyug, *Diocese of Barcelona*, 241–42 n. 577; Baucells, "Pia Almoina," 104.

32. Batlle Prats, "Inventari dels Bens," 68–76.

33. See his *Historia occidentalis*, cap. 29, 147.

34. In the Italian municipal hospital of Brescia in the 16th century, for example, many members of the staff had been children of the house, including the goatherd and the porters. See Brian Pullan, "Orphans and foundlings in early modern Europe," in *Poverty and Charity*, 3:23.

35. The Order of the Holy Spirit, for example, is estimated to have had fourteen establishments throughout Iberia in the thirteenth century, growing to thirty during the next two centuries. See B. Rano, "Ospitalieri di Santo Spirito," *Dizionario degli istituti di perfezione* (hereafter, *DIP*), 6:1005. In the thirteenth century, the Trinitarians had perhaps ten hospitals in Iberia, of which three were in Catalonia (Lleida, Tortosa, and Anglesola) and another in Valencia city. See James W. Brodman, "The Trinitarian and Mercedarian Orders: A Study in Religious Redemptionism in the Thirteenth Century" (Ph.D.dissertation, University of Virginia, 1974), 211–29. Mercedarian hospitals, really hospices for recently ransomed captives, were found in Catalonia (Barcelona, Montblanc), Aragon (Saragossa, Sarrión, Huesca, Teruel), Valencia (Valencia City, Denia), the Balearics (Palma de Mallorca), and Occitania (Maleville). See James William Brodman, *Ransoming Captives in Crusader Spain: The Order of Merced on the Christian-Islamic Frontier* (Philadelphia, 1986), 12, 21, 25, 27–28, 30, 35–36, 78. Franciscans were bequeathed funds to operate hospitals in Barcelona and Valencia, although they actually did so only in the latter. They also briefly operated a leprosarium in Tàrrega. See Webster, *Els Menorets*, 94–96, 109.

36. Léon LeGrand, "Les Maisons-Dieu: Leurs Statuts au XIIIᵉ siècle," *Revue des questions historiques* 60 (1896): 104; Miller, "Knights of Saint John," 720.

37. A short version of a rule is contained in Innocent III's grant of June 19, 1204 (*PL* 215:377–80). The articulated code is found in "Regula ordinis S. Spiritus de Saxia," *PL* 217:1138–56. See also P. L. Hug, "Order of the Holy Spirit," in *New Catholic Encyclopedia*, 7:103–4; Rano, "Santo Spirito," *DIP* 6:1002.

38. Batlle, *L'assistència*, 41.

39. For a discussion of the Augustinian Rule in the context of hospitaller communities, see Miller, "Knights of Saint John," 715–16; and *Statuts d'Hôtels-Dieu*, vi–viii.

40. Marquès, "Fundació d'un hospital a Organyà," 7–8.

41. In addition to the chaplain-brothers, there were, in the visitation of 1364, eight sisters who cared for the sick and poor, a number of lay brothers (who in the fifteenth century were replaced with maidservants), four secular chaplains to serve the church and chapels, and a host of lay servants who served as cooks, brewers, laundresses, and so on. Cullum, *Cremetts and Corrodies*, 7.

42. Specifically, members of these communities were to take vows of poverty, chastity, and obedience to the bishop, wear a religious habit, move on to another

place if their numbers exceeded the population of the poor to be assisted, use donated goods for the poor, not for themselves; married couples who entered the community were thenceforth to lead chaste lives in religious habits. *Statuts d'Hôtels-Dieu*, xi–xii, xxiii. See also Miller, "Knights of Saint John," 720–22.

43. For example, the administrator of the hospital, *frare* Jacme Just, was accused of heresy in 1353. Agustín Rubio Vela and Mateu Rodrigo Lizondo, "Els beguins de València en el segle XIV. La seua casa-hospital i els seus llibres," *Miscel.lània Sanchis Guarner* 1 (Valencia, 1984): 330–34.

44. Martínez García, *Hospital del Rey*, 60–61.

45. Durán, *Hospital de Somport*, 60–61, 86–90.

46. Tarragó, *Lérida*, 22–24.

47. Batlle, *L'assistència*, 58.

48. The Hospital of En Marcús, at the same time, had a rector, a *donat*, and two *donatas* (Pifarré, "Dos visitas," 2:84–89).

49. Pérez Santamaría, "San Lázaro," 105–7.

50. Pifarré, "Dos visitas," 2:85–86; Pérez, Santamaría, "San Lázaro," 1:104–13; Gallent Marco, "Hospital de la Reyna," 81–82. At Saint Leonard's in medieval York, the ratio was in the range of five or six to one, but since only eight actually served the inmates, the real ratio was closer to twenty-six to one. See Cullum, *Cremetts and Corrodies*, 8. At En Clapers in 1388, a female servant, Na Dolça, served the sick for no pay (Rubio Vela, *Pobreza, enfermedad y asistencia*, 118).

51. Rubio Vela, *Pobreza, enfermedad y asistencia*, 102. This evidence is corroborated by the experience of Burgos's Hospitals del Rey and San Lucas where the cost of patient care did not exceed fifteen percent of the budget (Martínez García, "Asistencia material," 356).

52. For a discussion of *donats* and the confusion between them and serving brothers/sisters and other inmates, see Mundy, "Charity and Social Work in Toulouse," 267–70. In Florence, where wives were often twenty years older than their husbands, widowed women were known to take religious vows at some sort of charitable institution where, in return for their estates, the hospital would guarantee them employment and care. At the fifteenth-century foundling hospital, such women were known as *commessi*; similar contracts are extant for single men and married couples (Gavitt, *Charity and Children*, 115–16).

53. Antonio Durán Gudiol, *Colección diplomática de la catedral de Huesca* (Saragossa, 1965–69), 2:533–34, no. 560; 497–98, no. 519.

54. Tarragó, *Lérida*, 22–24.

55. Vilaseca, *Hospitales medievals de Reus*, 31–32, 64.

56. Pere's two sons, daughter-in-law, and nephew assented to the arrangement, probably by way of relinquishing their claim to the amount being given Sant Martí (Tarragó, *Noves aportacions*, 14–15). For a discussion of corodies, that is, contracts that exchanged property for care, support, and burial, see Mundy, "Charity and Social Work in Toulouse," 258–65. For Joan Colom, see Batlle, *L'assistència*, 36.

57. Ollich, "Les entitats eclesiastiques de Vic," 97; Junyent, *Vic*, 87–88. Cap. 76 states that such girls would have the choice of service, under the three vows of religion, in which instance they would receive support for life, or else they could choose marriage. "Regula ordinis S. Spiritus," *PL* 217: 1151.

58. In the fourteenth and fifteen centuries, elderly who had children frequently joined their households. On average, Russell's studies suggest that between 1275 and 1450 the elderly represented between 8.5 and 12.5 percent of the population (Josiah C. Russell, "How Many of the Population Were Aged?" in *Aging and the Aged*, 124–25). On the institution of the corodies, see Cullum, *Cremetts and Corrodies*, 8–10, 20–28; on its practice in Florence, see Gavitt, *Charity and Children*, 116.

59. Sankt Nicholaus Spital (1458) in Kues of Germany's Mosel region housed thirty-three men over the age of fifty; Saint Jan's Hospital in Bruges provided rooms for pensioners who had property to give the hospital; but pilgrim hospices like Saint Jacques in Valenciennes specifically excluded the old. Luke Demaitre, "The Care and Extension of Old Age in Medieval Medicine," in *Aging and the Aged*, 13. All in all, the terminology used to describe the inhabitants of hospitals is imprecise. Cullum's study of Saint Leonard's of York, for instance, describes a wide variety of status: serving sisters who tended the poor; corodians and livery-holders who paid for varying levels of care; and livery and corody holders who wore the *habitum sororis*, who for a price were able to dress as the serving sisters and who may or may not have worked alongside them. Furthermore, corodies were priced at a level to enable the hospital to support the inmate for about a decade (Cullum, *Cremetts and Corrodies*, 21, 26–27).

60. For example, female superiors were appointed by the male master. Discipline also displayed a gender bias. Errant sisters were to be punished severely and, if necessary, denounced to the pope and turned over to civil authority. Brothers, however, were to be given several chances at reform, being subject to escalating penalties of prayer, defrocking, and imprisonment, but with the proviso that repentance would bring forgiveness ("Regula ordinis S. Spiritus," *PL*, 217: 1146, 1148–49, 1151, 1154, caps. 42, 62, 67, 80, 99).

61. Cullum, *Cremetts and Corrodies*, 15.

62. Rubio Vela, *Pobreza, enfermedad y asistencia*, 118–19.

63. See his *Historia occidentalis*, 148, cap. 29.

64. The *baciners* who worked for Barcelona's leper hospital, for example, begged at several of the city's churches on Sundays and on major feasts, but on minor feasts went to only one location. Pérez Santamaría, "San Lázaro," 94. López Alonso, *Pobreza en la España medieval*, 466. In general, the custom at Barcelona was to permit alms-seekers of all sorts access to churches on Sundays and feasts, except for those feasts specifically designated for the cathedral building fund, when only collectors from the see could make their appeal. See privileges extended in this regard to the Orders of Roncesvalles, the Holy Spirit and Saint Anthony (Gyug, *Diocese of Barcelona*, 331–32, n. 878; 337, n. 893; 344, n. 913).

65. Batlle, *L'assistència*, 42; Utterback, *Pastoral Care*, 114–15; Roca, *Sant Macià*, 6–7.

66. Tarragó, *Noves aportacions*, 28–29; *Ordinacions*, xvii.

67. *Ordinacions*, xxvi, xlii; Danon, *Visió històrica*, 157. On Majorca, caritative institutions evidently relied on the diligence of executors for the reception of pious legacies. During the plague years, however, when these legacies became difficult to collect, due both to the death of executors and the sudden impoverishment of the testator, the bishop attempted to appoint two priests to claim such gifts until re-

strained by royal intervention. López, "Documentos acerca de la peste negra," 369–70, no. 87 (January 19, 1350).

68. *Ordinacions*, ix–xl; Danon, *Visió històrica*, 57–58.

69. Rubio Vela, *Pobreza, enfermedad y asistencia*, 165.

70. Ibid., 36, 77–78.

71. Bed counts, however, are not always a reliable method for estimating capacity. While hospitals like Valencia's Hospital de la Reyna permitted only one inmate per bed, others allowed as many as two or three in a bed. Gallent Marco, "Hospital de la Reyna," 82.

72. Or, 15 to 23 places per 10,000 of population (García Ballester, *Medicina a la València*, 110). See also Gallent Marco, "Hospital de la Reyna," 82. In contrast, modern authorities recommend just for medical care upwards of 100 to 120 beds per 10,000 of population: Aragó, *Hospitals a Catalunya*, 45. Rubio Vela, *Pobreza, enfermedad y asistencia*, 87, 132.

73. Burgos's other major hospitals, those of the Emperador, with twelve beds, and that of Santa María la Real with eighteen spaces, more closely approximated Catalan conditions (Martínez, "Asistencia material," 351–52). At Toulouse, in 1256, the Hospital of Saint-Raymond had fifty-six beds, a size matched by only two of the other thirteen hospitals in the city (Mundy, "Charity and Social Work in Toulouse," 253). By contrast, contemporary estimates, doubtlessly exaggerated, of the patient population at the Hospital of Saint John in Jerusalem range from one to two thousand (Miller, "Knights of Saint John," 719). Saint Leonard's had a population of some two hundred inmates, making it a large hospital for England. By contrast, Saint John the Baptist, Canterbury, supported sixty, and Saint Cross, Winchester, only thirteen (Cullum, *Cremetts and Corrodies*, 2). In Paris, the principal hospital, the Hôtel-Dieu at Notre Dame, had 279 beds that could accommodate up to three patients each, and a lying-in room with 24 beds, but in the fifteenth century the average population was far below capacity, perhaps four hundred to five hundred persons at a time (Geremek, *Margins of Society*, 175–76). Florence in the fifteenth century had thirty-three hospitals, of which six housed fewer than ten inmates, seven had space for up to twenty, another could accommodate up to thirty, two others up to forty, one up to fifty, and five more than fifty. The largest were Santa Maria Nuova with 230 beds, and the foundling hospital of the Innocenti which could house as many as 700 (Henderson, *Piety and Charity*, 375–77).

74. At the Hospital del Rey at Burgos, for example, the hostel for women contained eight beds, while that for men had twenty-nine, that of the Emperador had three for women and nine for men, and of the original ten beds at Santa María la Real all were designated for males (Martínez, "Asistencia material," 350–52). In Catalonia, the Hospital of Sant Joan at Reus had fifteen beds for men and only four for women (Vilaseca, *Hospitales medievals de Reus*, 55–58).

75. Tarragó, *Noves aportacions*, 33; Batlle, *Urgell medieval*, 126–32, 157; Junyent, *Vic*, 124.

76. Pifarré, "Dos visitas," 2:83–89.

77. Batlle and Casas, "Caritat privada," 1:141–44.

78. Roca, *Sant Macià*, 4–12.

79. Marquès, "Fundació d'un hospital a Organyà," 8.

80. These descriptions seem fairly typical and may be compared with that of

Valencia's En Clapers, which was located in a central building, with a front porch for the inmates, and a central atrium off of which were located separate wards, with eighteen beds for men and sixteen for women, a chapel, kitchen, servants' quarters, administrator's room, dispensary, and loft. The central patio contained the hospital's water source, and a cypress tree. Rubio Vela, *Pobreza, enfermedad y asistencia*, 85–89.

81. In contrast, the Knights of Saint John, by their statutes of 1182, promised each patient not only bedding but also a coverlet, a cap and cloak, and slippers (Miller, "Knights of Saint John," 731).

82. The rector of Sant Llorenç received one hundred sous per year for his services, or about half of what was budgeted for physician care (Rubio Vela, *Pobreza, enfermedad y asistencia*, 127).

83. Batlle Prats, "Inventari dels Bens," 65–76; *Ordinacions*, lxxviii, lxxxiii–lxxxv; Vilaseca, *Hospitales medievals de Reus*, 55. Desvilar, in his will, directed that each inmate be fed daily with a ration of bread, wine, meat/cheese/eggs/fish, and accompaniments. The absence of an elaborate kitchen suggests either a failure to carry out these wishes, or perhaps just the simplicity of the preparation (Batlle, *L'assistència*, 51). Rubio Vela has published an inventory of the Hospital of En Clapers in Valencia that was taken in 1384, in which he also notes the presence of gardening tools. See his *Pobreza, enfermedad y asistencia*, 80–81; 187–91, n. 23.

84. Hospitals like En Clapers, however, would distribute alms to the needy, with which they could buy food (Rubio Vela, *Pobreza, enfermedad y asistencia*, 136).

85. López Alonso, *Pobreza en la España medieval*, 429–31.

86. Rubio Vela, *Pobreza, enfermedad y asistencia*, 37–38, 176; Danon, *Visió històrica*, 78.

87. Saint Leonard's in York had both types of corodians, those who purchased their place and those who received their place through crown appointment. See Cullum, *Cremetts and Corrodies*, 8–10, 22–23; and Burns, *Crusader Kingdom*, 1:285–89.

88. Batlle and Casas, "Caritat privada," 1:135–37, 178–80, no.7; Batlle, *L'assistència*, 51.

89. Batlle, *L'assistència*, 36.

90. Rubio Vela, *Pobreza, enfermedad y asistencia*, 129.

91. López Alonso, *Pobreza en la España medieval*, 415, 423–24.

92. A ration of bread was provided on Fridays, and a small meal of bread, fish, beans, and vegetables during Lent. Santa María la Real, another pilgrim hospice, also provided no food, but did dispense over fifty pairs of shoes to guests as replacements for worn-out footwear; during Lent, in addition, thirteen poor (five fewer than the number of available beds) were fed (Martínez, "Asistencia material," 351–52). Rodrigo Ximénez de Rada gives this contemporary account of the services provided by the Hospital del Rey: "And he [King Alfonso VIII of Castile] constructed buildings and houses for a hospital . . . which he enriched with so much wealth that at all hours of the day necessities were administered to all pilgrims, and no sufferer was turned away. Through a marvelous [system], beds were constantly made ready for all wishing to spend the night. Also for the sick, even [those] close to death, everything necessary to restore them to pristine health was used by the hands of merciful men and women." See his *De rebus Hispaniae*, bk. 7, caps. 13–14, 173–74.

93. López Alonso, *Pobreza en la España medieval*, 415.

94. Batlle Prats, "Inventari dels Bens," 78–79.

95. Rubio Vela, *Pobreza, enfermedad y asistencia*, 132.

96. *Ordinacions*, v.

97. Rubio Vela, *Pobreza, enfermedad y asistencia*, 133–34; Danon, *Visió històrica*, 78.

98. Pifarré, "Dos visitas," 2:87.

99. Batlle, *Urgell medieval*, 125–33.

100. Burying the dead was especially crucial during times of plague. In May 1375, the Hospital de la Reyna in Valencia was given by the municipal council a special allotment of thirty pounds for the purchase of burial shrouds (Rubio Vela, *Pobreza, enfermedad y asistencia*, 52). During the period 1473–91, Santa Creu admitted 5,027 patients, of whom 2,459 died (Danon, *Visió històrica*, 82).

101. Roca, *Sant Macià*, 8–9, 25–29.

102. Rubio Vela, *Pobreza, enfermedad y asistencia*, 133–34.

103. Danon, *Visió històrica*, 158.

104. For example, at Valencia in the late fourteenth century the initial twenty-pound endowment of the Hospital de la Reyna had fallen below the minimum necessary to keep its doors open, and the leper hospital of Sant Llàtzer in 1380 was said to be in "great need and misery" because of "the high prices of the things necessary for the sick" (Rubio Vela, *Pobreza, enfermedad y asistencia*, 71–72). In England, many rural hospitals, whose income was derived chiefly from land, disappeared after 1350, following the collapse of land values. See Miri Rubin, "Imagining Medieval Hospitals: Considerations on the Cultural Meanings of Institutional Change," in *Medicine and Charity before the Welfare State* (London, 1991), 20. On the complaints against older hospitals, see Pullan, *Renaissance Venice*, 204; and his "Support and Redeem," 5: 190.

105. The Hospital of Bernat Marcús, on the verge of bankruptcy in 1339, was turned over to Barcelona's council, and in Valencia the Hospital de la Reyna for the same reason became a municipal responsibility in 1379. While remaining independent, the Trinitarian hospital of Sant Guillem began to receive periodic subsidies toward its operating expenses from the municipal council. Assumption of responsibility for hospitals could also provide some advantage to municipal councils. Rubio Vela, for example, has discovered that at Valencia several hospitals were compelled by the council to invest in municipal bonds at below market rates in order to enable the city to pay off higher cost obligations. Similar studies have not been done for Barcelona, but parochial alms funds at parishes like Santa Maria del Pi and Sant Just did invest in municipal bonds. See Rubio Vela, *Pobreza en el Valencia*, 52–59, 63–64, 72–73; Batlle, *L'assistència*, 52–59. For England, see Clay, *Mediaeval Hospitals*, 212, 229.

106. Mundy, "Charity and Social Work in Toulouse," 278 n; Gavitt, *Charity and Children*, 11; Pullan, *Renaissance Venice*, 203–7; Pullan, "Support and Redeem," 5:191–92.

107. López Alonso, *Pobreza en la España medieval*, 450, 455–57; Antonio Contreras Mas and Ramón Rosselló, *La asistencia publica a los leprosos en Mallorca* (Majorca, 1990), 42; García Ballester, *Medicina a la València*, 111–12. In the Italian regions of Tuscany and Lombardy, the tendency to establish large general hospitals

also dates from the late fourteenth century. Some, like those of Santa Maria Nuova in Florence and Santa Maria della Scala of Siena, were reorganizations of much older institutions, while others in Brescia (1447) and Milan (1448) were new establishments (Gavitt, *Charity and Children*, 10–11).

108. Lara and Trenchs, "Hospital de Pedro Moliner," 59.

109. The merged hospital closed for a decade in 1452, and the building was turned into a town hall. Efforts to construct a new edifice were delayed until 1460 due to difficulty in raising money. The new building opened in 1462. Batlle, *Urgell medieval*, 149–55.

110. For example, in Tarragona the city hospital was merged with that of Santa Tecla, and in Montblanc Santa Magdalena acquired the assets of the Hospital of Sant Bartolomeu. Adell i Gisbert, "Montblanc," 246.

111. López Alonso, *Pobreza en la España medieval*, 455–56; Danon, *Visió històrica*, 21–22; 145–55.

112. Santa Creu's architectural style contrasted with a more domestic style typical of crowded urban neighborhoods, in which small rooms were constructed around a small, central patio. The monumental style was more typically found in less built-up areas (Adell i Gisbert, "Montblanc," 243–44). The inventory of Santa Creu from 1564 contains about 126 beds and 211 mattresses. For a general description of Santa Creu, see Danon, *Visió històrica*, 23–35; 88–89.

113. Danon, *Visió històrica*, 82; *Ordinacions*, xiii–xv.

114. *Ordinacions*, xi, xvi, xx–xxi, xxxii–xxxiii.

Chapter 5. Hospitals and Disease in the Medieval City

1. For a discussion this problem, see Cullum, *Cremetts and Corrodies*, 2.

2. For example, in 1397, the apothecary Francesc Conill of Valencia left his goods to endow such a hospital for the sick and others (Rubio Vela, *Pobreza, enfermedad y asistencia*, 38).

3. There are scattered references to lepers in northern France and England during the eleventh century; the first reference in Aragon is Pedro I's grant in 1096 of revenues "for the support of the poor and of lepers" (Ubieto Arteta, "Pobres y marginados," 21). See also Moore, *Persecuting Society*, 50. To the argument that leprosy was introduced into Europe by returning crusaders, Dols argues that there is no evidence that Muslims spread leprosy into Europe either during the era of Islamic conquest, or during the era of the Crusades, principally because Western polemical literature of the era makes no such charge. He does allow that sub-Saharan Africa was an important source for leprosy, and that there is little evidence of the disease in North Africa or Spain before the era of Muslim government. The first known leper hospital in North Africa, the Dimnah Hospital in Ifriqiyah, dates from circa 930; in al-Andalus, there was a leprosarium in ninth-century Córdoba in an orchard on the western edge of the city. The disease was prevalent in Palestine and Syria during the crusading era, and the increase in traffic between East and West might well have aggravated the disease in Europe. Michael W. Dols, "The Leper in Medieval Islamic Society," *Speculum* 58 (1983): 898, 905–8.

4. For Canon 23, see Bériac, *Lépreux*, 155–61. Most frequently the invocation was that of Saint Lazarus, whom medieval people tended to identify as both the brother of Mary and Martha and the pauper at the gate of Dives (Cullum, *Hospitals in Medieval Yorkshire*, 32).

5. Ward E. Bullock, "Leprosy (Hansen's Disease)," in *Cecil Textbook of Medicine*, ed. J .B. Wyngaarden and L. H. Smith (7th ed.; Philadelphia, 1985), 1634–35.

6. Cullum, "Hospitals," 23; Peter Richards, *The Medieval Leper and His Northern Heirs* (Cambridge, 1977), viii. Twelfth-century doctors, for example, dropped cold water on the skin of suspected lepers to watch how it ran, a test that is capable of identifying leprosy (Moore, *Persecuting Society*, 47). Other techniques of diagnosis included examination of the extremities for sensation and of the face for signs of deformation; less effective was the examination of how the patient's urine and blood reacted when mixed (David Nirenberg, *Communities of Violence: Persecution of Minorities in the Middle Ages* [Princeton, N.J., 1966], 94–96).

7. Nirenberg, *Communities of Violence*, 105; McVaugh, *Medicine before the Plague*, 218–23; Jacquart and Thomasset, *Sexuality and Medicine*, 184–86. On leprosy as a sign of sin, or as an expiation for sin, see Moore, *Persecuting Society*, 60–65. Luke Demaitre, citing the desire of Jordanus (a master at the University of Montpellier) for "the benefit of the commonwealth," argues that the lepers' plot may well have motivated his *Notes on Leprosy*; see Demaitre's "The Relevance of Futility: Jordanus de Turre (fl. 1313–1335) on the Treatment of Leprosy," *Bulletin of the History of Medicine* 70 (1996): 28.

8. Merovingian legislation did, on the other hand, call for such segregation. The Council of Lyons (583), for example, ordered bishops to provide lepers with "alimenta et necessaria vestimenta," but at the same time to deny them any permission "per alias civitates vagandi" (Loren C. MacKinney, *Early Medieval Medicine With Special Reference to France and Chartres* [Baltimore, 1937], 178). Many have argued that Western Christian society segregated lepers to a greater extent than did Muslims, or even Western crusaders in Palestine, because lepers were feared not only as a source of contagion but also as a source of religious impurity. Leprosy, it is argued, was more than a disease; it was a punishment inflicted on individuals who were damned by God. For a discussion, see Dols, "The Leper in Medieval Islamic Society," 912–16; Richards, *Medieval Leper*, 41–42, 48–49; Shulamith Shahar, "Des lépreux pas comme les autres. L'ordre de Saint-Lazare dans le royaume latin de Jérusalem," *Revue historique* 267 (1979): 22, 40–41. But, as the following discussion illustrates, the segregation actually practiced in the West differed little, if at all, from that found in the contemporary Middle East or North Africa; and the moral regime demanded in Christian asylums for lepers does not appear to give them up as damned. Indeed, Richards acknowledges that leprosy in the thirteenth century was an offense under English common law, as well as Scandinavian law, only if the leper insisted on continued residence in town and attendance at church and neighborhood affairs (Richards, *Medieval Leper*, 49–50). See also McVaugh, *Medicine before the Plague*, 218–19; Henderson, *Piety and Charity*, 244.

9. Various artistic depictions show lepers with short tunics in the twelfth century, but in long garments in the fourteenth. The diocese of Coutances prescribed a closed, hooded cape, as did the leprosaria of Lisieux (in 1256) and Chartres (in

1264). The Council of Lacaur in 1368 stated that lepers must wear closed garb that was neutral in color and which bore a distinctive insignia. See Bériac, *Lépreux*, 185–91; Geremek, *Margins of Society*, 174–75. "Regula ordinis S. Spiritus," *PL* 217: 1146, cap. 51. For Oviedo, see López Alonso, *Pobreza en la España medieval*, 434. For a survey of practices of segregation, see Moore, *Persecuting Society*, 55–60.

10. Medieval Toulouse, for example, had seven leprosaria, the earliest in existence by 1167, with the last having its first mention in 1246 (Mundy, "Charity and Social Work in Toulouse," 227–30). Moore's compilation of first references to leprosaria shows that in England the most active period of foundation was 1175 to 1200, followed by 1225 to 1250, with a gradual falling off thereafter. For the region around Paris, foundations begin a rapid development in the era of 1175 to 1200 and peak between 1225 and 1250. See Moore, *Persecuting Society*, 52.

11. The Franciscans, the Order of the Holy Spirit, and the Hospitalers of Saint John cared for lepers here and there, but more by way of accident than intention. See Webster, *Els menorets*, 186; Bériac, *Lépreux*, 233–34. The Order of Saint Lazarus, itself, was founded in Jerusalem during the 1120s as a confraternity that cared for the sick and lepers; Malcolm Barber argues that the order became an honorable refuge for Latin colonists in Palestine who had contracted leprosy. In Palestine, particularly under Baldwin IV of Jerusalem, the leper king, it acquired military responsibilities, and its grand master up until 1253 was required to be a leper. The order was introduced into France after the Second Crusade by Louis VII who is said to have given it a hospital in Paris to care for lepers, although others assert that even this institution remained under the jurisdiction of the bishop of Paris. Mutel's recent study of the order's commanderies in Normandy indicates that property management, initially for the benefit of the brethren in the Near East, and not the care of lepers, was their primary function, and the leprosarium of Saint-Lazare in Montpellier was a laic foundation with no connection to the order. In the Crown of Aragon, towns like Valencia, Girona, and Lleida had Hospitals of Sant Llàtzer, but their connection to the Order is uncertain. Studies of similar hospitals in the region of Asturias show no affiliation to the Order of Saint Lazarus. In August 1265, Pope Clement IV issued a bull that placed all lepers in Christendom under the care and protection of the order, but practical barriers to such a sweeping reform guaranteed that it came to naught. See Tolivar Faes, *Leprosos en Asturias*, 261; Burns, *Crusader Kingdom*, 1:242; W. G. Rödel, "San Lazzaro, di Gerusalemme," *DIP* 8:579; Gautier de Sibert, *Histoire de l'Ordre Militaire et Hospitalier de Saint-Lazare de Jérusalem* (1772; Paris, 1983), 48–63; Charles Moeller, "Lazarus, Saint, Order of," *The Catholic Encyclopedia* (New York, 1910), 9:96–97; André Mutel, "Recherches sur l'ordre de Saint-Lazare de Jérusalem en Normandie," *Annales de Normandie* 33 (1983): 121–42; Marcel Baudot, "La gestation d'une léproserie du XIVᵉ siècle: La maladrerie Saint-Lazare de Montpellier," *Actes du 110ᵉ Congrès national des sociétés savantes* (Paris, 1987), 1:411; Malcolm Barber, "The Order of Saint Lazarus and the Crusades," *Catholic Historical Review* 80 (1994): 443–44, 454.

12. Bériac, *Lépreux*, 163–66.

13. Cullum, "Hospitals," 20–26.

14. Mundy, "Charity and Social Work in Toulouse," 253.

15. López Alonso, *Pobreza en la España medieval*, 439–40.

16. Toliver Faes, *Leprosos en Asturias*, 251–54.

17. Martínez García, "Asistencia material," 353.

18. Sanchez Herrero, "Cofradías," 41; Carmona García, *Hospitalidad publica en Sevilla*, 26; García del Moral, *Hospital Mayor*, 39–40.

19. Pérez Santamaría, "San Lázaro," 1:77–89, 105–6, 114–15; Battle and Casas, "Caritat privada," 1:144; Batlle, *L'assistència*, 67–69.

20. Pérez Santamaría, "San Lázaro," 92–93. In contrast, during a similar period, 1374–75 to 1396–97, the Hospital of En Clapers in Valencia derived 66.5 percent of its income from land rents, 22 percent from various rights of lordship, 6.5 percent from municipal bonds, and only 5 percent from such variable sources as the sale of surplus food, the effects of deceased inmates, and alms (Rubio Vela, *Pobreza, enfermedad y asistencia*, 92–93).

21. For example, the statutes permitted two diners to be spent per day on each staff member for food, while inmates were allotted only twelve diners per week. On feast days, a single diner could be spent on each leper and staff member, but the administrator and chaplains were to receive food worth three diners each (Pérez Santamaría, "San Lázaro," 99–100).

22. Besides the administrator and chaplains, the staff included a porter, three individuals who collected bread as alms for the hospital (whose subsequent sale represented 30 percent of the hospital's income), a slave, a laundress, and the attendant (Pérez Santamaría, "San Lázaro," 99–100; 104–6). At Valencia's leper hospital, inmates were cautioned not to exceed their daily quota of wine and not to give any food to their friends or relatives. There is no evidence of any staff to provide care and it seems that inmates were expected to cook their own meals (Rubio Vela, *Pobreza, enfermedad y asistencia*, 165).

23. Tarragó, *Lérida*, 31, 36, 69.

24. Guilleré, *Girona medieval*, 89; idem, "Charité à Gérone," 1:196.

25. Batlle, *Urgell medieval*, 139–41.

26. Ollich, "Les entitats eclesiastiques de Vic," 97; Junyent, *Vic*, 87–88.

27. Nirenberg, *Communities of Violence*, 101; Danon, *Visió històrica*, 16; Duran, *Llibre de Cervera*, 213–14.

28. On the leper plot and the property confiscations within the Aragonese Crown, see Nirenberg, *Communities of Violence*, 93–108. See also J. R. Webster, "La reina doña Constanza y los hospitales de Barcelona y Valencia," *Archivo Ibero-Americano* 51 (1991): 378; and Webster, *Els Menorets*, 55, 186. Duran adds that the hospital was reconstructed with two hundred pounds left by the merchant Joan Llop in his will of 1377, and the church with money willed by another merchant, Bertran dels Archs, in 1389. *Llibre de Cervera*, 214–15. The decline in leprosy suggested by the Catalan evidence is also reflected in sources from England where many leper houses began to fall into disuse or else were converted into shelters for non-lepers during the fourteenth century (Cullum, *Cremetts and Corrodies*, 4).

29. Contreras and Rosselló, *Leprosos en Mallorca*, 21–22, 42, 57–59.

30. Burns, *Crusader Kingdom*, 1:242; Rubio Vela, *Pobreza, enfermedad y asistencia*, 54, 165; Mercedes Gallent Marco, "Instituciones hospitalarias y poderes públicos en Valencia," *Saitabi* 34 (1984): 82.

31. Local prejudice, however, was not so easily assuaged; Bernat was expelled a second time only to be declared healthy again by the doctors of Sant Llàtzer. The matter ultimately came before the king (Nirenberg, *Communities of Violence*, 106).

32. The ritual of civil death was practiced in England; for an example of the rite, see Richards, *Medieval Leper*, 123–24.

33. López Alonso, *Pobreza en la España medieval*, 435–36.

34. This prioritization is contained in statutes promulgated in 1326 (Pérez Santamaría, "San Lázaro," 88–89).

35. My own study of medieval wills in Spain shows that, for the most part, families would automatically inherit all of a decedent's real property and up to 80 percent of his personal property, with the remainder disposable at the testator's wish. See James W. Brodman, "What is a Soul Worth? *Pro anima* Bequests in the Municipal Legislation of Reconquest Spain," *Medievalia et Humanistica*, new series, no. 20 (1994): 20–21. In France, the customs of Beauvais in effect gave the leprosarium the family's right to a leper's property, leaving the disposition of only a fifth of those goods to the leper. See Bériac, *Lépreux*, 226.

36. For example, a leper at Castelsarrasias gave six pounds in 1300 for his admission, while in 1280 a father promised his daughter's future inheritance to the commander of the leprosarium at Capdenac (Bériac, *Lépreux*, 226).

37. Ibid., 228–31; Pérez Santamaría, "San Lázaro," 88, 92–93, 111; Rubio Vela, *Pobreza in la Valencia*, 165; McVaugh, *Medicine before the Plague*, 224.

38. Mundy, "Charity and Social Work in Toulouse," 249. The leper hospital at Chartres, the Grand Beaulieu, imposed its statutes, based loosely upon the Rule of Saint Augustine, on both healthy and leprous, although these were separated by condition as well as by gender. Since this hospital was successful and of note, its usages were imitated by other leprosaria, such as that of Saint Gilles, established in 1135 in the Norman town of Pont-Audemer. See Simone C. Mesmin, "Waleran of Meulan and the Leper Hospital of S. Gilles de Pont-Audemer," *Annales de Normandie* 32 (1982): 8–11.

39. Rubio Vela, *Pobreza, enfermedad y asistencia*, 165. While both Christian and Muslim medical authorities allowed that leprosy might be communicated through sexual intercourse, concern for containing the disease within a society already infected could hardly have been the reason for this call to chastity. For ideas concerning communicability, see Barber, "Saint Lazarus," 444; Dols, "The Leper in Medieval Islamic Society," 897–98; and Richards, *Medieval Leper*, 54.

40. Bériac, *Lépreux*, 235–44, 249; Pérez Santamaría, "San Lázaro," 89; Rubio Vela, *Pobreza, enfermedad y asistencia*, 165.

41. Bériac, *Lépreux*, 84, 262.

42. The physician's charge was three sous per visit, suggesting, *inter alia,* an economic motive for avoiding medical care (Pérez Santamaría, "San Lázaro," 112–13). Records at Urgell show that lepers were administered oakum or tow, perhaps as a kind of bandage (Batlle, *Urgell medieval*, 1300). Jordanus de Turre, a master at the University of Montpellier in the 1320s, diagnosed three stages in the progression of leprosy and, in his *De lepra nota*, prescribed a regimen of care for each stage, hoping for a cure in its earlier phases and greater comfort for the patient in its terminal period. There are no indications, however, that Jordanus's advice had an

impact on the character of care actually dispensed in Catalan leprosaria (Demaitre, "Relevance of Futility," 30–46).

43. Matthew J. Ellenhorn and Donald G. Barceloux, *Medical Toxicology: Diagnosis and Treatment of Human Poisoning* (New York, 1988), 1317–18; *A Companion to Medical Studies*, ed. R. Passmore and J. S. Robson, 3 vols. (Philadelphia, 1970), 2:13.1–2. Mary Matossian argues that some victims of ergotism, because of their hallucinogenic behavior and spasms, were accused of witchcraft; see her *Poisons of the Past: Molds, Epidemics and History* (New Haven, Conn., 1989), 9–14, 57.

44. For example, the statutes of the Hospital of Saint Jean at Angers forbade the admission of both lepers and those who suffered from ergotism, in addition to paralytics and young children (Moore, *Persecuting Society*, 55).

45. I. Ruffino, "Canonici Regolari di Sant'Agostine di Sant'Antonio, di Vienne," *DIP*, 2:134–41; J. F. Hinnebusch, in Jacques de Vitry, *Historia Occidentalis*, 281.

46. Duran, *Llibre de Cervera*, 209–11. Before moving to Barcelona, the brothers were nonetheless active there seeking alms for their order, as evidenced by a privilege of June 3, 1349, allowing them to announce indulgences in the city to their benefactors (Gyug, *Diocese of Barcelona*, 331–32 n. 878).

47. Mutgé, *Ciudad de Barcelona*, 49; Duran, *Llibre de Cervera*, 209.

48. Tarragó, *Lerida*, 65–66.

49. Burns, *Crusader Kingdom*, 1:244; Rubio Vela, *Pobreza, enfermedad y asistencia*, 35, 45–46.

50. The Valencian institution, however, does not seem to have been fully utilized because in 1493 its administrators petitioned that other poor be accepted as well. See García Ballester, *Medicina a la Valencia*, 111; López Alonso, *Pobreza en la España medieval*, 440–44; Cullum, *Cremetts and Corrodies*, 3; Rubio Vela, *Pobreza, enfermedad y asistencia*, 44; McVaugh, *Medicine before the Plague*, 225–35; Katherine Park, "Medicine and society in Early Medieval Europe, 500–1500," in *Medicine and Society: Historical Essays*, ed. Andrew Wear (Cambridge, 1992), 88–90; and George Rosen, "The Mentally Ill and the Community in Western and Central Europe during the Late Middle Ages and Renaissance," *Journal of the History of Medicine* 19 (1964): 377–83.

51. Or, one could argue, the medieval era witnessed the reprofessionalization of medicine, since hospitals or *xenodochia* of the late Roman period had also associated the two elements. Paul the Deacon described the sixth-century hospital established by Bishop Masona at Mérida: "He built a *xenodochium* and endowed it with a large patrimony, and he ordered that, with the appointment of ministers or physicians (*medici*), it serve the needs of the sick and pilgrims." Likewise, in southern France, Bishop Praeiectus of Avernus founded a hospital "where he established medical men or strenuous men, who had charge of care, to always tend to twenty sick people, and to provide them with an allotment of food there; but after they get well, they give their places to others." For the Latin texts, see MacKinney, *Early Medieval Medicine*, 170, 177. The first medical school in medieval Spain was recognized by Alfonso VIII of Castile in 1209 at Palencia, but evidence suggests that this had disappeared by 1250 (Hergueta, "Noticias," 424–25). Alfonso X, in his legal works, acknowledged the importance of physicians and medicine, but his interest

seems to have been in the social, rather than the scientific aspects of medicine. The University of Salamanca, for example, was given an endowment for two chairs in medicine in 1254, yet there is no evidence for an active medical faculty there until the early fifteenth century. See Luis García Ballester, "Medical Science in Thirteenth-Century Castile: Problems and Prospects," *Bulletin of the History of Medicine* 61 (1987): 188–90; Marcelino V. Amasuno Sarraga, *La escuela de medicina del estudio salmantino (siglos XIII–XV)* (Salamanca, 1990), 14–32. Outside of Iberia, the fourteenth century likewise marked the appearance of physicians at hospitals. The first surgeon, for example, was appointed to the Holy Spirit Hospital at Frankfurt am Main in 1377 (Rosen, "Historical Sociology," 17).

52. Physicians generally treated internal or systemic illness, while the surgeon dealt with fractures, wounds, abscesses, skin ailments, and external complaints. The apothecary could recommend as well as prepare medication. He could also sell wax and candles for funerals and other types of merchandise. Barbers bled patients and also shaved, cut hair, and pulled teeth. Being relatively low paid, they often engaged in a number of unrelated occupations and also attempted to infringe upon the domain of the surgeon. McVaugh cites several cases in which individuals moved from calling themselves barbers to being surgeons, and of others who claimed dual competence. See McVaugh, *Medicine before the Plague*, 38–40; 123–25.

53. Montpellier became a center of medical activities in the mid-twelfth century, and medical instruction had begun there before 1200. A "university" of both medical masters and students was subsequently established, whose statutes received papal approval in 1220. See Nancy G. Siraisi, *Medieval and Early Renaissance Medicine: An Introduction to Knowledge and Practice* (Chicago, 1990), 59.

54. Roger II of Sicily (1130–54) had mandated that practitioners be examined by royal officials; in 1231, the Emperor Frederick II entrusted this function to the masters of the University of Salerno, although contemporaries lamented that such regulations were not well-observed. See Siraisi, *Medieval and Early Renaissance Medicine*, 17–18. See also Luis García Ballester, Michael R. McVaugh, and Agustín Rubio Vela, *Medical Licensing and Learning in Fourteenth-Century Valencia* (Philadelphia, 1989), 2–4; James M. Powell, "Greco-Arabic Influences on the Public Health Legislation in the Constitutions of Melfi," *Archivio storico pugliese* 31 (1978): 80, 88–89. At Toulouse, as the result of complaints about unqualified practitioners, those who wished to practice were required to be examined by the bishop, with the assistance of experienced physicians. The masters of the university questioned the bishop's competence and stated that inept individuals continued to practice. As a result, the town council transferred this function to the masters, and the king in 1411 upheld the requirement: Philippe Wolff, "Recherches sur les médecins de Toulouse aux XIVe et XVe siècles," in *Assistance et assistés jusqu'à 1610. Actes du 97e congrès national des sociétés savantes, Nantes, 1972* (Paris, 1979), 534–35. See also McVaugh, *Medicine before the Plague*, 69–71.

55. García Ballester, McVaugh and Rubio Vela, *Medical Licensing*, 6–8; McVaugh, *Medicine before the Plague*, 95–96; López, "Documentos acerca de la peste negra," 305, no. 18.

56. For an account of the foundation and history of medical study at Lleida, see McVaugh, *Medicine before the Plague*, 83–87.

57. Danon, *Visió històrica*, 130.

58. For earlier decades, the numbers are even smaller: two in the 1300s, five in the 1310s, three in the 1320s, and four in the 1330s; see McVaugh, *Medicine before the Plague*, 81.

59. The sentiments concerning the importance of experience in surgery were expressed in November 1389 by two Valencian medical masters, Pere Giguerola and Guillem Ça-Fàbrega, in the report of their examination of the surgeon Johan de Sena. See García Ballester, McVaugh, and Rubio Vela, *Medical Licensing*, 15–17, 34–39, 54. As late as the sixteenth century, for example, half of the practitioners in London were unlicensed (Siraisi, *Medieval and Early Renaissance Medicine*, 20, 188–89). In Toulouse, physicians as early as 1306 were required to be examined, but such a requirement for barbers is not found earlier than their guild's new statutes of 1457 (Wolff, "Médecins de Toulouse," 534, 537).

60. In Italy, a medical guild was established in Florence in 1293. In 1314, it divided itself into three branches to represent *medici*, apothecaries, and barbers. University-trained physicians established their own association in 1393. Venice had a College of Physicians in 1316 (Siraisi, *Medieval and Early Renaissance Medicine*, 18).

61. This was suppressed, along with most other confraternities, early in the reign of Jaume II but permitted to reform in 1311. Other such bodies appear in early fourteenth-century Aragon (Calatayud and Huesca). These bodies assumed some regulatory authority over their members; elsewhere, in places like Lleida and Barcelona, the regulation was municipal. Much of the concern was centered on enforcing a prohibition against practice on Sundays and feasts, although Barcelona, in also regulating bleeding, recognized the barber's medical functions. See McVaugh, *Medicine before the Plague*, 125–27.

62. García Ballester, *Medicina a la Valencia*, 58–67; Guilleré, *Girona medieval*, 73. At Toulouse, barbers organized themselves into a guild sometime between 1363 and 1391, and by 1404 they had adopted a set of *consuetudines* that were modified and amplified in 1442. The first required that barbers be residents of the town, while the second more precisely insisted that the practitioner reside in a house with his family, maintain only one location of practice, attend to his patients in person, and not delegate his responsibilities to anyone less qualified (Wolff, "Médecins de Toulouse," 535–36). See also McVaugh, *Medicine before the Plague*, 118.

63. García Ballester, McVaugh and Rubio Vela, *Medical Licensing*, 39–40; Siraisi, *Medieval and Early Renaissance Medicine*, 22.

64. These statistics also hold true for the longer interval of 1320–70, during which sixty-one apothecaries have been identified as practicing in Girona, along with twenty-nine barbers, twenty-three surgeons, and eleven physicians (Guilleré, *Girona al segle XIV*, 2:362–65). See also Guilleré, "Le milieu médical géronais au XIVᶜ siècle," in *Actes du 110ᵉ Congrès*, 1:265–66, 269–70; and Richard W. Emery, "The Black Death of 1348 in Perpignan," *Speculum* 42 (1967):619–20.

65. A smaller town like Manresa, on the other hand, was served from 1320 to 1345 by a single physician and two surgeons, all of whom were exempted by the town from the payment of taxes on the understanding that they remain and practice in the town. See McVaugh, *Medicine before the Plague*, 44, 108; the figures, based on fewer sources, are lower in García Ballester, McVaugh and Rubio Vela, *Medical Licensing*, 37.

66. McVaugh counts 201 practitioners of all types in Barcelona, from 1300 to 1340, and 197 for Valencia, or 20 and 22.7 per 10,000 of population. See his *Medicine before the Plague*, 42–49.

67. Their count of the names of healers from the fourteenth century preserved in the archives yields some two thousand names for the Crown of Aragon, and only two dozen for the entire Crown of Castile (García Ballester, "Medical Science," 185).

68. Florence, for example, in 1379 had seventy medical practitioners of all kinds for a population of about fifty thousand (Siraisi, *Medieval and Early Renaissance Medicine*, 23). Toulouse, in 1405, had only three local physicians and twenty-two barbers. Wolff, however, estimates that nonresidents raised the total closer to thirty or thirty-five. See his "Médecins de Toulouse," 533. See also McVaugh, *Medicine before the Plague*, 64–67.

69. McVaugh, *Medicine before the Plague*, 49.

70. Ibid., 43–45.

71. The sharp difference in mortality rates between the closely situated towns of Girona and Perpignan is undoubtedly due to the time of the year when each community was infected. Perpignan was hit during the spring, when the bacillus was most active, while Girona was saved by the hot temperatures of the Mediterranean summer that inhibited the disease. See Guilleré, "Milieu médical," 268; and Emery, "Black Death," 612, 619–20. For Xàtiva, see López, "Documentos acerca de la peste negra," 411–12, no. 132 (February 23, 1352).

72. Siraisi, *Medieval and Early Renaissance Medicine*, 24.

73. Indeed, García Ballester and McVaugh have argued that an important motivation in the establishment of licensing requirements for medical practitioners was to take medicine out of the hands of unbelievers and place it into Christian hands, since only Christians would have access to the university training demanded by the law. See García Ballester, McVaugh and Rubio Vela, *Medical Licensing*, 42, 49; see also McVaugh, *Medicine before the Plague*, 96–103. The Rule of the Hospitaller Order of the Holy Spirit, in describing the manner of how the poor ought to be received into its hospitals, manifests this concern by mandating that before they are fed or shown to a bed they should be confessed by a priest ("Regula ordinis S. Spiritus," *PL* 217:1141, cap. 13).

74. Synodal legislation (1354) at Barcelona forbade Christian physicians to begin treatment before the parish priest had been summoned to confess the patient and give him communion and also forbade the use of a Jewish doctor unless he had a Christian assistant on penalty of excommunication. Various exceptions, however, suggest that this was not strictly enforced (Utterback, *Pastoral Care*, 39). One such convert was Mosse Falcó, who became Francesc Pendralbes and subsequently served as a consulting physician to two hospitals in Barcelona, Sant Macià and Santa Creu (Danon, *Visió històrica*, 130).

75. The phenomenon is found elsewhere. Twenty-five female surgeons are known to have practiced in Naples between 1273 and 1410; in Frankfurt, between 1387 and 1497, fifteen women, most of whom were Jewish, have similarly been identified. While any statistics on the number of female medical practitioners are problematical, nevertheless, one estimate is that women in late medieval France constituted 1.5 percent of all medical practitioners, and 1.2 percent of those in England

(Siraisi, *Medieval and Early Renaissance Medicine*, 27). See also Muriel Joy Hughes, *Women Healers in Medieval Life and Literature* (Freeport, N.Y., 1968), 82–96.

76. García Ballester, *Medical Licensing*, 21–32. Cullum, in her study of Saint Leonard's of York, in England, discovers female nurses like Ann, who in 1276 is described as a *medica*. She argues that women, as nurses, must have accumulated a body of medical knowledge, probably based on traditional herbal medicine, that they used in the absence of physicians to treat patients. This included even minor surgery (*Cremetts and Corrodies*, 13–15). On the important role of Jewish physicians within the Crown of Aragon, see McVaugh, *Medicine before the Plague*, 55–64; on women, see 103–7. The accounts of Valencia's Hospital of En Clapers of the late fourteenth century contain entries showing payment to *metgesses* called in to care for children, for example, one florin paid in 1396–97 for setting the fracture for an illegitimate child. See Agustín Rubio Vela, "La asistencia hospitalaria infantil en la Valencia del siglo XIV: Pobres, huérfanos y expósitos," *Dynamis* 2 (1982): 180.

77. The appointment of municipal physicians can be found outside of Catalonia. In 1377, a physician at Frankfurt am Main treated without charge all municipal employees and patients in the town hospital. The Emperor Sigismund in the 1430s issued a number of reform proposals that, *inter alia*, recommended that each municipality have a physician, and that physicians should treat the poor without charge (Rosen, "Historical Sociology," 17–18). Monarchs like Jaume II routinely appointed physicians, as well as barbers and apothecaries, to positions at court and at relatively high salaries (McVaugh, *Medicine before the Plague*, 4–34).

78. Albert's contract required him to live within Girona's walls, not to leave the city if any member of the chapter currently was ill, and to treat the canons free of further charge anywhere within the boundaries of the diocese. There are also examples of individuals entering into similar lump-sum contracts with physicians, including members of the royal army who typically yielded the equivalent of a day's pay to a contract physician in return for guaranteed medical care (McVaugh, *Medicine before the Plague*, 174–76).

79. In Italy, the practice of appointing town doctors, or *medici condotti*, dates from the 1210s and became almost universal in the fourteenth century. At first these *medici* were surgeons charged with the treatment of wounds and fractures, but after 1300 physicians were also under contract. Between 1333 and 1377, Venice on average kept seven physicians and ten surgeons under contract to reside in the city, treat the poor free of charge, and give medical advice and testimony. In France, the phenomenon was later, coming toward the end of the fourteenth and beginning of the fifteenth century. See McVaugh, *Medicine before the Plague*, 190–91; Siraisi, *Medieval and Early Renaissance Medicine*, 38.

80. López Alonso, *Pobreza en la España medieval*, 474; Guilleré, "Milieu médical," 266–68; McVaugh, *Medicine before the Plague*, 191–200; Santamaría, "Asistencia a los pobres en Mallorca," 394–95.

81. For example, in the 1370s, Castelló sued Jacme Maderes, a master of arts and medicine and medical examiner of Valencia, for contractual violations. Those in Alzira, in 1351, lamented, "There was no one to cure the sick or to help the poor" (García Ballester, *Medicina a la Valencia*, 83–86). The village of Fortià, in northern Catalonia, acquired its barber in 1308 by sending a native son, Bernat Leto, as an

apprentice to Castelló d'Empúries, from which he was obligated to return on Fridays to cut hair. After the expiration of his two-year apprenticeship, he moved back home as a resident barber (McVaugh, *Medicine before the Plague*, 46).

82. The town of Castelló d'Empúries, for example, contracted with a series of town doctors in the first quarter of the fourteenth century to inspect the urine of town residents, to provide advice on bloodletting and diet, and to provide two house calls to any sick resident of the town who requested service (McVaugh, *Medicine before the Plague*, 138–39).

83. The association between physicians and hospitals occurred earlier in the East than in the West. Not only did Saint John's have four physicians, but it also provided, according to a papal letter of 1184, four surgeons as well. The hospital, or Xenon, of the Pantocrator monastery in Constantinople, perhaps the richest in the Byzantine Empire, was even better endowed. It possessed ten clinics that housed sixty-five beds, served by some thirty-five doctors. See Miller, "Knights of Saint John," 719, 730; and Demetrios Constantelos, *Byzantine Philanthropy and Social Welfare* (2nd ed. rev.; New Rochelle, N.Y., 1991), 129. In Florence, for example, the Hospital of Santa Maria Nuova, established in the 1280s, grew to contain some three hundred beds in the late fifteenth century, at which time it employed nine resident practitioners; three other Florentine hospitals (San Paolo, San Giovanni and San Mateo), with capacities that ranged between fifty and seventy-five, also employed physicians, surgeons, and pharmacists. See Siraisi, *Medieval and Early Renaissance Medicine*, 39; Park, "Healing the Poor," 32. The Hôtel-Dieu of Paris had a surgeon from at least 1231. There is evidence of *medici* with some sort of affiliation with English hospitals in the later twelfth and early thirteenth centuries, but even London hospitals had no permanent physicians until the sixteenth century. In Italy, however, they were a regular fixture after 1350, perhaps as a consequence of the plague (Cullum, *Cremetts and Corrodies*, 3; McVaugh, *Medicine before the Plague*, 229).

84. Burns acknowledges that the Hospitallers may have operated the first hospital within Christian Valencia but concedes that it was soon squeezed out by the growth of the brothers' church and cemetery. Elsewhere, and located principally in the rural locales as castellans and property managers, the Hospitallers do not seem to have taken up this work with any seriousness. See Burns, *Crusader Kingdom*, 1:186–89; María Luisa Ledesma Rubio, *Templarios y Hospitalarios en el Reino de Aragón* (Saragossa, 1982), 104–5.

85. Within the Kingdom of Castile, the addition of medical care seems to have come later. At Valladolid's Hospitals of Esgueva and Todos Santos, for example, the first evidence of such care dates from the mid-fifteenth century (Rucquoi, "Hospitalisation et charité à Valladolid," 400).

86. Rubio Vela, *Pobreza, enfermedad y asistencia*, 71, 122–23, 185–86, no. 21. In contrast, a grateful King Pere the Ceremonious in 1350 paid the physician Berenguer de Torrelles two thousand sous for successfully treating his children during the recent outbreak of the plague. See López, "Documentos acerca de la peste negra," 383–84, no. 101 (April 15, 1350).

87. Guilleré, "Milieu médical," 268.

88. McVaugh, *Medicine before the Plague*, 230; Roca, *Sant Macià*, 12, 15–17; *Ordinacions*, xxxii–xxxiii.

89. In the fourteenth century, among Valencia's Christian population, between fifteen and twenty-three received hospital care per thousand of population (García Ballester, *Medicina a la Valencia*, 100–110; Rubio Vela, *Pobreza, enfermedad y asistencia*, 125). Evidently the use of women as medical personnel in hospitals was widespread. In Florence's Hospital of Santa Maria Nuova, for example, several of the resident staff of laywomen or *servae* are described in the documents also as *medicae* or doctors (Park, "Healing the Poor," 32).

90. In subsequent years, Pere Garbí's stipend fell to as low as a hundred and ten sous, perhaps reflecting fewer consultations. The physician Pere de Coll was paid forty florins (about six hundred sous) in 1411 and twenty florins in each of the succeeding two years. Francesc Pedralbes, a converted Jew, got two hundred and eighty sous in 1412, about three hundred in both 1413 and 1414 (Danon, *Visió històrica*, 129–30). See also Gallent Marco, "Hospital de la Reyna," 81.

91. *Ordinacions*, xxxii–xxxiii.

92. Rubio Vela, *Pobreza, enfermedad y asistencia*, 124–26.

93. Gallent Marco, "Hospital de la Reyna," 84; Rubio Vela, *Pobreza, enfermedad y asistencia*, 134–36.

94. Danon, *Visió històrica*, 76–77. The character of disease is remarkably similar to statistics from Florence's Hospital of San Paolo in 1587–88: 55 percent with fevers (or infections), 15 percent with skin diseases, 8 percent with wounds and fractures, 4 percent with syphilis. Death rates for men were lower, about 10 percent, than the figures from Barcelona, but mortality rates for women were significantly higher (Park, "Healing the Poor," 35–36; Henderson, *Piety and Charity*, 398).

95. Contemporary medical writers, citing Galen's dictum — *omnium natura operatrix, medicus vero minister* — believed the processes of healing were natural, or as Niccolò Falcucci expressed it, "the art [of medicine] is the image of nature and her follower" (Park, "Healing the Poor," 37).

96. Rubio Vela, *Pobreza, enfermedad y asistencia*, 142. For prayer, see the statutes of the Hospital del Rey in Burgos that required that the sick, upon admission, be confessed, take communion, and execute a will. Only then would they be visited by a physician (Martínez García, "Asistencia material," 354).

97. Roca, *Sant Macià*, 11; *Ordinacions*, xiii, xvi, xx.

98. For a discussion of medieval theories of medicine and their sources, see Siraisi, *Medieval and Early Renaissance Medicine*, 141–52; for a general description of the confections, syrups, and drugs used in medieval Catalonia, see McVaugh, *Medicine before the Plague*, 158–58.

99. Rubio Vela, *Pobreza, enfermedad y asistencia*, 136–38, 197–246. In order to assist the apothecary in the proper formulation of medicine, whether prescribed by himself or a physician, various recipe books like the *Antidotarium Nicolai*, a thirteenth-century composition that became a text at the University of Paris in the 1270s, circulated within the Crown of Aragon (McVaugh, *Medicine before the Plague*, 119–20). Records from the Hospital del Rey in Burgos show that the apothecary stocked almonds, sugar, raisins, quince, mint, cassia-fruit, dates and, more exotic ingredients like amber, musk, rhubarb, and agaric (Martínez García, "Assistencia material," 354). Those of Santa Creu in Barcelona speak of the apothecary producing syrups, compounds, and conserves from a supply of oils, sugars, and other materials

(Ordinacions, xxiii–xxiv). Among the most commonly administered medications at the Hospital de la Reyna in the fifteenth century were: syrups and extracts derived from dates, lilies, and other sources, mixed with sweeteners and herbs; distilled waters made from honey, copper, and sage, or from orange blossoms and water, or rose water; ointments confected from substances like herbs, roses, and other flowers, walnuts, turpentine, soap and honey, or sheepshead; and purgatives made from rose or meat extracts (Gallent Marco, "Hospital de la Reyna," 84–85).

100. *Ordinacions*, xxxii–xxxiv.

101. Park, "Healing the Poor," 37; *Ordinacions*, xxxi–xxxii.

102. Rubio Vela, *Pobreza, enfermedad y asistencia*, 132, 151–53, 166–67 n. 4.

103. Park, "Healing the Poor," 28. Another indication of the severity of the plague was the shortage of cemetery space. The vicar general of the Barcelona diocese, for example, noted in 1349 that the plague had necessitated that many be buried in unconsecrated ground (Utterback, *Pastoral Care*, 109).

Chapter 6. The Care of Women and Children

1. The Hospital of Santa Creu maintained a separate ward for females, under the supervision of a woman. But the routine of care—tending to the needs of patients, keeping them clean, dispensing food and medicine — differs not at all from that of the male ward: *Ordinacions*, xx.

2. For reasons that have yet to be adequately examined, medieval shelters, wherever they were located, generally allocated more beds to men than to women. For instance, in Burgos, the Hospital del Rey housed twenty-nine men and twelve women, and that of the Emperador had nine and three (Martínez García, "Asistencia material," 350–51). Sant Macià in Barcelona had twenty-two for men and only six for women (Roca, *Sant Macià*, 4–15). In Italy, Florence's Hospital of Santa Maria Nuova contained one hundred beds in the male ward, and seventy in the women's section, despite the fact that the latter area seems to have been more crowded (Park, "Healing the Poor," 36). The large Constantinopolitan hospital of the Pantocrator reserved only twelve of sixty-one beds for women, and assigned two of the thirty-five staff physicians to their service (Constantelos, *Byzantine Philanthropy*, 129–30). The evidence of the alms fund for Barcelona's parish of Santa Maria del Pi suggests that doles were allocated on the basis of class and gender, that is, widows of notable personages received larger allotments than other women, and men were given more money than women (Cabestany and Claramunt, "Santa María del Pí," 166–67). The Order of the Holy Spirit established such a hospital in Lleida in 1214, to serve single mothers and abandoned children (Tarragó, *Lérida*, 49–50). In larger cities like Paris, on the other hand, the situation was more complicated. Here the large general shelter, the Hôtel-Dieu of Notre Dame, housed pregnant women and orphans, alongside poor cripples, the mentally ill, and the sick, but shelters specifically reserved for women also existed, such as the Hôpital Sainte-Madeleine, established in 1316, as a shelter for homeless women, or the Hôpital Sainte-Avoie and Les Haudriettes for widows, or the Hôpital de Sainte-Catherine. Florence had the Orbatello, a shelter established by a wealthy merchant in 1370 to

house several dozen widows (and their children) of honorable estate in separate apartments. See Geremek, *Margins of Society*, 171; and Richard C. Trexler, "A Widow's Asylum of the Renaissance: The Ortabello of Florence," in *Old Age in Preindustrial Society*, ed. Peter N. Stearns (New York, 1982), 119–49. On Santa Creu, see Danon, *Visió històrica*, 82.

 3. For a general discussion of the evolution of the dowry in Catalan society, see Bensch, *Barcelona*, 260–76.

 4. For skilled and unskilled workers, the dower payment could represent as much as two years' wages or more. In 1414 a municipal official in Barcelona complained to the city council that his salary was insufficient for him to support his sons and dower his daughter Constança. See Teresa-María Vinyoles i Vidal, "Ajudes a donzelles pobres a maridar," in *La pobreza*, 1:297–98; Guilleré, *Girona al segle XIV*, 2:436–40; Bensch, *Barcelona*, 356. Ramon Llull, in the *Blanquerna*, argues that poor women had two alternatives to prostitution: a position as a servant or the gift of a dowry (*Blanquerna: A Thirteenth-Century Romance*, trans. E. Allison Peers [London, 1926], 283–84). See also Batlle, *Urgell medieval*, 143. While there is no comprehensive study of the geographical origins of Barcelona's prostitutes, studies in southeast France show that for the most part they were girls of local origin, pushed as teenagers into prostitution by the loss of a parent, public rape, or the poverty of their family. See Jacques Rossiaud, *Medieval Prostitution*, trans. Lydia G. Cochrane (Oxford, 1988), 32. Vinyoles, however, argues that the situation in Barcelona was markedly different — that pimps and prostitutes were mostly outsiders. But the evidence that she cites is less than clear. Of the twenty-one pimps expelled from the city on August 20, 1404, for example, only three are identified as being non-Catalan, with five others from the Catalan towns of Tarragona, Tortosa, and Terrassa. She cites anecdotal examples from the same era of prostitutes from Seville, Galicia, Lisbon, and Sicily, but undertakes no general survey of women who plied this trade. The evidence for Valencia is similarly ambiguous. Of the 676 women, whose origins are identifiable and who were charged before the Valencian court between 1367 and 1399 with offenses related to prostitution, fully 92.8 percent were non-Valencian. Of these, 53 percent came from Castile. But this number represents only 12.3 percent of the entire sample; over 87 percent of these women cannot be identified geographically. Thus, these studies do not invalidate the argument that Catalans had concern that poor, local girls might turn to prostitution. See Vinyoles, *Vida quotidiana*, 120, 124–25; and M. Carmen Peris, "La prostitución valenciana en la segunda mitad del siglo XIV," in *Violència i marginació en la societat medieval, Revista d'història medieval* 1 (1990): 191–92.

 5. These small bequests have not been collated or studied, but they do appear in the lists of pious bequests made by Barcelonan testators as *puellas maritandas* or *puellis maritandis*. As examples, see the will of Larrentius, a canon of Barcelona, redacted in 1267, or that of Guillem, a shoemaker, in 1305 (ASPP, carp. 24, perg. 333; ACB, calaix 32-B, perg. 157). See also Ana Magdalena Lorente, "El Plato de los Pobres Vergonzantes de la parroquia de Santa María del Mar," in *La pobreza*, 2:168. This charity is also found in Jewish wills. See the will of Sayt Mill of 1377 that bequeathed the substantial sum of two hundred pounds for the dowries of two needy Jewish girls (Pons, *Judios del reino*, 2:134). For Vic, see Ollich, "Les entitats eclesiastiques de Vic," 94.

6. At Urgell, of 127 wills dated from 1287–91 studied by Batlle, only 5 left money for this cause, but several more remembered the daughters of specific friends, neighbors, or relatives (Batlle, *Urgell medieval*, 143). See also Batlle and Casas, "Caritat privada," 1:157; Vinyoles, "Donzelles a maridar," 1:328–35; 355; Batlle, "San Justo," 1:64.

7. Steven Epstein, *Wills and Wealth in Medieval Genoa, 1150–1250* (Cambridge, Mass., 1984), 185–86; and his *Genoa and the Genoese, 958–1528* (Chapel Hill, 1996), 185–86. Between 1376 and 1400, Sienese testators gave more money for dowries than they had in the previous 170 years, and in the fifteenth century the amounts grew. In 1400 this charity represented 6.8 percent of pious bequests, 11.6 percent in 1425, and 11.9 percent in the years after 1475 (Jeremy Cohn, *Death and Property in Siena, 1205–1800* [Baltimore, 1988], 28). In Florence after the plague, dowries also became the favorite charity of charitable confraternities like the Orsanmichele, which in the 1350s is said to have assisted in as many as 20 percent of all marriages (Henderson, *Piety and Charity*, 340).

8. A certain amount of this charity was private and individual, wherein decedents empowered executors to distribute a sum of money to needy girls whom they knew. An example is the will of Master Larrentius, a canon of Barcelona's cathedral. His will of 1267 left the residue of his estate to orphans, widows, captives, and girls of marriageable age, the money to be handed out by his manumissors (ASPP, carp. 25, no. 333). Cabestany and Claramunt, "Santa María del Pí," 1:171; Vinyoles, "Donzelles pobres a maridar," 1:319. At Urgell, young ladies also received partial subsidies. Here the amount of assistance ranged between twenty sous and one hundred sous, at a time when dowries began in the range of two to three hundred sous (Batlle, *Urgell medieval*, 143).

9. Utterback, *Pastoral Care*, 181.

10. Pere III's largest grant of eight hundred sous went to the daughter of the royal scribe; two hundred sous were given to a poor relation of the powerful Morell family. See Vinyoles, "Donzelles pobres a maridar," 1:300–10.

11. Vinyoles, "Donzelles pobres a maridar," 1:322–23.

12. Agustín Rubio Vela, "Infancia y marginación. En torno a las instituciones trecentistas valencianas para el socorro de los huérfanos," in *Violència i marginació en la societat medieval, Revista d'història medieval* 1 (1990): 120–26.

13. Canon law defined a prostitute as one who offered her body in return for remuneration, or any woman who made any sort of public display of herself, who dressed extravagantly, or who simulated love. See Katherine L. Jansen, "Mary Magdalen and the Mendicants: The Preaching of Penance in the Late Middle Ages," *Journal of Medieval History* 21 (1995): 20. In Dijon, for example, women in bordellos were typically around twenty-eight years old, while those who freelanced or worked in private brothels were between seventeen and twenty. For a discussion of the types of prostitutes, see Geremek, *Margins of Society*, 215–28; and Rossiaud, *Medieval Prostitution*, 5–8, 33; for Barcelona usages, Mutgé, *Ciudad de Barcelona*, 62; for Valencia, see Peris, "Prostitución valenciana,"180, 188–89.

14. Vinyoles, *Vida quotidiana*, 121. The principal taboo for Muslims, Jews as well as Christian authorities involved sex with a woman of another religion. Jews and Muslims were absolutely forbidden sex with Christian prostitutes. Christian men who sinned with a Muslim woman risked whipping, and burning for sex with a

Jewish woman. Nirenberg argues that a gallows was erected just outside the Valencian brothel as a warning to those who might be tempted to cross an interfaith boundary (*Communities of Violence*, 136–46).

15. Many prostitutes in Paris had married as a way of assuming some of the external signs of respectability. See Geremek, *Margins of Society*, 231. Barcelona's prostitutes, on the other hand, were exempt from sumptuary laws that prohibited decent women from wearing pearls, silver jewelry, and silk. Indeed, given the association in canon law between *luxuria* and prostitution, such rich display would mark women as prostitutes. In Valencia, the council passed an ordinance in 1334 that, like that of Barcelona, forbade prostitutes to wear capes or other wraps; but in 1384 it also forbade luxurious adornments like furs. See Vinyoles, *Vida quotidiana*, 125; Jansen, "Mary Magdalen and the Mendicants," 20; and Peris, "Prostitución valenciana," 184.

16. For complaints that the Franciscans of Daroca, Huesca, Saragossa and Valencia made to the king in the early fourteenth century, see Webster, *Els menorets*, 80, 147. The problem, however, was evidently of long standing, for as early as 1247 King Jaume I was asked by the Dominicans of Majorca to issue an injunction forbidding prostitutes of the city from congregating outside their house. See *Documentos de Jaime I de Aragón*, ed. Ambrosio Huici Miranda and María Desamparados Cabanes Pecourt (Valencia, 1976–88), 2:265–66, no. 461 (June 7, 1247).

17. Mutgé, *Ciudad de Barcelona*, 162–64.

18. Vinyoles, *Vida quotidiana*, 120–23.

19. In Valencia, 15.8 percent of those arrested for offenses related to prostitution between 1367 and 1399 were charged with working outside the *bordell*. See Vinyoles, "Donzelles pobres a maridar," 1:316; Peris, "Prostitución valenciana," 183–84, 186; Vicente Graullera, "Los hosteleros del Burdel de Valencia," in *Violència i marginació in la societat medieval*, *Revista d'història medieval* 1 (1990): 201. In France, Louis IX issued a number of edicts ordering that prostitutes be expelled from all towns and villages, but in 1256 allowed that at a minimum such persons should be kept out of good neighborhoods and away from ecclesiastical establishments. Later in the century, districts for prostitution became established in Languedoc. Hot Street was established in Montpellier in 1285; similar red-light districts existed in Toulouse at the end of the century, and in Narbonne in 1334. Between 1350 and 1450 most towns of southeast France, including Dijon, Orange, Lyons and Arles, established a *prostibulum publicum*, a brothel that was actually owned by the municipality or other local authority and leased out to a manager. Paris, as early as 1226, had established a shelter for former prostitutes, called the convent of Filles-Dieu; Louis IX subsequently gave it a substantial endowment worth four thousand pounds a year; in 1360, it was joined to the shelter for homeless women, the Hôpital de Sainte-Madeleine. See Geremek, *Margins of Society*, 171, 212–15; Otis, *Prostitution in Medieval Society*, 27–34; Rossiaud, *Medieval Prostitution*, 4–5, 59–61. The numbers of prostitutes in Valencia, to judge by the level of fines actually collected, seems to have been quite substantial. The majority of these were Muslim, suggesting that it was far easier for Christian men to cross the boundary of religion than it was for Muslim men. See John Boswell, *The Royal Treasure: Muslim Communities under the Crown of Aragon in the Fourteenth Century* (New Haven, Conn., 1977), 70–71, 349–50.

20. There was the House for Repentant Prostitutes of Saint Mary Magdalene in Avignon, established in 1280, and significantly expanded in the later fourteenth century. It received former prostitutes, aged twenty-five or older, who were still capable of attracting men to "voluptuous pleasures" (Rossiaud, *Medieval Prostitution*, 202–4). Other institutions of various types existed widely throughout France; some had a profoundly religious character, some were shelters, and a few even were more like prisons. See Otis, *Prostitution in Medieval Society*, 72–76; Jansen, "Mary Magdelan and the Mendicants," 21.

21. Elsewhere, the mendicant friars demonstrated a particular interest in rehabilitating "Mary Magdelenes," but, in the Crown of Aragon, no evidence of this apostolate survives in the records of the Franciscans who, to the contrary, frequently complained about prostitutes loitering near their convents. See Rossiaud, *Medieval Prostitution*, 47; and Webster, *Els menorets*, 147, 186–87.

22. This might have been a refuge of last resort for women who survived in the brothel until the age of forty or so, and who were not able to ascend to the position of *hostelero* in the *bordell*. See Rubio Vela and Rodrigo Lizondo, "Els beguins de València," 330; Peris, "Prostitución valenciana," 197–98; and Graullera, "Los hostaleros del Burdel," 203, 210.

23. This custom appears to have imitated practices in neighboring Languedoc. In 1357, for example, the consuls of Uzès decreed that five prostitutes from the municipal brothel were to be taken by town officials to spend Holy Week in the local hospital of the poor. At Toulouse, in the early sixteenth century, such women were required to stay at some house other than their brothel from Palm Sunday until the Tuesday after Easter. Prostitutes in Perpignan during the Holy Week of 1442 were less fortunate in their relocation, to the municipal leper house! Albi, Dijon, and Arles, on the other hand, seem to have preferred paying public women to refrain from their activities during Holy Week to sequestering them. The Hospitaller Order of the Holy Spirit, whose houses were widespread throughout Europe, provided shelter for prostitutes during both Holy Week and the Octave of Easter. In southeast France, the leases of municipal brothels frequently expired at the beginning of Lent, so that the period of penance could be used to settle in the new tenants who presumably would open for business just after Easter. See Otis, *Prostitution in Medieval Society*, 85–87; "Regula ordinis S. Spiritus," *PL*, 217:1146, cap. 46; and Rossiaud, *Medieval Prostitution*, 8, 63.

24. Vinyoles, *Vida quotidiana*, 125–26; and Vinyoles, "Donzelles pobres a maridar," 1:320.

25. Guilleré, *Girona medieval*, 53. Girona's demographic profile was similar to that of Florence, where families in 1325 seem also to have averaged two children: Henderson, *Piety and Charity*, 263.

26. Philippe Ariès, for example, has argued from artistic evidence that childhood was not regarded as a separate stage in life until the seventeenth century, when children were first subjected to a special regime of discipline. Until that time, he argues, families avoided developing any special attachments to children, probably because of high levels of infant and child mortality. See his *Centuries of Childhood*, 33–49. His general thesis has been accepted by writers like Lawrence Stone, Edward Shorter, and François Lebrun, as well as by popularizers like Elisabeth Badinter. For a critique of the "indifference and neglect" school, see Stephen Wilson, "The Myth

of Motherhood a Myth: The Historical View of European Child-rearing," *Social History* 9 (1984): 181–98. Other writers like Shulamith Shahar disagree with the neglect interpretation; see her *Childhood in the Middle Ages*, 2–3. For an overview of the discussion, see Gavitt, *Charity and Children*, 19.

27. Shahar, *Childhood in the Middle Ages*, 22; *Furs de València*, ed. G Colon and A. Garcia (Valencia, 1980–   ), 2:215, 2.13.1.

28. For a discussion of infanticide, see Shahar, *Childhood in the Middle Ages*, 126–39.

29. This story is not found in any thirteenth-century documentation and undoubtedly is apocryphal (see *PL*, 215:377–80; 217:1131–36); instead it is based on a fifteenth-century illustration discovered in Dijon (Boswell, *Kindness of Strangers*, 416).

30. See Richard C. Trexler, "Infanticide in Florence: New Sources and First Results," *History of Childhood Quarterly* 1 (1973): 100–101; Mary McLaughlin, "Survivors and Surrogates: Children and Parents from the Ninth to the Thirteenth Centuries," in *The History of Childhood*, ed. Lloyd de Mause (New York, 1974), 122. Cemetery evidence from eastern Europe, for example, shows medieval male/female sex ratios to be between 112 and 122 to 100, as opposed to an expected ratio of 105 to 100. Some limited German evidence has a ratio as high as 147 to 100. In Spain, the Kingdom of Aragon had similarly high ratios in the twelfth century, and a study of two regions in the Aragonese Pyrenees in 1429 and 1470 documents the existence, respectively, of 77 male children to 20 female, and 76 to 20, which extrapolates to figures of 385 and 380 to 100! See Josiah C. Russell, *The Control of Late Ancient and Medieval Population* (Philadelphia, 1985), 190, 211–12. See also Heath Dillard, *Daughters of the Reconquest: Women in Castilian Town Society, 1100–1300* (Cambridge, 1984), 209.

31. Otherwise unexplained deaths brought a sentence of excommunication, which then presumably could be lifted after some sort of inquiry (Utterback, *Pastoral Care*, 38, 162–63). There were also accidents. The Hospitaller statutes of 1181, for example, require that "little cradles should be built for the babies of women pilgrims born in the House, so that they might lie separate, and that the baby in its own bed may be in no danger from the restlessness of its mother." *The Rule, Statutes and Customs of the Hospitallers, 1099–1310*, ed. and trans. E. J. King (London, 1934), 35.

32. See Pullan, "Orphans and Foundlings," 3: 10.

33. Boswell, *Kindness of Strangers*, 274–76. Interestingly enough, the institution of prostitution was not viewed as a serious cause of unwanted children, probably because of the widely held belief that prostitutes, for various reasons, were sterile (Jacquart and Thomasset, *Sexuality and Medicine*, 25, 64, 81, 190).

34. Of the foundlings whose parentage is known, 60 percent had a mother who was a slave or servant. See Boswell, *Kindness of Strangers*, 336–40; and Gavitt, *Charity and Children*, 20, 207. In another study in Florence, of the 7,584 children identified as being abandoned in Florence between 1385 and 1484, 1,096 or 14 percent were the children of a slave: Jacques Heers, *Esclaves et domestiques au moyen âge* (Paris, 1981), 228.

35. Teresa M. Vinyoles i Vidal and Margarida González Betlinski, "Els infants abandonats a les portes de l'Hospital de Barcelona (1426–1439)," in *La pobreza*, 2:273.

36. Teresa-Maria Vinyoles i Vidal, "La violència marginal a les ciutats medievals (exemples a la Barcelona des volts del 1400)," in *Violència i Marginació en la societat medieval, Revista d'història medieval* 1 (1990): 161–62; Vinyoles and González, "Infants abandonats," 2:215–20, 273, 278; Guilleré, *Girona medieval*, 53; Rubio Vela, "La asistencia hospitalaria infantil," 172–73.

37. Italian orphanages, for example, had a revolving box, or shelf, called the *ruota* or *tour* or *scaffetta*, into which foundlings could be placed out of sight of hospital personnel. Pullan, "Orphans and Foundlings," 3: 9.

38. In Norway, abandoning children was forbidden, but for practical not intrinsic reasons. Evidently the sparseness of churches, the usual point of abandonment, raised concerns that children would be left far from the ministrations of clergy and thus would not be baptized (Boswell, *Kindness of Strangers*, 292). Among Castilian towns of the twelfth century, children were evidently too valuable a resource for abandonment to become a serious problem; only the *fuero* of Soria, which prescribes the death penalty, addresses the issue. See Dillard, *Daughters of the Reconquest*, 209.

39. Such a ruling is found among the decretals of Pope Gregory IX; it also appears a few decades later in Alfonso X's *Fuero real* (ed. Gonzalo Martínez Diez [Avila, 1988], 4.23.1, p. 501), and in his *Siete Partidas*, 4.20.4. See also Boswell, *Kindness of Strangers*, 325–27; and Shahar, *Childhood in the Middle Ages*, 126.

40. See *Las Siete Partidas*, 4.17.8; 4.19.2–5; 4.20.4.

41. Boswell, *Kindness of Strangers*, 326–31. *Fuero real*, 4.23.3, p. 502.

42. Shahar, *Childhood in the Middle Ages*, 124; Lloyd de Mause, "The Evolution of Childhood," in *The History of Childhood*, ed. Lloyd de Mause (New York, 1974), 28; Boswell, *Kindness of Strangers*, 277; McLaughlin, "Survivors and Surrogates," 121.

43. Baptism, preferably within one week of birth, was generally regarded, despite the development of the idea of limbo by twelfth-century theologians, as necessary to the salvation of a child who might die. Furthermore, many believed that a baptized child had a better chance for survival in this life. For a discussion of medieval practices of infant baptism, see Shahar, *Childhood in the Middle Ages*, 45–52; and Boswell, *Kindness of Strangers*, 323, 362.

44. *Statuts d'Hôtels-Dieu*, 14; "Regula ordinis S. Spiritius de Saxia," *PL*, 217: 1146; *Rule, Statutes and Customs of the Hospitallers*, 38.

45. Orphanages in Florence have been particularly well studied. In addition to San Gallo, the asylum of Santa Maria della Scala was established for the poor sick and infants in 1316 and Santa Maria degli Innocenti just for foundlings in 1445. See McLaughlin, "Survivors and Surrogates," 122; Boswell, *Kindness of Strangers*, 415–17; Heers, *Esclaves*, 227; Nicholas Terpstra, "Apprenticeship in Social Welfare: From Confraternal Charity to Municipal Poor Relief in Early Modern Italy," *Sixteenth Century Journal* 25 (1994): 103.

46. Among the earlier foundling homes in France was one at Marseilles, and another, the Hôpital du Saint-Esprit-en-Grève (1363), in Paris; in Germany, there were those at Ulm, Freiburg. and Nuremberg. See Boswell, *Kindness of Strangers*, 361, 415; Rubio Vela, "Infancia y marginación," 121; *Statuts d'Hôtels-Dieu*, 25, 115, 124; Heers, *Esclaves*, 226; Leah L. Otis, "Municipal Wet Nurses in Fifteenth-Century Montpellier," in *Women and Work in Preindustrial Europe*, ed. Barbara A.

Hanawalt (Bloomington, Ind., 1986), 83; Vinyoles and González, "Infants abandonats," 2:192; Paule Bavoux, "Enfants trouvés et orphelins du XIVᵉ au XVIᵉ siècle,"
in *Assistance et assistés jusqu'à 1610. Actes du 97ᵉ congrès national des sociétés savantes.
Nantes, 1972* (Paris, 1979), 359–69. Foundling homes were very rare in medieval
England; children instead were included within the inmate population of hospitals
and other shelters (Cullum, *Hospitals*, 192). For student hostels, see J. M. Reitzel,
"The Medieval Houses of Bons-Enfants," *Viator* 11 (1980): 179–207. In 1334, four
Italian residents of Paris established a shelter for "poor Italian scholars" who were
studying in the faculties of arts and theology (Manno Tolu, "Pauperum scolarium,"
49–56).

47. Sanchez Herrero, "Cofradías," 28–29; Maureen Flynn, *Sacred Charity:
Confraternities and Social Welfare in Spain, 1400–1700* (Ithaca, N.Y., 1989), 58.

48. Vinyoles and González, "Infants abandonats," 2:192; Rubio Vela, "Infancia
y marginación," 121, 127, 133; Tarragó, *Lerida*, 50; Sanahuja, *Beneficencia en Lérida*,
29; Santamaría, "Asistencia a los pobres en Mallorca," 386. The municipal council of
Valencia in 1473 attempted to consolidate care for foundlings at the Hospital de la
Reyna, but in 1476 abandoned the effort and resumed sending children to En
Clapers (Gallent Marco, "Instituciones hospitalerias," 83). Childcare was an important activity at En Clapers; accounts indicate that between 1374 and 1397 this
activity consumed between 15 and 20 percent of the total budget (Rubio Vela, "La
asistencia hospitalaria infantil," 164, 167).

49. Rubio Vela, "Infancia y marginación," 128–33, 144; Ubieto Arteta, "Pobres
y marginados," 8.

50. See Gavitt, *Charity and Children*, 20, 188, 204, 207, 210. Boswell to some
degree disagrees with Gavitt in arguing that the population of abandoned children
in Florence was split roughly equally between those who were illegitimate and those
whose parents had suffered some sort of social catastrophe (famine, poverty, war,
death of a spouse, and so on); see his *Kindness of Strangers*, 419.

51. Children of mixed religious heritage, for example Christian-Muslim or
Christian-Jewish, were assumed legally to be Christian. Nirenberg argues that the
stigma that attached itself to converts in later centuries simply did not exist in the
Crown of Aragon in the fourteenth century. See his *Communities of Violence*, 150.

52. Older children seem to have had handicaps with which parents were unwilling or unable to cope. For example, Martina, who was mute and disturbed, was
left in 1437 when she was seven, and another without a name was abandoned in
1428 at the age of five with similar afflictions. Joan de València, however, admitted at
the age of five in 1428, was just poor, the illegitimate son of a beggar. The child
evidently resisted abandonment and had to be chained to a tree. Fragmentary records from the 1420s and 1430s show an average of 3.3 abandonments per month,
with March (3.8), April (4.4) and July (4.4) having the most, and June (2.2) and
February (2.4) the fewest. Vinyoles y González, "Infants abandonats," 2:202, 204–
6, 240–54. For Valencia, see Rubio Vela, "La asistencia hospitalaria infantil," 165.

53. The surviving *Llibres d'expòsits* contain admission records for five complete
years, with the indicated number of entries: 1427 (48), 1428 (45), 1436 (33), 1437
(36), 1438 (40). Economic distress, for example, likely caused Pere de Mura, a
candlemaker, to abandon his son at birth, and improving conditions likely explain

his reclamation two years later. Similarly, a leather worker, Francesc Vallès, left Antonia, his daughter, at Santa Creu in 1428 and reclaimed her in 1430. Vinyoles and González, "Infants abandonats," 2:207, 215–21, 239–54. Valencia's principal hospital, En Clapers, received on average twenty children each year during the second half of the fourteenth century; in one sample, over 85 percent of these were either illegitimate and/or abandoned (Rubio Vela, "La asistencia hospitalaria infantil," 163, 166–67, 172–73). Castile's *Siete Partidas* (4.20.4) forbade the return of any children to parents who had deliberately abandoned them, but such a custom evidently did not exist in Catalonia or in the Italian communes. For a discussion of foundlings and illegitimacy, see Pullan, "Orphans and Foundlings," 3: 10, 16–18; and Joan Sherwood, *Poverty in Eighteenth-Century Spain: The Women and Children of the Inclusa* (Toronto, 1988), 95–124.

54. The Hospital of Sant Joan in Perpignan in 1456 employed some fifty wet nurses to feed the children of slaves; a complaint of 1455 made the point that most of the revenues of this hospital served the illegitimate offspring of the town's well-to-do citizens. Italian institutions also served such populations. Genoa, for example, had a hospice for freed captives and their children and another that cared for the children and orphans of former Greek slaves. See Heers, *Esclaves*, 227–28; Miguel Gual Camarena, "Una confradia de negros libertos en el siglo XV," *Estudios de edad media en la Corona de Aragón* 5 (1952): 457–66.

55. Vinyoles and González, "Infants abandonats," 2:217; evidently the stricture contained in the *Siete Partidas* (4.20.4) that automatically freed any slave child who was abandoned by his master did not pertain in Catalonia or else was difficult to enforce. For domestic slavery in Barcelona, see Bensch, "Slavery in Catalonia and Aragon," 80–85.

56. Heers, *Esclaves*, 230. At Florence, between 1434 and 1446, Stefano Moronti sent four infants whom he had fathered by slaves to the Hospital of Santa Maria della Stella because as free children they could not easily be pressed into domestic service; for other examples, see Christiane Klapisch-Zuber, "Women Servants in Florence during the Fourteenth and Fifteenth Centuries," in *Women and Work in Preindustrial Europe*, ed. Barbara Hanawalt (Bloomington, Ind., 1986), 69–70.

57. The savings are apparent from the fact that the 16 percent who were aided in this fashion consumed only 2.7 percent of the amount expended on childcare, despite the fact that the subsidy was often equivalent to what would be paid to a wet nurse for a few months. For example, Sant Macià gave twenty-two sous in one month, and eleven sous in another to a woman for her daughter Antinoga; and between twenty and thirty sous to Campderá for her girl Eulalia. In one of the rare instances when En Clapers was able to ferret out a mother's identity, she turned out to be a mentally disturbed emigrant from Majorca, scarcely able to cope with her child. But, in another instance, where the child was the illegitimate offspring of a father who had died and a mother who had fled from Valencia, the hospital was able to identify the father's family and force it to support the child. Rubio Vela, "La asistencia hospitalaria infantil," 165, 171–72, 186; Roca, *Sant Macià*, 26. A variation of the subsidy has been documented in prerevolutionary France, where mothers, desperately poor, abandoned their children but arranged to be hired by the foundling home to nurse their own children (Wilson, "European Child-rearing," 196).

58. While abandoned children might have diverse backgrounds, in order to receive care in Barcelona's hospitals, they would have to be Christian. In a similar vein, decrees of the provincial synod at Tarragona in 1330 forbade Christian women to serve as nurses or wet nurses for the children of Jews on penalty of excommunication, an enactment that in effect forbade Christian orphanages and shelters to serve Jewish children. Utterback, *Pastoral Care*, 75.

59. The presence of salt and evidence in a note were possible signs of baptism. Boswell, *Kindness of Strangers*, 420; Gavitt, *Charity and Children*, 187–88; Vinyoles and González, "Infants abandonats," 2:193–201; Rubio Vela, "La asistencia hospitalaria infantil," 167–70; Shahar, *Childhood in the Middle Ages*, 48; *Ordinacions*, xii.

60. This meant, of course, that the greatest number of children were nursed by their own mothers (Wilson, "European Child-rearing," 195). The alternative to nursing, that is, feeding children animal milk, was exceedingly rare in the Middle Ages, because children so nourished were thought to have little chance for survival. Nonetheless, there are instances of bottle-feeding when breast milk for various reasons was not available. For example, the records of Barcelona's Hospital of Sant Macià have several examples of the administrator purchasing a goat when a wet nurse could not be found for a child (Roca, *Sant Macià*, 26). The Italian Hospital of Brescia in the 1580s employed a dozen nurses to feed nineteen children, supplementing their human milk with that of twelve goats (Pullan, "Orphans and Foundlings," 3:9).

61. The nurses were to be of good family, well formed, healthy, with good habits, and a calm disposition. Beauty and grace would allow them better to control the children; above all they should have abundant milk. See *Las Siete Partidas* 2.7.3, 11.

62. For an overview, see Shahar, *Childhood in the Middle Ages*, 59–64.

63. A study of wet nurses here in the middle decades of the fifteenth century shows that 99 percent of the women were town residents, and 88 percent were married (another 9 percent were widows), the wives of carpenters, bakers, masons, tailors, and dyers. For these women, this was not a regular source of income since 91 percent were never assigned more than one child. Approximately a fifth of the children were kept between one and three years, another fifth for three to five years, and a tenth over five years. The remainder nursed their children for less than a year, suggesting a high rate of mortality (Otis, "Municipal Wet Nurses," 84–87).

64. Gavitt, *Charity and Children*, 163–67; 189.

65. Joseph F. O'Callaghan, *The Learned King: The Reign of Alfonso X of Castile* (Philadelphia, 1993), 100; Dillard, *Daughters of the Reconquest*, 207. Elsewhere, restrictions were aimed against Christian women who nursed Jewish children (Shahar, *Childhood in the Middle Ages*, 58, 279 n. 30).

66. Gavitt, *Charity and Children*, 217, 237; Vinyoles and González, "Infants abandonats," 2:232–33; Rubio Vela, "La asistencia hospitalaria infantil," 181; Shahar, *Childhood in the Middle Ages*, 35, 149. A recent study of Madrid's foundling home, the Inclusa, for the eighteenth century shows that 58 percent of children died before they were sent out to nurse, and only 11 percent of the children survived until the age of seven (Sherwood, *Poverty in Eighteenth-Century Spain*, 174).

67. Thirty months or so seems to have been the norm for wet-nursing in Barcelona, but slight variations were likely caused by the varying circumstances of

the individual children and of their wet nurses. Three newborns were each received into Santa Creu in October 1426 (Joan Cristòfol, Joan Robí and Agnès Valterra), and each had the good fortune to survive and be returned to the hospital between March 29 and May 2, 1429, indicating terms of thirty or thirty-one months of nursing. Antònia Magdalena, abandoned on January 6, 1427, had twenty-seven months, and Cristina, received on February 15, 1427, enjoyed thirty-three months (Vinyoles and González, "Infants abandonats," 2:223–24, 240–41). The shuffling around of children can also be seen in the records of the smaller Hospital of Sant Macià. For example, a child was discovered on May 20, 1389, at the cathedral. It was unclear whether the girl had been baptized, and so the rite was performed at the nearby parish church of Santa Maria del Pi. Margarida, as she called, was then nursed within the hospital for twenty-three days, during which her background was investigated. After it had been determined that her origins were foreign and thus she had no local family to be located, she was given out to nurse, first to Na Puig who kept her for the month of August, and then to Na Ladona who gave the child to her slave to suckle. See Roca, *Sant Macià*, 29.

68. Saint Vicent Ferrer, in one of his sermons, recommended that when a child turned three his mother ought to tempt him with grapes, cherries, figs, and bread (Rubio Vela, "La asistencia hospitalaria infantil," 174–79).

69. Among the causes of contamination were believed to be sexual intercourse and bad diet. See Dillard, *Daughters of the Reconquest*, 178–79, 209.

70. The Hospital of Sant Macià at times had a live-in nurse. In 1386, for example, the administrator rented from Bartolomeu Poal of Martorell his slave Maria for seven months at a cost of seven pounds (Roca, *Sant Macià*, 25). See also Trexler, "Infanticide in Florence," 100; Gavitt, *Charity and Children*, 228–31; Otis, "Municipal Wet Nurses," 88–89; Vinyoles and González, "Infants abandonats," 2:225, 229.

71. Trexler, "Infanticide in Florence," 101–3; Gavitt, *Charity and Children*, 210–14. At Barcelona there are examples of both girls and boys being restored to their parents. Digna, an infant of three months, was left at the hospital and reclaimed by her father thirteen months later, while Pere Bertran, a newborn abandoned in January 1435, was not reclaimed by his father until mid-1437; see Vinyoles and González, "Infants abandonats," 2:221–22, 244, 249.

72. Shahar, *Childhood in the Middle Ages*, 305–6 n. 51.

73. Vinyoles and González, "Infants abandonats," 2:229, 233–34; Rubio Vela, "La asistencia hospitalaria infantil," 181–82.

74. Castilian law established the age of three as an important point of demarcation in a child's life. Up until that age, the baby was to be under the tutelage of the mother, presumably to be nursed, but afterward the child was under the jurisdiction of the father. See *Las Siete Partidas* 4.19.3. For royal children, see McVaugh, *Medicine before the Plague*, 19.

75. Shahar, *Childhood in the Middle Ages*, 121. The children's diet of bread, meat, legumes, and cheese at Florence would appear to have been more appetizing than the porridge and meat that constituted the diet at Barcelona. Vinyoles and González, "Infants abandonats," 2:225, 228, 230; Gavitt, *Charity and Children*, 172–73, 189; *Ordinacions*, xx–xxi.

76. On June 24, 1374, for example, sixteen sick adults and two children were in residence (Rubio Vela, "La asistencia hospitalaria infantil, 175).

77. Rubio Vela, "Infancia y marginación," 133.

78. As an example, Agnes, the widow of Ramon de Vall, a citizen of Barcelona, took on two eight-year-olds, Joan-Pere and Gràcia-Ventura. The former she promised to teach to read, while the latter was to be given twenty-five pounds as dowry (Vinyoles and González, "Infants abandonats," 2:235–36, 241–42; Gavitt, *Charity and Children*, 248–50, 257). The unwanted children of slaves could in similar fashion be given out by their masters. In 1394, for example, a merchant of Barcelona gave Gabriela, the six-year-old daughter of his Muslim slave Marguerita, to another merchant; and in 1412 Elisenda, the widow of the merchant Jaume Texander, gave the infant daughter of her slave Magdalena to a Barcelona resident named Francesca on the understanding that the girl remain in service until the age of twenty, when she would be given a dowry to marry (Heers, *Esclaves*, 229–30). Children in general seem to have been a source of cheap domestic help for society's elite. The 1427 census at Florence, for example, reveals that 41.5 percent of male servants and 34.2 percent of female servants were children between the ages of eight and seventeen (Shahar, *Children in the Middle Ages*, 240). The French houses of *bons-enfants*, which in some ways functioned as training schools for future clergy, typically housed youths between the ages of nine and sixteen (Reitzel, "Bons-Enfants," 189).

79. Shahar, *Childhood in the Middle Ages*, 227–40; Guilleré, *Girona al segle XIV*, 1:314. There was evidently no great consistency to apprenticeships, for the evidence from medieval Montpellier is different still. Here there is no direct correlation between the length of the apprenticeship contract and the particular craft; furthermore, children typically entered their training even later than in Catalonia, around age fourteen for boys and twelve for girls. See Kathryn L. Reyerson, "The Adolescent Apprentice/Worker in Medieval Montpellier," *Journal of Family History* 17 (1992): 355–56.

80. For a general discussion of apprenticeship, see Shahar, *Childhood in the Middle Ages*, 232–37.

81. Rubio Vela, "Infancia y marginación," 134–43; idem, "La asistencia hospitalaria infantil," 183–85. Apprenticeships for the boys of Girona, for example, commenced generally between the ages of twelve and fourteen and lasted for terms of two years (hatters, bag makers, and shoemakers), three years (apothecaries, blacksmiths, and tanners), four years (furriers and sword makers), and six years (silversmiths and blanket makers) (Guilleré, *Girona medieval*, 80–81).

82. The social acceptance of prostitution might be tied to the medieval idea that it was sexuality without consequence, that is, that because prostitutes were considered to be sterile there could be no children (Jacquart and Thomasset, *Sexuality and Medicine*, 154).

Chapter 7. Late Medieval Assistance

1. See Mollat, *Poor in the Middle Ages*, chapters 3, 6, 8, 12.

2. See López Alsonso, *Pobreza en la España medieval*, 479–84.

3. Barcelona's population, for example, is estimated to have grown from 25,000 to 40,000 between 1213 and 1349; Perpignan had a population of some 13,000, Lleida 12,000. Towns in the range of 6,000 included Tortosa, Tarragona, Girona, and Puigcerdà; between 2,000 and 6,000 were Cervera, Montblanc, Vilafranca del Penedès, Manresa, Berga, and Valls. Towns like Urgell and Vic perhaps had a thousand residents. Michael Mollat argues that the explosion of hospital construction in the thirteenth century was set off by a subsistence crisis at the end of the twelfth century that precipitated an exodus from countryside to town and the development of widespread vagabondage. In Catalonia, the agricultural regime is generally described as being prosperous, but the years after 1190 saw an institutionalization of serfdom which may have had some of the same effect. See Michel Mollat, "Hospitalité et assistance au début du XIIIᵉ siècle," in *Poverty in the Middle Ages*, ed. David Flood (Paderborn, 1975), 37, 40–45; Batlle, *L'expansió baixmedieval*, 90–91, 119–23; Paul Freedman, *The Origins of Peasant Servitude in Medieval Catalonia* (Cambridge, 1991), 89–118.

4. Josep M. Salrach, *El procés de feudalització (segles III–XII)*, vol. 2 of *Història de Catalunya*, ed. Pierre Vilar (Barcelona, 1987), 421–26, 433–38; Charles-E. Dufourcq and Jean Gautier-Dalché, *Historia económica y social de la España cristiana en la edad media*, trans. Federico Revilla (Barcelona, 1983), 120–23; Paul Freedman, *The Diocese of Vic: Tradition and Regeneration in Medieval Catalonia* (New Brunswick, N.J., 1983), 80–81.

5. Caroline Walker Bynum, *Docere Verbo et Exemplo: An Aspect of Twelfth-Century Spirituality* (Missoula, Mont., 1979), 195–97.

6. For a discussion, see Jean Becquet, "Chanoines réguliers et érémitisme clérical," *Revue d'ascétique et de mystique* 48 (1972): 361–70; Toubert, "La vie commune," 11–26; Bynum, *Jesus as Mother*, 9–12; Bynum, *Docere verbo*, 4–5.

7. In the Kingdom of León, for example, only two, albeit the poorest, of twelve chapters accepted the Rule of Saint Augustine. See R. A. Fletcher, *The Episcopate in the Kingdom of León in the Twelfth Century* (Oxford, 1978), 144–45. In Saragossa, the chapter, newly created in 1119, abandoned the common life in 1139. See María Rosa Gutiérrez Iglesias, *La mensa capitular de la iglesia de San Salvador de Zaragoza en el pontificado de Hugo de Mataplana* (Saragossa, 1980), 18. At Vic, despite its foundation as a reformed chapter in 816 and later efforts to enact the Rule of Saint Augustine, canons led essentially private lives (Freedman, *Diocese of Vic*, 41–42). Bishop Bernat de Berga (1172–88) of Barcelona led efforts to keep reforming monks out of the principality (Bensch, *Barcelona*, 54–55).

8. Stephen Bensch argues that municipal institutions developed later in Catalonia than in Italy because the Catalan patriciate, for the most part, was only formed after the economic revival of the 1140s and had not coalesced into a self-confident group when the count-kings reasserted their power in the city in the later twelfth century (*Barcelona*, 82–84; 192–93).

9. Early municipal legislation in Barcelona, for example, dealt with the regulation of inns, meat and poultry prices, and the quality of craft production. For an overview of municipal development, see Batlle, *Expansió baixmedieval*, 78–82; Guilleré, *Girona al segle XIV*, 1:152ff; Bensch, *Barcelona*, 314–17.

10. In fifteenth-century Valladolid, for example, two of the three largest hospi-

tals were operated by confraternities (Rucquoi, "Hospitalisation et charité à Valladolid," 400).

11. André Vauchez argues that confraternities flourished especially during the fourteenth and fifteenth centuries, when practically every parish had at least one, and it would not be uncommon even for rural villages to have several. They were institutions of social integration, with most containing mixed memberships of men and women, young and old. In terms of function, most also demonstrated multiple purposes: simple religious devotions, mutual association, and works of internal and external charity. Some, like the *Laudesi* in Italy or Franciscan tertiaries, emphasized devotion; others works of piety. See André Vauchez, "Conclusion," in *Le mouvement confraternel au Moyen Âge: France, Italie, Suisse* (Rome, 1987), 398–402.

12. Cullum, "Hospitals," 317; Miri Rubin, *Charity and Community in Medieval Cambridge* (Cambridge, 1987), 146–47.

13. Gavitt, *Charity and Children*, 47.

14. López Alonso, *Pobreza en la España medieval*, 453, 472–74.

15. Rubio Vela, *Pobreza, enfermedad y asistencia*, 34, 40–44.

16. Llull, *Blanquerna*, 81–95.

17. Batlle, *L'expansió baixmedieval*, 429–37.

18. Batlle, *Urgell medieval*, 126–27; Guilleré, "Charité à Gérone," 1:197–99.

19. Batlle Prats, "Inventari dels Bens," 59.

20. Guilleré has shown that some 78 percent of rural wills and 35 percent of urban ones left a legacy for the *elemosina panis* ("La peste noire à Gérone," 132).

21. Epstein, *Wills and Wealth*, 169–70; Rubin, "Imagining Medieval Hospitals," 21; Geremek, *Margins of Society*, 190 ff.

22. Barnes critiques James R. Banker, *Death in the Community: Memorialization and Confraternities in an Italian Commune in the Late Middle Ages* (Athens, Ga., 1988); Christopher Black, *Italian Confraternities in the Sixteenth Century* (Cambridge, 1989); and less directly Brian Pullan, *Renaissance Venice*. See Barnes, "Poor Relief and Brotherhood," 603–11. See also Black, *Italian Confraternities*, 4–12, 176–78.

23. Rubin, "Imagining Medieval Hospitals," 16–17; Park, "Healing the Poor," 28; Sandra Cavallo, "The Motivations of Benefactors: An Overview of Approaches to the Study of Charity," in *Medicine and Charity before the Welfare State*, ed. Jonathan Barry and Colin Jones (London, 1991), 46, 59–60; Barry and Jones, introduction to *Medicine and Charity*, 1–2. Brian Tierney, in surveying the development of canonist theory and its implementation between the twelfth and early seventeenth century, argues that in England there was "a single developing tradition without any sudden break or reversal of policy" (*Medieval Poor Law*, 132). Cissie C. Fairchilds, *Poverty and Charity in Aix-en-Provence, 1640–1789* (Baltimore, 1976), 55, 160.

24. Elsewhere, however, where care was the responsibility of organized religious communities, secularized hospitals tended to remain religious houses, served by sisters living under a rule (Rosen, "Historical Sociology," 10).

25. Tierney, *Medieval Poor Law*, 86; Pérez Santamaría, "San Lázaro," 1:86–87, 90.

26. See above, Chapter 3, note 64. There is the further example of the *consell* of Valencia joining with the bishop to conduct a joint visitation and inspection of each

of the city's hospitals in 1341. Muncipalities, in principle, seemed to have resisted the appointment of clerical administrators, lest their rights of supervision be diminished, as demonstrated by the failure of the Jeronymite friar Joan de Conca to succeed his brother as hospitaller of Valencia's Hospital de la Reyna. See Rubio Vela, *Pobreza, enfermedad y asistencia*, 59–61, 168.

27. McVaugh acknowledges that medicine in fact became a secular profession in the fourteenth century, but argues that the reasons were purely practical and related to the growing esteem in which the profession was held; see his *Medicine before the Plague*, 72–75.

28. Rubio Vela, *Pobreza, enfermedad y asistencia*, 40.

29. See above, Chapter 6, note 59; *Ordinaciones de Santa Creu*, xiii. Late fourteenth-century records of Barcelona's Sant Macià, for example, cite cases of the hospital collecting money to provide for the dead, not only for shrouds but for masses. See above, Chapter 5, note 96; Roca, *Sant Macià*, 8. See above, Chapter 6, note 23.

30. Rosen, "Historical Sociology," 9–10, 18.

31. For a discussion of this position, see Tierney, *Medieval Poor Law*, 47–49. Older histories saw this as a fundamental distinction in the sixteenth century between Catholic and Protestant approaches to social welfare. While more recent works have effectively disputed the notion that Catholic charity was not discriminating, authors such as J.-P. Gutton have attempted to argue that Catholic Spain practiced indiscriminate charity well into the Hapsburg era. See Pullan, *Renaissance Venice*, 11–12, 197–99; Linda Martz, *Poverty and Welfare in Hapsburg Spain: The Example of Toledo* (Cambridge, 1983), 1–3.

32. See above, Chapter 1, note 12, Chapter 2, notes 63–68, and Chapter 4, note 94.

33. The arguments of Penyafort and the *Glossa ordinaria* are echoed in an English treatise which distinguishes between those who are *honestus* and *inhonestus*. See Tierney, *Medieval Poor Law*, 60, 150 n. 43.

34. Peter Rycraft, "The Late Medieval Catalan Death-bed," in *God and Man in Medieval Spain: Essays in Honour of J. R. L. Highfield*, ed. Derek W. Lomax and David Mackenzie (Warminster, 1989), 123, 127. The fifteenth-century archbishop of Florence, Antoninus, argued that it was more of a sin to assist a scoundrel than it was a means to achieve grace (Henderson, *Piety and Charity*, 357–58). Eiximenis felt that blind people could make things with their hands; lame folks could carry burdens on the shoulders; and those without feet could teach, write, or sell (Martín, "La pobreza y los pobres," 594).

35. *Ordinacions*, xvii, xxiv–vi, xlii.

36. Gallent Marco, "Hospital de la Reyna," 79; Rubio Vela, *Pobreza, enfermedad y asistencia*, 52, 72–73, 186–87. See also Webster, *Els Menorets*, 94–96.

37. Danon, *Visió històrica*, 61, 63.

38. Batlle, *Urgell medieval*, 149–50.

39. Rubio Vela, *Pobreza, enfermedad y asistencia*, 73; Bertrán, "Almoina de la Seu de Lleida," 352–53.

40. During the fourteenth century, the municipal council of Venice encouraged hospitals in that city to move their investments from property into government

bonds in order to avoid the high costs of property management. Like Barcelona, however, the collapse of the bond market in the next century revealed the strategy to be faulty. See Brian Pullan, "Houses in Service of the Poor in the Venetian Republic," in *Poverty and Charity*, 10: 4. Rubio Vela, *Pobreza, enfermedad y asistencia*, 68–69; Claramunt, "Los ingresos," 375; and Freedman, *Peasant Servitude*, 161–63.

41. Pifarré, "Dos visitas," 2:88–89; Rubio Vela, *Pobreza, enfermedad y asistencia*, 92–93; Claramunt, "Los ingresos," 1:388; Aramayona, "Santa María del Mar," 2:188; see also above, Chapter 5, note 20. This is in sharp contrast to charitable confraternities. For example, the Orsanmichele of Florence in 1329 received 57 percent of its income from money offerings and another 27 percent from the sale of candles at its devotions, but even this institution came increasingly to rely on investment income after wills of 1348, the year of the plague, swelled its endowment (Henderson, *Piety and Charity*, 200, 208–9, 233).

42. At Urgell, for example, she argues that the typical legacy to the municipal hospital in the late thirteenth and early fourteenth centuries ranged up to thirty sous, or else consisted of the decedent's bed and bed linen. Batlle, *Urgell medieval*, 133; Batlle, *L'expansió baixmedieval*, 429; Batlle and Casas, "Caritat privada," see the charts following 1:182.

43. On the capitalization of alms and legacies, see examples in Batlle, *Urgell medieval*, 135–37; Lorente, "Plato de los Pobres," 2:165.

44. For example, at the hospitals of Santa Maria Nuova and San Matteo only 32 percent and 27 percent of recorded deaths are those of Florentines. At the foundling hospital of the Innocenti, only 34 percent of the children were born in Florence. As many as a fifth of all hospital inmates belonged to the servant class. Henderson notes that, although the hospitals were the richest institutions in the city, they nonetheless were in debt and, like their compeers elsewhere in Europe, suffered an economic crisis in the fifteenth century. Henderson, *Piety and Charity*, 376–78, 393, 399–400, 407, 422.

45. Claramunt, "Los ingresos," 1:384, 388; Aramoyona, "Santa María del Mar," 2:186.

46. Pérez Santamaría, "San Lázaro," 1:88–89; Batlle Prats, "Inventari dels Bens," 78–79.

47. In 1401, King Martí and Queen Maria donated fifteen thousand sous to the construction fund; there must also have been an active campaign to raise money from others to judge by a papal indulgence granted in 1403 to contributors to the building fund; a privilege of 1433 suggests that collectors were dispatched to churches in the region for the purpose of collecting monies (Danon, *Visió històrica*, 25, 78, 157–58).

48. Nirenberg, *Communities of Violence*, 200 ff., 150.

49. Mutgé, *Ciudad de Barcelona*, 317; Vinyoles, *Vida quotidiana*, 119.

50. Rubio Vela, "Infancia y marginación," 129–30.

51. An example from 1391 of a funeral of a Barcelonan merchant had twelve poor folk acting as pallbearers, with four fools acting as acolytes (Vinyoles, "Violència marginal," 158–69).

52. Rubio Vela, "La asistencia hospitalaria infantil," 166.

53. Martz, *Poverty and Welfare*, 74–75.

54. See their introduction to *Medicine and Charity*, 2.

55. Fairchilds, *Poverty and Charity in Aix-en-Provence*, 160; Martz, *Poverty and Welfare*, 7–44; Flynn, *Sacred Charity*, 141–45. Similarly, Brian Pullan's study of charity in early modern Venice affirms the importance of religious motivations (*Renaissance Venice*, 631).

Bibliography

Actes du 110ᵉ Congrès national des sociétés savantes. 3 vols. Paris: Editions du C.T.H.S., 1987.

Adell i Gisbert, Joan-Albert. "L'hospital de pobres de Santa Magdalena de Montblanc i l'arquitectura hospitalària medieval a Catalunya." *Acta historica et archaeologica mediaevalia* 4 (1983): 239–63.

Aging and the Aged in Medieval Europe: Selected Papers from the Annual Conference of the Centre for Medieval Studies, University of Toronto, held 25–26 February and 11–12 November 1983. Edited by Michael M. Sheehan, C.S.B. Toronto: Pontifical Institute of Mediaeval Studies, n.d.

Alimentació i societat a la Catalunya medieval. Anuario de estudios medievales, Anex 20. Barcelona: C.S.I.C., 1988.

Altisent, Agustí. *L'Almoina reial de la cort de Pere el Cerimoniós. Estudi i edició dels manuscrits de l'almoiner Fra Guillem Duedé, monjo de Poblet (1378–1385).* Scriptorium Populeti, 2. Abbey of Poblet, 1969.

Amasuno Sarraga, Marcelino V. *La escuela de medicina del estudio salmantino (siglos XIII–XV).* Acta Salmanticensia, Historia de la Universidad, 52. Salamanca: Universidad, Servicio de Public, 1990.

A pobreza e a assistência aos pobres na península ibérica durante a idade média. Actas das 1.ᵃˢ jornadadas luso-espanholas de história medieval, Lisboa, 25–30 de Setembro de 1972. 2 vols. Lisbon: Instituto de Alta Cultura, 1973.

Aragó, Ignasi. *Els hospitals a Catalunya.* Barcelona: Imp. Altés, 1967.

Aramayona Alonso, Guillermo. "El cuaderno de 1421 del «Bací dels Pobres Vergonyants» de la parroquia de Santa María del Mar, de Barcelona." In *La pobreza y la asistencia a los pobres en la Cataluña medieval.* Edited by Manuel Riu, 2:173–89. Barcelona: C.S.I.C, 1980–82.

Ariès, Philippe. *Centuries of Childhood: A Social History of Family Life.* Translated by Robert Baldick. New York: Vintage Books, 1962.

Assistance et assistés jusqu'à 1610. Actes du 97ᵉ congrès national des sociétés savantes. Nantes, 1972. Paris: Bibliothèque nationale, 1979.

Assistance et charité. Edited by M.-H. Vicaire. Cahiers de Fanjeaux, 13. Toulouse: Privat, 1978.

Banker, James R. *Death in the Community: Memorialization and Confraternities in an Italian Commune in the Late Middle Ages.* Athens: University of Georgia Press, 1988.

Barber, Malcolm. "The Order of Saint Lazarus and the Crusades." *Catholic Historical Review* 80 (1994): 439–56.

Barnes, Andrew. "Poor Relief and Brotherhood." *Journal of Social History* 24 (1991): 603–11.

Barry, Jonathan, and Colin Jones, eds. *Medicine and Society Before the Welfare State*. London: Routledge, 1991.

Batlle i Gallart, Carme. *L'assistència als pobres a la Barcelona medieval (s. XIII)*. Episodis de la Història. Barcelona: Editorial Rafael Dalmau, 1987.

———. "La ayuda a los pobres en la parroquia de San Justo de Barcelona." In *A pobreza e a assistência aos pobres na península ibérica durante a idade média*, 1:59–71. Lisbon: Instituto de Alta Cultura, 1973.

———. *L'expansió baixmedieval (segles XIII–XV)*. Vol. 3 of *Història de Catalunya*. Edited by Pierre Vilar. Barcelona: Edicions 62, 1988.

———. "La Seu d'Urgell a la segona meitat del segle XIII." *Urgellia* 3 (1980): 369–417.

———. *La Seu d'Urgell medieval: La ciutat i els seus habitants*. Barcelona: Editorial Rafael Dalmau, 1985.

Batlle i Gallart, Carme, and Montserrat Casas. "La caritat privada i les institucions benèfiques de Barcelona (segle XIII)." In *La pobreza y la asistencia a los pobres en la Cataluña medieval*. Edited by Manuel Riu, 1:117–90. Barcelona: C.S.I.C., 1980–82.

Batlle Prats, Luis. "Inventari dels Bens de l'Hospital de la Seu de Girona." *Estudis Universaris Catalans* 19 (1934): 58–80.

Baucells i Reig, Josep. "L'església de Catalunya." *Acta historica et archaeologica mediaevalia* 13 (1992): 427–42.

———. "Gènesi de la Pia almoina de la Seu de Barcelona: els fundadors." In *La pobreza y la asistencia a los pobres en la Cataluña medieval*. Edited by Manuel Riu, 1:17–75. Barcelona: C.S.I.C., 1980–82.

———. *El maresme i la Pia Almoina de la Seu de Barcelona: Catàleg del fons en pergamí de l'Arxiu Capitular de la Catedral de Barcelona*. Barcelona: Generalitat de Catalunya, 1987.

———. "La Pia Almoina de la seo de Barcelona. Origen y desarrollo." In *A pobreza e a assistência aos pobres na península ibérica durante a idade média*, 1:73–135. Lisbon: Instituto de Alta Cultura, 1973.

Baudot, Marcel. "La gestion d'une léproserie du XIVe siècle: la maladrerie Saint-Lazare de Montpellier." In *Actes du 110e Congrès national des sociétés savantes*, 1:411–26. Paris: Editions du C.T.H.S., 1987.

Bavoux, Paule. "Enfants trouvés et orphelins du XIVe au XVIe siècle à Paris." In *Assistance et assistés jusqu'à 1610*, 359–70. Paris: Bibliothèque nationale, 1979.

Bayerri y Bertomeu, Enrique. *Historia de Tortosa y su comarca*. 8 vols. Tortosa: Imprenta de Algueró y Barges, 1933–1960.

Becker, Marvin B. *Medieval Italy: Constraints and Creativity*. Bloomington: Indiana University Press, 1981.

Becquet, Jean. "Chanoines réguliers et érémitisme clérical." *Revue d'ascétique et de mystique* 48 (1972): 361–70.

Bensch, Stephen P. *Barcelona and its Rulers, 1096–1291*. Cambridge: Cambridge University Press, 1995.

———. "From Prizes of War to Domestic Merchandise: The Changing Face of Slavery in Catalonia and Aragon, 1000–1300." *Viator* 25 (1994): 63–93.

Bériac, Françoise. *Histoire des lépreux au Moyen Âge, une société d'exclus*. Paris: Éditions Imago, 1988.

Bermúdez Aznar, Agustín. "La abogacía de pobres en la España medieval." In *A pobreza e a assistência aos pobres na península ibérica durante a idade média*, 1:135–55. Lisbon: Instituto de Alta Cultura, 1973.

Bertrán i Roigé, Prim. "La alimentación de los pobres de Lérida en el año 1338." In *Manger et boire au Moyen Âge*, 1:361–73. Paris: Belles lettres, 1984.

———."L'Almoina de la Seu de Lleida a principis del segle XV." In *La pobreza y la asistencia a los pobres en la Cataluña medieval*. Edited by Manuel Riu, 2:347–68. Barcelona: C.S.I.C., 1980–82.

———. "El menjador de l'almoina de la catédral de Lleida. Notes sobre l'alimentació dels pobres lleidatans al 1338." *Ilerda* 40 (1979): 89–124.

Black, Christopher. *Italian Confraternities in the Sixteenth Century*. Cambridge: Cambridge University Press, 1989.

Bofarull y de Sartario, Manuel de, ed. *Gremios y cofradías de la antigua Corona de Aragón*. Colección de documentos inéditos del Archivo General de la Corona de Aragón. Vols. 40, 41. Barcelona, 1876–1910.

Boix Pociello, J. "Les persones pobres e miserables a la Ribagorça medieval." *Acta historica et archaeologica mediaevalia* 5–6 (1984–85): 185–210.

Bonenfant, Paul. "Hôpitaux et bienfaisance publique dans les anciens Pays-Bas des origines à la fin du XVIIIᵉ siècle." *Annales de la Société Belge d'Histoire des Hôpitaux* 3 (1965): 1–195.

Bonnassie, Pierre. *La Catalogne du milieu du Xᵉ à la fin du XIᵉ siècle, croissance et mutations d'une société*. 2 vols. Toulouse: Université de Toulouse — Le Marail, 1975–77.

Boswell, John. *The Kindness of Strangers: The Abandonment of Children in Western Europe from Late Antiquity to the Renaissance*. New York: Pantheon Books, 1988.

———. *The Royal Treasure: Muslim Communities under the Crown of Aragon in the Fourteenth Century*. New Haven, Conn.: Yale University Press, 1977.

Brodman, James William. *Ransoming Captives in Crusader Spain: The Order of Merced on the Christian-Islamic Frontier*. Philadelphia: University of Pennsylvania Press, 1986.

———. "The Trinitarian and Mercedarian Orders: A Study in Religious Redemptionism in the Thirteenth Century." Ph.D. dissertation, University of Virginia, 1974.

———. "What Is a Soul Worth? *Pro anima* Bequests in Municipal Legislation of Reconquest Spain." In *Medievalia et Humanistica: Studies in Medieval and Renaissance Culture*. Edited by Paul Maurice Clogan, 15–23. New Series, no. 20. Lantham, Maryland: Rowman and Littlefield, 1994.

Broida, Equip. "El àpats funerais segons els testaments vers al 1400." In *Alimentació i societat a la Catalunya medieval*, 263–69. Barcelona: C.S.I.C., 1988.

Bullock, Ward E. "Leprosy (Hansen's Disease)" In *Cecil Textbook of Medicine*. Edited by J. B. Wyngaarden and L. H. Smith, 7th ed., 1634–38. Philadelphia: Saunders, 1985.

Burns, Robert I., S.J. *The Crusader Kingdom of Valencia: Reconstruction on a Thirteenth-Century Frontier*. 2 vols. Cambridge, Mass.: Harvard University Press, 1967.

————. "Los hospitales del reino de Valencia en el siglo XIII." *Anuario de estudios medievales* 2 (1965): 135–54.

Bynum, Caroline Walker. *Docere Verbo et Exemplo: An Aspect of Twelfth-Century Spirituality*. Missoula, Mont.: Scholars Press, 1979.

————. *Jesus as Mother: Studies in the Spirituality of the High Middle Ages*. Berkeley: University of California Press, 1982.

Cabestany, Joan-F., and Salvador Claramunt. "El «Plat dels pobres» de la parroquia de Santa María del Pi de Barcelona (1401–1428)." In *A pobreza e a assistência aos pobres na península ibérica durante a idade média*, 1:157–81. Lisbon: Instituto de Alta Cultura, 1973.

Caille, Jacqueline. "Assistance et hospitalité au Moyen Âge." *Bulletin de la Société des Etudes Littéraires, Scientifiques et Artistiques du Lot* 102 (1981): 295–301.

Cardoner Planas, A. "El 'hospital para judios pobres' de Barcelona." *Sefarad* 22 (1922): 373–75.

Carlé, María del Carmen. "Alimentación y abastecimiento." *Cuadernos de historia de España* 61–62 (1977): 246–341.

Carmona García, Juan Ignacio. *El sistema de hospitalidad publica en la Sevilla del antiguo Regimen*. Seville: Diputacion Provincial, 1979.

Cartulari de Poblet: Edicio del manuscrit de Tarragona. Barcelona: Institut d'Estudis Catalans, 1938.

Cartulario de «Sant Cugat» del Vallés. Edited by José Rius Serra. 3 vols. Barcelona: C.S.I.C., 1945–47.

Castillón Cortada, Francisco. "El limosnero de la catedral de Roda de Isábena (Huesca)." *Cuadernos de Aragón* 21 (1990): 63–100.

Cateura Bennasser, Pablo. *Sobre la fundación y dotación del Hospital de San Andres, en la Ciudad de Mallorca, por Nuño Sans*. Palma: Centro Asociado de Baleares, 1980.

Cavallo, Sandra. "The Motivations of Benefactors: An Overview of Approaches to the Study of Charity." In *Medicine and Charity before the Welfare State*. Edited by Jonathan Barry and Colin Jones, 46–62. London: Routledge, 1991.

Chenu, M.-D. *La théologie au douzième siècle*. Paris: J. Vrin, 1966.

Claramunt, Salvador. "Dos aspectos de l'alimentació medieval: Dels canonges a les «miserabiles personae»." In *Alimentació i societat a la Catalunya medieval*, 167–72. Barcelona: C.S.I.C., 1988.

————. "Los ingresos del «Bací o Plat dels Pobres» de la parroquia de Santa María del Pí de Barcelona, de 1434 a 1456." In *La pobreza y la asistencia a los pobres en la Cataluña medieval*. Edited by Manuel Riu, 1: 373–90. Barcelona: C.S.I.C., 1980–82.

————. "Una primera aproximación para establecer un plano de la pobreza vergonzante en el arrabal de la Rambla, de Barcelona, a lo largo del siglo XV." In *La pobreza y la asistencia a los pobres en la Cataluña medieval*. Edited by Manuel Riu , 2:369–82. Barcelona: C.S.I.C., 1980–82.

Clay, Rotha Mary, *The Mediaeval Hospitals of England*. [1909 ed.] London: Methuen, 1966.

Cohn, Jeremy. *Death and Property in Siena, 1205–1800*. Baltimore: Johns Hopkins University Press, 1988.

Colección diplomática de la catedral de Huesca. Edited by Antonio Durán Gudiol. 2 vols. Saragossa: C.S.I.C., 1965–69.

Coll Julià, Núria. "Documentación notarial relativa a los pobres en la Cataluña del siglo XV." In *La pobreza y la asistencia a los pobres en la Cataluña medieval.* Edited by Manuel Riu, 2: 287–311. Barcelona: C.S.I.C., 1980–82.

A Companion to Medical Studies. Edited by R. Passmore and J. S. Robson. 3 vols. Philadelphia: Davis, 1970.

Contreras Mas, Antonio, and Ramón Rosselló. *La asistencia publica a los leprosos en Mallorca: Siglos XIV al XIX.* Majorca: En Tall, 1990.

Constable, Giles. "Renewal and Reform in the Religious Life: Concepts and Realities." In *Renaissance and Renewal in the Twelfth Century.* Edited by Robert L. Benson and Giles Constable, 37–67. Cambridge, Mass.: Harvard University Press, 1982.

Constantelos, Demetrios J. *Byzantine Philanthropy and Social Welfare.* 2nd edition revised. New Rochelle, N. Y.: Aristide D. Caratzas, 1991.

Costa i Paretas, Maria-Mercè. "Els antics ponts de Girona." *Anales del instituto de Estudios Gerundenses* 22 (1974–75): 131–48.

Cullum, Patricia Helen. *Cremetts and Corrodies: Care of the Poor and Sick at St. Leonard's Hospital, York, in the Middle Ages.* York: Borthwick Papers, 79, 1991.

———. "Hospitals and Charitable Provision in Medieval Yorkshire, 936–1547." D. Phil. thesis, University of York, 1989.

Danon, Josep. *Visió històrica de l'Hospital General de Santa Creu de Barcelona.* Barcelona: Editorial Rafael Dalmau, 1978.

Demaitre, Luke. "The Care and Extension of Old Age in Medieval Medicine." In *Aging and the Aged in Medieval Europe.* Edited by Michael M. Sheehan, 3–22. Toronto: Pontifical Institute of Mediaeval Studies, n.d.

———. "The Relevance of Futility: Jordanus de Turre (fl. 1313–1335) on the Treatment of Leprosy." *Bulletin of the History of Medicine* 70 (1996): 25–61.

de Mause, Lloyd. "The Evolution of Childhood." In *The History of Childhood.* Edited by Lloyd de Mause, 1–73. New York: The Psychohistory Press, 1974.

Dillard, Heath. *Daughters of the Reconquest: Women in Castilian Town Society, 1100–1300.* Cambridge: Cambridge University Press, 1984.

Documentos de Jaime I de Aragón. Edited by Ambrosio Huici Miranda and María Desamparados Cabanes Pecourt. 5 vols. Valencia and Saragossa: Anubar, 1975–88.

Dols, Michael W. "The Leper in Medieval Islamic Society." *Speculum* 58 (1983): 891–916.

Dufourcq, Charles-E., and Jean Gautier-Dalché. *Historia económica y social de la España cristiana en la edad media.* Translated by Federico Revilla. Barcelona: Ediciones Albir, 1983.

Durán Gudiol, Antonio. *El hospital de Somport entre Aragón y Béarn (siglos XII y XIII).* Colección diplomática. Saragossa: Guara Editorial, 1986.

Duran i Sanpere, Agustí. *Llibre de Cervera.* Barcelona: Curial, 1977.

Echániz Sans, María. "La alimentación de los pobres asistidos por la Pia Almoina de la catedral de Barcelona según el libro de cuentas de 1283–1284." In *Alimentació i societat a la Catalunya medieval*, 173–261. Barcelona: C.S.I.C., 1988.

Ellenhorn, Matthew J., and Donald G. Barceloux. *Medical Toxicology: Diagnosis and Treatment of Human Poisoning*. New York: Elsevier, 1988.

Emery, Richard W. "The Black Death of 1348 in Perpignan." *Speculum* 42 (1967): 611–23.

Epstein, Steven. *Genoa and the Genoese, 958–1528*. Chapel Hill: University of North Carolina Press, 1996.

———. *Wills and Wealth in Medieval Genoa, 1150–1250*. Cambridge, Mass.: Harvard University Press, 1984.

Fairchilds, Cissie C. *Poverty and Charity in Aix-en-Provence, 1640–1789*. Baltimore: Johns Hopkins University Press, 1976.

Feliu, Lluís G. "L'hospital de Santa Eulàlia del Camp." *Analecta sacra Terraconensia* 11 (1935): 291–306.

Ferreira de Almeida, C .A., "Os caminhos e a assistência no norte de Portugal." In *A pobreza e a assistência aos pobres na península ibérica durante a idade média*, 1:39–57. Lisbon: Instituto de Alta Cultura, 1973.

Fletcher, R. A. *The Episcopate in the Kingdom of León in the Twelfth Century*. Oxford: Oxford University Press, 1978.

Flynn, Maureen. *Sacred Charity: Confraternities and Social Welfare in Spain, 1400–1700*. Ithaca, N.Y.: Cornell University Press, 1989.

Fort i Cogul, E. "Sant Bernat Calvó i l'hospital de pobres de Santes Creus." In *Miscel.lània Històrica Catalana: Homenatge al Pare Jaume Finestres, Historiador de Poblet*. Scriptorim Populeti 3, 181–213. Abadia de Poblet, 1970.

Freedman, Paul. *The Diocese of Vic: Tradition and Regeneration in Medieval Catalonia*. New Brunswick, N.J.: Rutgers University Press, 1983.

———. *The Origins of Peasant Servitude in Medieval Catalonia*. Cambridge: Cambridge University Press, 1991.

Fuero real. Edited by Gonzalo Martínez Diez. Avila: Fundación Sanchez Albornoz, 1988.

Furs de València. Edited by G. Colon and A. Garcia. 6 vols. to date. Valencia: Editorial Barcino, 1980– .

Gallent Marco, Mercedes. "Aproximación a un modelo medieval de institución sanitaria: El Hospital de la Reyna." *Saitabi* 31 (1981): 73–87.

———. "Instituciones hospitalerias y podres públicos en Valencia." *Saitabi* 34 (1984): 75–88.

García Ballester, Luis. "Medical Science in Thirteenth-Century Castile: Problems and Prospects." *Bulletin of the History of Medicine* 61 (1987): 183–202.

———. *La medicina a la Valencia medieval: Medicina i societat en un país medieval mediterrani*. Valencia: Institució Valenciana d'Estudis i Investigació, 1988.

Garcia Ballester, Luis, Michael R. McVaugh, and Agustín Rubio-Vela. *Medical Licensing and Learning in Fourteenth-Century Valencia*. Philadelphia: American Philosophical Society, 1989.

García del Moral, Antonio. *El Hospital Mayor de San Sebastian de Córdoba: Cinco siglos de Asistencia Médico-sanitaria Institucional (1363–1816)*. Córdoba: Diputacion Provincial, 1984.

Gavitt, Philip. *Charity and Children in Renaissance Florence: The Ospedale degli Innocenti, 1410–1536*. Ann Arbor: University of Michigan Press, 1990.

Geremek, Bronislaw. *Les marginaux parisiens aux XIVe et XVe siècles.* Paris: Flammarion, 1976.

———. *The Margins of Society in Late Medieval Paris.* Translated by Jean Birrell. Cambridge: Cambridge University Press, 1987.

———. *Poverty: A History.* Translated by Agnieszka Kolakowska. Oxford: Blackwell, 1994.

Graullera, Vicente. "Los hostaleros del Burdel de Valencia." In *Violència i marginació en la societat medieva. Revista d'història medieval* 1 (1990): 201–13.

Gual Camarena, Miguel. "La asistencia a los pobres en la corte de Pedro IV, el Ceremonioso." In *A pobreza e a assistência aos pobres na península ibérica durante a idade média*, 1:455–81. Lisbon: Instituto de Alta Cultura, 1973.

———. "Una cofradia de negros libertos en el siglo XV." *Estudios de edad media en la Corona de Aragón* 5 (1952): 457–66.

Guilleré, Christian. "Assistance et charité à Gérone au début du XIVe siècle." In *La pobreza y la asistencia a los pobres en la Cataluña medieval.* Edited by Manuel Riu, 1: 191–204. Barcelona: C.S.I.C., 1980–82.

———. *Diner, poder i societat a la Girona del segle XIV.* Girona: Ajuntament de Girona, 1984.

———. *Girona al segle XIV.* Translated by Núria Mañé. 2 vols. Barcelona: Publicacions de l'Abadia de Montserrat, 1993–94.

———. *Girona medieval. L'etapa d'apogeu, 1285–1360.* Girona: Diputacio de Girona, 1991.

———. "Le milieu médical géronais au XIVe siècle." In *Actes du 110e Congrès national des sociétés savantes*, 1:263–81. Paris: Editions du C.T.H.S., 1987.

———. "La peste noire à Gerone." *Annals de l'Institut d'Estudis Gironins* 27 (1984): 87–161.

———. "Une institution charitable face aux malheurs du temps: La Pia Almoina de Gerone (1347–1380)." In *La pobreza y la asistencia a los pobres en la Cataluña medieval.* Edited by Manuel Riu, 2:313–45. Barcelona: C.S.I.C., 1980–82.

Gutiérrez Iglesias, María Rosa. *La mensa capitular de la iglesia de San Salvador de Zaragoza en el pontificado de Hugo de Mataplana.* Saragossa: Institución «Fernando el Católico», 1980.

Gyug, Richard. *The Diocese of Barcelona during the Black Death: The Register Notule Communium 15 (1348–1349).* Subsidia mediaevalia, 22. Toronto: Pontifical Institute of Mediaeval Studies, 1994.

Hanawalt, Barbara A., ed. *Women and Work in Preindustrial Europe.* Bloomington: Indiana University Press, 1986.

Heers, Jacques. *Esclaves et domestiques au Moyen Âge.* Paris: Fayard, 1981.

Henderson, John. *Piety and Charity in Late Medieval Florence.* Oxford: Clarendon Press, 1994.

Hergueta, Narciso. "Noticias históricas del maestre Diego de Villar, médico de los reyes Alfonso VIII, Doña Berenguela y San Francisco, de los hospitales y hospederías que hugo en la Rioja en los siglos XII y XIII, y de la villa de Villar de Torre." *Revista de Archivos, Bibliotecas y Museos* 11 (1904): 126–32, 423–34.

Hernández Iglesias, Fermin. *La beneficencia en España*, 2 vols. Madrid: Tipografía de Manuel Minuesa, 1876.

Hernando, Josep. "Els moralistes i l'alimentació a la baixa edat mitjana." In *Alimentació i societat a la Catalunya medieval*, 271–93. Barcelona: C.S.I.C., 1988.

Hillgarth, J. N., and Guilio Silano. *The Register* NOTULE COMMUNIUM 14 *of the Diocese of Barcelona (1345–1348)*. Toronto: Pontifical Institute of Mediaeval Studies, 1983.

Horden, Peregrine. "A Discipline of Relevance: The Historiography of the Later Medieval Hospital." *Social History of Medicine* 1 (1988): 359–74.

Hug, P. L. "Order of the Holy Spirit." *New Catholic Encyclopedia*, 7:103–4. New York: McGraw-Hill, 1967.

Hughes, Muriel Joy. *Women Healers in Medieval Life and Literature*. Freeport, N.Y.: Books for Libraries Press, 1968.

Imbert, Jean. *Les hôpitaux en droit canonique*. Paris: J. Vrin, 1947.

Jacquart, Danielle, and Claude Thomasset. *Sexuality and Medicine in the Middle Ages*. Translated by Matthew Adamson. Princeton, N.J.: Princeton University Press, 1988.

Jacques de Vitry. *The* Historia occidentalis *of Jacques de Vitry: A Critical Edition*. Edited by J. F. Hinnebusch, O.P. Freibourg: University Press, 1972.

Jansen, Katherine L. "Mary Magdalen and the Mendicants: The Preaching of Penance in the Late Middle Ages." *Journal of Medieval History* 21 (1995): 1–25.

Jugnot, Gérard. "Deux fondations augustiniennes en faveur des pèlerins: Aubrac et Roncevaux." In *Assistance et charité*. Cahiers de Fanjeaux, 13, 321–41. Toulouse: Privat, 1978.

Junyent, Eduard. *La ciutat de Vic i la seva història*. Barcelona: Documents de Cultura Curial, 1976.

Kealey, Edward J. *Medieval Medicus: A Social History of Anglo-Norman Medicine*. Baltimore: Johns Hopkins University Press, 1981.

Klapisch-Zuber, Christiane. "Women Servants in Florence during the Fourteenth and Fifteenth Centuries." In *Women and Work in Preindustrial Europe*. Edited by Barbara Hanawalt, 56–80. Bloomington: Indiana University Press, 1986.

Lara Peinado, Federico, and José Trenchs Odena. "Documento inedito sobre la venta del Hospital de Pedro Moliner de la ciudad de Lerida (1459)." *Ilerda* 37 (1976): 58–68.

Ledesma Rubio, María Luisa. *Templarios y Hospitalarios en el Reino de Aragón*. Saragossa: Guara Editorial, 1982.

LeGrand, Léon. "Les Maisons-Dieu: Leurs statuts au XIIIᵉ siècle." *Revue des questions historiques* 60 (1896): 95–134.

Little, Lester K. *Religious Poverty and the Profit Economy in Medieval Europe*. Ithaca, N.Y.: Cornell University Press, 1978.

Lladonosa i Pujol, Josep. *Història de la ciutat de Lleida*. Barcelona: Curial, 1980.

——. *La pediatria als antics hospicis de Lleida*. Lleida: Primer Congrès de Pediatres de Llengua Catalan, 1978.

Llibre del Repartiment de València. Edited by Antoni Ferrando i Francés. Valencia: Vicent García Editores, 1979.

Llompart, Gabriel. "La hostelería mallorquina en el siglo XIV." In *XIII Congrés d'història de la Corona d'Aragó, Comunicacions*, 2:83–93. Palma de Mallorca, 1990.

Llull, Ramon. *Blanquerna: A Thirteenth-Century Romance.* Translated by E. Allison Peers. London: Jarrolds, 1926.

López Alonso, Carmen. *La pobreza en la España medieval.* Madrid: Ministerio de Trabajo y Seguridad, 1986.

López de Meneses, Amada. "Documentos acerca de la peste negra en los dominios de la Corona de Aragón." *Estudios de la edad media en la Corona de Aragón* 6 (1956): 291–447.

Lorente, Ana Magdalena. "El Plato de los Pobres Vergonzantes de la parroquia de Santa María del Mar." In *La pobreza y la asistencia a los pobres en la Cataluña medieval.* Edited by Manuel Riu, 2:153–71. Barcelona: C.S.I.C., 1980–82.

MacKinney, Loren C. *Early Medieval Medicine with Special Reference to France and Chartres.* Baltimore: Johns Hopkins Press, 1937.

Mane, P. "L'alimentation des paysans en France et en Italie aux XIIe et XIIIe siècles à travers l'iconographie des calendriers (sculpture, fresques, mosaïques et vitrail)." In *Manger et boire au Moyen Âge,* 1:319–33. Paris: Belles lettres, 1984.

Manger et boire au Moyen Âge: Actes du colloque de Nice, 15–17 octobre 1982. 2 vols. Paris: Belles lettres, 1984.

Manno Tolu, Rosalia. "La «Domus pauperum scolarium Italorum» a Parigi nel 1334." *Archivo Storico Italiano* 146 (1988): 49–56.

Marquès, B. "Fundació d'un hospital a Organyà en 1156." *Església d'Urgell* 108 (1982): 7–8.

Martín, José Luis, "La pobreza y los pobres en los textos literarios del siglo XIV." In *A pobreza e a assistência aos pobres na península ibérica durante a idade média,* 2:587–635. Lisbon: Instituto de Alta Cultura, 1973.

Martinell, César. "Els hospitals medievals catalans." *Pratica medicina* (1935): 109–32.

———. "L'antic hospital de santa Tecla de Tarragona." *Butlleti arqueologic [Bolétin Arqueologico] de Tarragona* 3, no. 49 (1934): 388–96.

Martínez García, Luis. *La asistencia a los pobres en Burgos en la baja edad media. El hospital de Santa Maria la Real, 1341–1500.* Burgos: Diputación Provincial de Burgos, 1981.

———. "La asistencia material en los hospitales de Burgos a fines de la Edad Media." In *Manger et boire au Moyen Âge,* 1: 349–60. Paris: Belles lettres, 1984.

———. *El Hospital del Rey de Burgos: Un señorío medieval en la expansión y en la crisis (siglos XIII y XIV).* Burgos: Ediciones J.Garrido Garrido, 1986.

Martínez San Pedro, Rafael. *Historia de los hospitales en Alicante.* Alicante: Instituto de Estudios Alicantinos, 1974.

Martínez Sopena, P., and María J. Carbajo Serrano. "L'alimentation des paysans castillans du XIe au XIIIe siècle d'après les «fueros»." In *Manger et boire au Moyen Âge,* 1: 335–47. Paris: Belles lettres, 1984.

Martz, Linda. *Poverty and Welfare in Hapsburg Spain: The Example of Toledo.* Cambridge: Cambridge University Press, 1983.

Matossian, Mary A. *Poisons of the Past: Molds, Epidemics, and History.* New Haven, Conn.: Yale University Press, 1989.

McCrank, Lawrence J. "Restoration and Reconquest in Medieval Catalonia: The

Church and the Principality of Tarragona, 971–1177." Ph.D. dissertation, University of Virginia, 1974.

McLaughlin, Mary Martin. "Survivors and Surrogates: Children and Parents from the Ninth to the Thirteenth Centuries." In *The History of Childhood.* Edited by Lloyd de Mause, 101–81. New York: The Psychohistory Press, 1974.

McVaugh, Michael R. *Medicine before the Plague: Practitioners and Their Patients in the Crown of Aragon, 1285–1345.* Cambridge: Cambridge University Press, 1993.

Mesmin, Simone C. "Waleran of Meulan and the Leper Hospital of S. Gilles de Pont-Audemer." *Annales de Normandie* 32 (1982): 3–19.

Miller, Timothy S. "The Knights of Saint John and the Hospitals of the Latin West." *Speculum* 53 (1978): 709–33.

Miquel Parellada, José María, and José Sánchez Real. *Los hospitales de Tarragona.* Tarragona: Instituto de Estudios Tarraconenses «Ramon Berenguer IV», 1959.

Moeller, Charles. "Lazarus, Saint, Order of." *The Catholic Encyclopedia,* 9:96–97. New York: Appleton, 1907–12.

Molénat, J. P. "Menus des pauvres, menus des confrères à Tolède dans la deuxième moitié du XVᵉ siècle." In *Manger et boire au Moyen Âge,* 1:313–18. Paris: Belles lettres, 1984.

Mollat, Michel, ed. *Études sur l'histoire de la pauvreté (Moyen Âge–XVIᵉ siècle).* 2 vols. Paris: Publications de la Sorbonne, 1974.

———. "Hospitalité et assistance au début du XIIIᵉ siècle." In *Poverty in the Middle Ages.* Edited by David Flood, 37–51. Paderborn: Werl/Westf, 1975.

———. *Les pauvres au moyen âge.* Paris: Hachette, 1978.

———. "Pauvres et assistés au moyen âge." In *A pobreza e a assistência aos pobres na península ibérica durante a idade média,* 1:11–27. Lisbon: Instituto de Alta Cultura, 1973.

———. "Pauvres et marginaux." *Acta historica et archaeologica mediaevalia* 5–6 (1984–85): 73–82.

———. *The Poor in the Middle Ages: An Essay in Social History.* Translated by Arthur Goldhammer. New Haven, Conn.: Yale University Press, 1986.

Moore, R. I. *The Formation of a Persecuting Society: Power and Deviance in Western Europe, 950–1250.* Oxford: Basil Blackwell, 1987.

Mundy, John H. "Charity and Social Work in Toulouse, 1100–1250." *Traditio* 22 (1966): 203–87.

Mutel, André. "Recherches sur l'ordre de Saint-Lazare de Jérusalem en Normandie." *Annales de Normandie* 33 (1983): 121–42.

Mutgé Vives, Josefina. *La ciudad de Barcelona durante el reinado de Alfonso el Benigno (1327–1336).* Anuario de estudios medievales, anejo no. 17. Madrid and Barcelona: C.S.I.C., 1987.

Neuman, Abraham A. *The Jews in Spain: Their Social, Political, and Cultural Life during the Middle Ages.* Vol 1., *A Political-Economic Study.* Vol. 2, *A Social-Cultural Study.* 1942. Reprint, New York: Octagon, 1969.

Nirenberg, David. *Communities of Violence: Persecution of Minorities in the Middle Ages.* Princeton, N.J.: Princeton University Press, 1996.

O'Callaghan, Joseph F. *The Learned King: The Reign of Alfonso X of Castile*. Philadelphia: University of Pennsylvania Press, 1993.

Ollich i Castanyer, Immaculada. "Les entitats eclesiastiques de Vic al segle XIII." *Ausa* 8, no. 84 (1976): 90–101.

Ordinacions del Hospital General de la Santa Creu de Barcelona (any MCCCCXVII): Copiades textualment del manuscrit original y prologodes. Edited by Joseph María Roca. Barcelona: Fidel Giró, 1920.

Orme, Nicholas. "Medieval Almshouse for the Clergy: Clyst Gabriel Hospital near Exeter." *Journal of Ecclesiastical History* 39 (1988): 1–15.

Orme, Nicholas, and Margaret Webster. *The English Hospital, 1070–1570*. New Haven, Conn.: Yale University Press, 1995.

Otis, Leah L. "Municipal Wet Nurses in Fifteenth-Century Montpellier." In *Women and Work in Preindustrial Europe*. Edited by Barbara A. Hanawalt, 83–93. Bloomington: Indiana University Press, 1986.

———. *Prostitution in Medieval Society: The History of an Urban Institution in Languedoc*. Chicago: University of Chicago Press, 1985.

Pagarolas i Sabaté, Laureà. *La comanda del Temple de Tortosa*. Tortosa: Institut d'Estudis Dertosenses, 1984.

Pardo Fernández, Miguel. "'El bací dels pobres vergonyants' de la parroquia de Santa Maria del Mar." *Estudis Històrics i Documents dels Arxius de Protocols* 8 (1980): 149–64.

Park, Katherine. "Healing the Poor: Hospitals and Medical Assistance in Renaissance Florence." In *Medicine and Charity before the Welfare State*. Edited by Jonathan Barry and Colin Jones, 26–45. London: Routlege, 1991.

———. "Medicine and Society in Medieval Europe, 500–1500." In *Medicine and Society: Historical Essays*. Edited by Andrew Wear, 59–90. Cambridge: Cambridge University Press, 1992.

Patrologiae cursus completus, series latina. Edited by Jacques-Paul Migne. 221 vols. Paris, 1844–85.

Pérez Santamaria, Aurora. "El hospital de San Lázaro o Casa dels Malalts o Masells." In *La pobreza y la asistencia a los pobres en la Cataluña medieval*. Edited by Manuel Riu, 1: 77–116. Barcelona: C.S.I.C., 1980–82.

Peris, M. Carmen. "La prostitución valenciana en la segunda mitad del siglo XIV." In *Violència i marginació en la societat medieval. Revista d'història medieval* 1 (1990): 179–99.

Pifarré Torres, Dolors. "Dos visitas de comienzos del signo XIV a los hospitales barceloneses d'en Colom y d'en Marcús." In *La pobreza y la asistencia a los pobres en la Cataluña medieval*. Edited by Manuel Riu, 2:81–93. Barcelona: C.S.I.C., 1980–82.

La pobreza y la asistencia a los pobres en la Cataluña medieval. Edited by Manuel Riu. 2 vols. Barcelona: C.S.I.C., 1980–82.

Pons, Antonio. *Los judios del reino de Mallorca durante los siglos XIII y XIV*. 2 vols. Palma de Mallorca: Miguel Font, 1984.

Pons Alós, Vicente. *El archivo histórico del Hospital "Major de Pobres" de Xàtiva: Catálogo y estudio*. Valencia: Consellera de Cultura, 1987.

Pourrière, Jean. *Les Hôpitaux d'Aix-en-Provence au Moyen Âge: XIIIe, XIVe et XVe siècles.* Aix-en-Provence: Paul Roubaud, 1969.

Powell, James M. "Greco-arabic Influences on the Public Health Legislation in the Constitutions of Melfi." *Archivio storico pugliese* 31 (1978): 77–93.

Prim Tarragó, Agustín. *Cosas viejas de Lérida.* Lleida: Casa provincial de Misericordia, 1893.

Puig y Puig, Sebastián. *Episcopologio de la sede barcinonense.* Barcelona: Biblioteca Balmes, 1929.

Pullan, Brian. "Houses in the Service of the Poor in the Venetian Republic." In *Poverty and Charity: Europe, Italy, Venice, 1400–1700*, 10:1–17. Aldershot, England: Variorum, 1994.

——. "Orphans and Foundlings in Early Modern Europe." In *Poverty and Charity: Europe, Italy, Venice, 1400–1700*, 3: 5–28. Aldershot, England: Variorum, 1994.

——. *Rich and Poor in Renaissance Venice: The Social Institutions of a Catholic State to 1620.* Cambridge, Mass.: Harvard University Press, 1971.

——. "'Support and Redeem': Charity and Poor Relief in Italian Cities from the Fourteenth to the Seventeenth Century." In *Poverty and Charity: Europe, Italy, Venice, 1400–1700*, 5: 177–208. Aldershot, England: Variorum, 1994.

Rano, B. "Ospitalieri di Santo Spirito." In *Dizionario degli istituti di perfezione.* Edited by G. Pellicia and G. Roca, 6:994–1014. Rome: Edizioni Paoline, 1974–88.

RB 1980: The Rule of St. Benedict. Edited by Timothy Fry. Collegeville, Minn.: Liturgical Press, 1981.

Reitzel, J. M. "The Medieval Houses of Bon-Enfants." *Viator* 11 (1980): 179–207.

Revest Corzo, Luis. *Hospitales y pobres en el Castellón de otros tiempos.* Castellón de la Plana: Sociedad castellonense de cultura, 1947.

Reyerson, Kathryn. "The Adolescent Apprentice/Worker in Medieval Montpellier." *Journal of Family History* 17 (1992): 353–70.

Ricci, Giovanni. "Naissance du pauvre honteux: Entre l'histoire des idées et l'histoire sociale." *Annales: économies, sociétés, civilisations* 38 (1983): 158–77.

Richards, Peter. *The Medieval Leper and His Northern Heirs.* Cambridge: D. S. Brewer, 1977.

Riu, Manuel. "Presentación." In *La pobreza y la asistencia a los pobres en la Cataluña medieval.* Edited by Manuel Riu, 1:7–16. Barcelona: C.S.I.C., 1980–82.

Roca, Joseph Maria. *L'hospital migeval de Sant Macià.* Barcelona: Vidua de Lluis Tasso, 1926.

Rödel, W.G. "San Lazzaro, di Gerusalemme." *Dizionario degli istituti di perfezione.* Edited by G. Pellicia and G. Roca, 8:579–82. Rome: Edizioni Paoline, 1974–88.

Rosen, George. "The Hospital: Historical Sociology of a Community Institution." In *The Hospital in Modern Society.* Edited by Eliot Freidson, 1–36. New York, 1963.

——. "The Mentally Ill and the Community in Western and Central Europe during the Late Middle Ages and Renaissance." *Journal of the History of Medicine*, 19 (1964): 377–88.

Rossiaud, Jacques. *Medieval Prostitution.* Translated by Lydia G. Cochrane. Oxford: Basil Blackwell, 1988.

Rouche, Michel. "La matricule des pauvres. Évolution d'une institution de charité du Bas Empire jusqu'à la fin du Haut Moyen Âge." In *Études sur l'histoire de la pauvreté*. Edited by Michel Mollat, 1:83–110. Paris: Publications de la Sorbonne, 1974.

Rubin, Miri. *Charity and Community in Medieval Cambridge*. Cambridge: Cambridge University Press, 1987.

———. "Imagining Medieval Hospitals: Considerations on the Cultural Meanings of Institutional Change." In *Medicine and Charity Before the Welfare State*. Edited by Jonathan Barry and Colin Jones, 14–25. London: Routledge, 1991.

Rubio Vela, Agustín. "La asistencia hospitalaria infantil en la Valencia del siglo XIV: Pobres, huérfanos y expósitos." *Dynamis* 2 (1982): 159–91.

———. "Infancia y marginación. En torno a las instituciones trecentistas valencianas para el socorro de los huérfanos." In *Violència i marginació en la societat medieval. Revista d'història medieval* 1 (1990): 111–53.

———. *Pobreza, enfermedad y asistencia hospitalaria en la Valencia del siglo XIV*. Valencia: Institución Alfonso el Magnanimo, 1984.

Rubio Vela, Agustín, and Mateu Rodrigo Lízondo. "El beguins de València en el segle XIV. La seua casa-hospital i els seus llibres." *Miscel.lànea Sanchis Guarner* 1 (Valencia, 1984): 327–41.

Rucquoi, Adeline. "Hospitalisation et charité à Valladolid." In *Les sociétés urbaines en France méridionale et en Péninsule Ibérique au Moyen Âge. Actes du Colloque de Pau, 21–23 Septembre 1988*, 393–408. Paris: Editions du C.N.R.S., 1991.

Ruffino, I. "Canonici Regolari di Sant'Agostino di Sant'Antonio, di Vienne." *Dizionario degli istituti di perfezione*. Edited by G. Pellicia and G. Roca, 2:134–141. Rome: Edizioni Paoline, 1974–88.

Ruiz, Juan. *The Book of True Love*. Translated by Saralyn R. Daly. Edited by Anthony Z. Zahareas. University Park, Pa.: Pennsylvania State University Press, 1978.

The Rule, Statutes and Customs of the Hospitallers, 1099–1310. Edited and translated by E. J. King. London: Methuen, 1934.

Rumeu de Armas, Antonio. *Historia de la previsión social en España: cofradías, gremios, hermandades, montepios*. Madrid: Editorial Revista de derecho privado, 1944.

Russell, Josiah C. "How Many of the Population Were Aged?" In *Aging and the Aged in Medieval Europe*. Edited by Michael Sheehan, 119–128. Toronto: Pontifical Institute of Mediaeval Studies, n.d.

———. *The Control of Late Ancient and Medieval Population*. Philadelphia: American Philosophical Society, 1985.

Rycraft, Peter. "The Late Medieval Catalan Death-bed." In *God and Man in Medieval Spain; Essays in Honour of J. R. L. Highfield*. Edited by Derek W. Lomax and David Mackenzie, 117–28. Warminster: Aris and Phillips, 1989

Salrach, Josep M. *El procés de feudalització (segles III–XII)*. Vol. 2 of *Història de Catalunya*. Edited by Pierre Vilar. Barcelona: Edicions 62, 1987.

Sanahuja, Pedro, O.F.M. *Historia de la Beneficencia en Lérida*. Lérida: Escuela Provincial, 1944.

Sanchez Herrero, José. "Cofradías, hospitales y beneficencia en algunas diócesis del valle del Duero, siglos XIV y XV." *Hispania* 34, no. 126 (1974): 5–51.

Santamaría, Alvaro. "La asistencia a los pobres en Mallorca en el bajomedievo." *Anuario de estudios medievales* 13 (1983): 381–406.

Ser Quijano, Gregorio del. "Algunos aspectos de la caridad asistencial altomedieval. Los primeros hospitales de la ciudad de León." *Studia historica* 3 (1985): 157–79.

Shahar, Shulamith. *Childhood in the Middle Ages*. London: Routledge, 1990.

——. "Des lépreux pas comme les autres. L'ordre de Saint-Lazare dans le royaume latin de Jérusalem." *Revue historique* 267 (1979): 19–41.

Sherwood, Joan. *Poverty in Eighteenth-Century Spain: The Women and Children of the Inclusa*. Toronto: University of Toronto Press, 1988.

Sibert, Gautier de. *Histoire de l'Ordre Militaire et Hospitalier de Saint-Lazare de Jérusalem*. 1772; Paris: Slatkine, 1983.

Las Siete Partidas. Translated by Samuel Parsons Scott. Chicago: Commerce Clearing House, 1931.

Siraisi, Nancy G. *Medieval and Early Renaissance Medicine: An Introduction to Knowledge and Practice*. Chicago: University of Chicago Press, 1990.

Sivilla, Tomas. "Apuntos históricos sobre el hospital de Barcelona." *Memorias de la Academia de Buenas Letras de Barcelona* 3 (1880): 43–70.

Statuts d'Hôtels-Dieu et de Léproseries. Recueil de textes du XIIᵉ au XIVᵉ siècle. Edited by Léon LeGrand. Paris: Alphonse Picard et Fils, 1901.

Tarragó Valentines, Josep F. *Hospitales en Lérida durante los siglos XII al XVI*. Lérida: Colegio oficial de medicos de la Provincia de Lérida, 1975.

——. *Noves aportacions a l'historia dels antics hospitals de Lleida*. Lleida: Anals del Col.legi Oficial de Metges de Lleida, 1977.

Terpstra, Nicholas. "Apprenticeship in Social Welfare: From Confraternal Charity to Municipal Poor Relief in Early Modern Italy." *Sixteenth Century Journal* 25 (1994): 101–20.

Tierney, Brian. *Medieval Poor Law: A Sketch of Canonical Theory and Its Application in England*. Berkeley and Los Angeles: University of California Press, 1959.

Tits-Dievaide, M.-J. "Les tables des pauvres dans les anciennes principautés belges au Moyen Âge." *Tijdschrift voor geschiedenis* 88 (1975): 562–58.

Tolivar Faes, J. *Hospitales de leprosos en Asturias durante las edades media y moderna*. Oviedo: Imprenta "La Cruz," Instituto de Estudios Asturianos, 1966.

Toubert, Pierre. "La vie commune des clercs aux XIᵉ–XII ᵉ siècles: Un questionnaire." *Revue historique* 231 (1964): 11–26.

Trenchs Odena, José, and Federico Lara Peinado. "La casa de caridad y la cofradia de los clerigos pobres, dos instituciones medievales leridanas." *Ilerda* 36 (1975): 7–36.

Trexler, Richard C. "Charity and the Defense of Urban Elites in the Italian Communes." In *The Rich, the Well Born and the Powerful: Elites and Upper Classes in History*. Edited by Frederic Cople Jaher, 64–109. Urbana: University of Illinois Press, 1973.

——. "Infanticide in Florence: New Sources and First Results." *History of Childhood Quarterly* 1 (1973): 98–116.

—— "A Widow's Asylum in the Renaissance: The Orbatello of Florence." In *Old Age in Preindustrial Society*. Edited by Peter N. Stearns, 119–49. New York: Holmes & Meier, 1982.

Ubieto Arteta, Antonio. "Pobres y marginados en el primitivo Aragón." *Aragon en el edad media* 5 (1983): 7–22.

Utterback, Kristine. *Pastoral Care and Administration in Mid-Fourteenth Century Barcelona: Exercising the "Arts of Arts."* Lewiston, N.Y.: Edwin Mellen Press, 1993.

Vauchez, André. "Conclusion." In *Le mouvement confraternel au Moyen Âge: France, Italie, Suisse. Actes de la table ronde organisée par l'Université de Lausanne avec le concours de l'École française de Rome et de l'Unité associée 1011 du CNRS «L'institution ecclésiale à la fin du Moyen Âge», Lausanne 9–11 mai 1985*, 395–405. Rome: École Française de Rome, 1987.

Verlinden, Charles. *L'esclavage dans l'Europe médiévale.* 2 vols. Bruges: De Tempel, 1955–77.

Vila i Comaposada, Marc-Aureli. *Tortosa al segle XIII: vida i costums dels tortosins.* Barcelona: El Llamp, 1986.

Vilaseca Anguera, Salvador. *Hospitales medievals de Reus.* Reus: Asociación de estudios Reusenses, 1958.

Vinyoles i Vidal, Teresa-María. "Ajudes a donzelles pobres a maridar." In *La pobreza y la asistencia a los pobres en la Cataluña medieval.* Edited by Manuel Riu, 1: 295–362. Barcelona: C.S.I.C., 1980–82.

———. *La vida quotidiana a Barcelona vers 1400.* Barcelona: Editorial Rafael Dalmau, 1985.

———. "La violència marginal a les ciutats medievals (exemples a la Barcelona dels volts del 1400)." *Violència i marginació en la societat medieval. Revista d'historia medieval* 1 (1990): 155–77.

Vinyoles i Vidal, Teresa-María, and Margarida González Betlinski. "Els infants abandonats a les portes de l'Hospital de Barcelona (1426–1439)." In *La pobreza y la asistencia a los pobres en la Cataluña medieval.* Edited by Manuel Riu, 2:191–285. Barcelona: C.S.I.C., 1980–82.

Violència i marginació en la societat medieval. Vol. 1 of *Revista d'història medieval.* Valencia, 1990.

Webster, Jill R. "La reina doña Constanza y los hospitales de Barcelona y Valencia." *Archivo Ibero-Americano* 51 (1991): 375–90.

———. *Els Menorats: The Franciscans in the Realms of Aragon from St. Francis to the Black Death.* Toronto: Pontifical Institute of Mediaeval Studies, 1993.

Wilson, Stephen. "The Myth of Motherhood a Myth: The Historical View of European Child-rearing." *Social History* 9 (1984): 181–98.

Witters, Willibrord. "Pauvres et pauvreté dans les coutumes monastiques du Moyen Âge." In *Études sur l'histoire de la pauvreté.* Edited by Michel Mollat, 1:117–216. Paris: Publications de la Sorbonne, 1974.

Wolff, Philippe. "Recherches sur les médecins de Toulouse aux XIVᵉ et XVᵉ siècles." In *Assistance et assistés jusqu'à 1610*, 531–49. Paris: Bibliothèque nationale, 1979.

Ximénez de Rada, Rodrigo. *Historia de rebus Hispanie sive Historia Gothica.* Edited by Juan Fernández Valverde. Corpus Christianorum, 72. Turnhout: Brepols, 1987.

Index

Navarre, 29, 113
new orders, 2
Nirenberg, David, 141, 196
nurses. *See* sisters

old age. *See* the elderly
Olesa de Bonesvalls, 35, 53, 126, 169
Organyà, 36, 55, 63
orphanages and foundling homes, 41, 51, 110–12, 120–21, 143, 195–96, 200
orphans, 4, 30, 35, 58, 69, 73, 102–3, 107, 110–11, 120–23, 127, 140–41, 151, 189
Oviedo, 29, 75, 179

Palencia, 77, 112, 182
Palestine, 84, 93, 174, 177–79, 187
Palou, Berenguer de (bishop of Barcelona), 9–10, 17, 32, 155
pare dels òrfens. See father of the poor
Paris, 29, 55, 62, 72, 75–76, 83, 87, 90, 93, 100, 111–12, 121, 133, 166, 174, 179, 187, 189–92, 195–96
parishes, 6, 19, 27, 29, 40, 61, 64, 101, 105, 111, 133, 158; parish alms funds, 6, 18–21, 102, 109, 130–31, 136–37, 140, 158, 176, 189
Park, Katherine, 98, 134
pauperes verecundi, 5, 17, 19–20, 27, 81, 102, 109, 114, 131–32, 136, 139–42, 153, 158
paupers. *See* the poor
Pedro I (king of Aragon), 177
Pedro I (king of Castile), 5, 152
Penyafort, Ramon de, 4, 136, 142
Pere II (III of Aragon), 45, 129
Pere III (IV of Aragon), 14, 18, 50, 60, 62, 85, 87, 89, 94, 102–4, 113, 166, 187, 191
Pérez de Ravidats, Guillem (bishop of Lleida), 10, 23, 39
Perpignan, 31, 87, 90, 129, 185, 193, 197, 201; corts of, 109
physicians, 61, 67, 71, 80–81, 83, 86–97, 181–89; town, 92–94, 186–87
pia almoina, 8–14, 26–27, 126, 140, 142–43, 154
pilgrims, 3–4, 9, 11, 17, 28–30, 32–33, 35–36, 38–39, 42–43, 62, 65–69, 77, 84–85, 140, 163, 166, 182, 194
Pisa, 111
plague, 12, 14, 39, 43–44, 50, 62, 66, 73, 80, 87, 89, 90–93, 95–96, 101–2, 119, 125, 137–38, 173, 185, 187, 189, 191, 203
Plegamans, family, 49, 52, 77, 155; Ramon de, 9, 52, 77, 155
Poblet, monastery of, 42, 66
poor, the, 2–4, 7–9, 14, 127–28, 141–42, 153, 156; advocates of, 3, 151; ordinary vs. extraordinary, 14–18, 142; worthy vs. unworthy, xii–xiii, 4–6, 26, 65, 126, 133, 136, 139, 141–42, 152, 203
poor of Christ, 2, 4–5, 31, 102, 133, 151–54, 157
poor clerics, 1, 37, 39, 42, 45, 64, 132, 166
Portugal, 29, 69, 122
poverty, xiii, 1–6, 127, 150, 152
prostitutes, 6–7, 30, 103, 123–24, 127, 135, 141, 143, 152, 190–93, 200; reform of, 100–101, 193; segregation of, 5, 104–6, 109–10, 192–93
public defender, 3
Puigcerdà, 92, 201
Pullan, Brian, 6, 68, 108, 133, 152–53, 205

quarantine, 62, 75–76, 80, 98

Ramon Berenguer I (count of Barcelona), 31
Ramon Berenguer IV (count of Barcelona), 10, 43
Reus, 19, 43, 58, 63–64, 126, 130, 168, 174
Reyna, hospital of La (Valencia), 45, 57, 62, 94, 112, 130, 137, 143, 159, 170, 174, 176, 189, 196, 203
Roda, 39, 154
Roger I (king of Sicily), 93
Roger II (king of Sicily), 86, 183
Rome, 30
Roncesvalles, Order of, 29, 44, 54, 66, 173
Rosen, George, 136
Rubin, Miri, 131, 133–34, 153
Rubio Vela, Agustín, xiii, 48–49, 52, 64, 86, 98, 114, 122, 131, 135, 176
Ruiz, Juan, 25

sailors, 33
Saint Lazarus, Order of, 76, 179
Salamanca, 29, 112, 183
salaries, wages and professional fees, 11, 51, 53, 57, 92–94, 118, 170–71, 175, 181, 187–88

DATE DUE

			Printed in USA